PLATE TO PODIUM

Recipes and Routines from 33 Elite Athletes

SASHA FEAR

ISBN: 9798851194337
Imprint: Independently published

Copyright @ Plate to Podium, Sasha Fear, 2022
All rights reserved in Canada. Copyright Certificate Registration 1198032. No part of this publication may be reproduced or transmitted in any form or by any means without the prior written permission of the publisher.

The use of Olympic-related designations and other content belonging to the International Olympic Committee (IOC) in this publication has been authorized by the IOC but their mere appearance does not constitute, and shall not be construed as, an endorsement by the IOC of this publication. In particular, the designations employed and the presentation of material throughout this publication do not imply the expression of any opinion whatsoever on the part of the IOC. The ideas, views and opinions expressed in this publication are those of the author of the publication only and do not necessarily represent those of the IOC.

Editor: *Cameron Kraemer*
Photographers: Alison Slattery (food and lifestyle); *athlete images (Charlie Booker, Olivier Braj, Jason Brown, Michael Burns, Guillaume Cizeron, Francesco Costa, Meryl Davis, Hailey Duff, Lilah Fear, Anna Fernstädt, Makayla Gerken Schofield, Lewis Gibson, Ryan Harnden, Jed Jacobsohn (Getty), Charlotte Kalla, Jaelin Kauf, Xavier Laine (Getty), Shaolin Liu and Shaoang Liu, Robert Michael (Getty), Manu Naef, Mercedes Nicoll, O/S, David Pearce, Mohd Rasfan, Ryan Regehr, Dawn Richardson Wilson, Susan Russell, Paul Shoebridge, Meghan Tierney, Michelle Uhrig, Fredrik Von Erichsen (Getty), Bree Walker, Noah Wallace, Amy Willams MBE, Josh Williamson, Neville Wright).*
Stylist: *Kerri Ahern*

Introduction *page 6-11*

Chapter 1
Meal Prep Like A Pro *page 12-30*

Chapter 2
The Breakfast Of Champions *page 31-71*

Chapter 3
Lunch Time, Crunch Time *page 72-103*

Chapter 4
Dinner like a Winner *page 104- 135*

Chapter 5
Elite Snacks and Sweets *page 136-173*

Chapter 6
Hydration Station *page 174-195*

Chapter 7
Training Tips *page 196-207*

Chapter 8:
Mental Preparation *page 208-219*

Chapter 9
Sleep + Recovery *page 220-233*

Acknowledgments

Introduction

Most people think Olympians are superheroes with powers that make them invincible and unstoppable. It's true—they are pretty freaking awesome! But beyond the capes are real humans who face physical, mental, and emotional challenges, all to compete for just one, single moment: one routine, one race, one gold medal. Their grit, determination, and dedication to the sport are the true superpowers.

Like anyone, Olympians need sources of strength, both physical and emotional. This cookbook will give you an inside look at how 33 different Olympians eat, mentally prepare, train, and recover for peak performance. It will also include tips on how to maximize your mornings and wind down to optimize your sleep. There are sample meal plans from different athletes so that you can mix and match to create your dream nutrition plan.

By Going for Gold and building elite-level habits, you too will be at peak performance for any sport, work, or play.

My skating story:

I started skating when I was 2 years old in London, England. I come from a skating family: my Uncle Xavier was a hockey player for Team Canada, and my mom figure skated competitively in her hometown of Fernie, British Columbia. Because of this, (and because it *is* super Canadian), she thought my sisters and I should give it a try. Since then, I've never looked back. From kindergarten all the way to high school graduation, we spent countless early mornings driving to ice rinks all over London before school, listening to the Ellen Degeneres Show and SNL skits to brighten our moods. Some mornings were so hectic that I even skated in my school uniform!

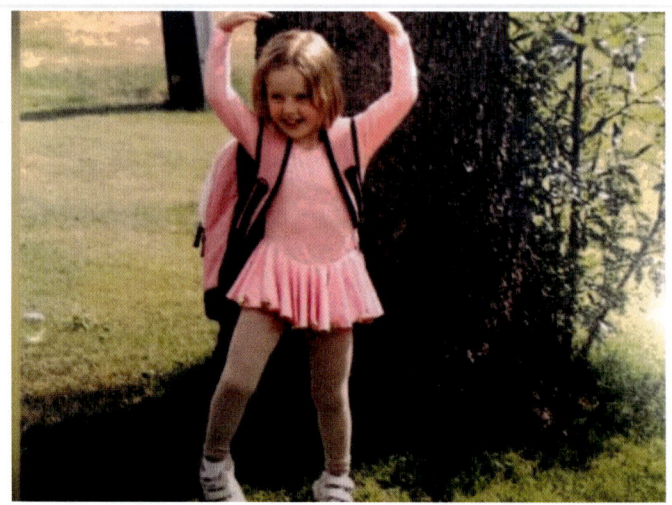

Baby Sasha learning to skate in Fernie, BC.

I started with both figure skating (which includes jumps and spins) and ice dancing (more artistic and technical), but I soon realized I wasn't a natural jumper. I found my first ice dance partner when I was 10, and his name was Jack Osman. I was completely mortified. I remember crying in the back of the car saying "Mommmmm, I don't want to skate with a boy!" We awkwardly held hands and barely looked at each other for the first few weeks. Eventually, though, we became close friends and skated together for three years, traveling to our first international competitions and Grand Prixs. After our first Junior Grand Prix in Courchevel, Jack realized he was losing his love for the sport and decided to stop skating. I was devastated: finding a partner can be difficult, and I didn't know if I would find another British partner.

However, I was lucky to find another British skater, Elliot Verburg, just two weeks later. If I could describe this partnership in one word it would be "whirlwind." As soon as we started skating together, we improved very quickly and were able to jump to the top of the British ranks and compete at our first Junior World Championships for Great Britain.

It was such an exciting year, and we achieved so much together. Unfortunately, I had an insane growth spurt and ended up being too tall for Elliot, so we had to go our separate ways.

After the split, I stayed in the UK and trained hard to work on my skating skills as I looked for a new partner. I got a call from my coach in Montreal, Romain Haganaeur, saying that George Waddell wanted to skate with me. George and I knew each other well because he trained in Toronto and I skated there every summer growing up. I thought it would be a great idea to try it out, especially because he, too, had a British passport. This would mean that we were eligible to compete at the Winter Olympics. He was also 6ft tall (growth spurt be damned!), and trained in Montreal where I had been training the last three summers. Physically we were perfectly matched and we had similar goals, so we decided to go for it! He was 18 at the time, and I was 15. For the first two years of our partnership, we trained in the UK as I was still in British high school, and then we transitioned to Montreal once I graduated.

Since then, we both moved full-time to Canada to train at the Ice Academy of Montreal among the best ice dancers in the world.

Our progression sky-rocketed after moving to Montreal and its familial, inspiring, and demanding training environment. Together we have competed at two Junior World Championships, the European Championships, and the 2022 World Figure Skating Championships. My ultimate goal is to compete at the 2026 Winter Olympics in Milan, and it would be a cherry-on-top to go alongside my sister Lilah and her partner, Lewis Gibson.

My food story:

The strong women in my life introduced me to cooking and baking. To me, cooking is therapeutic and rewarding because I love how great food brings people together, sparks joy, and creates memories.

My grandmothers are the most badass cooks and bakers I know. Well, I might be biased, but get back to me after you have tried Granny Harriet's desserts and Grandma Anne's meatloaf. My fondest memories in the kitchen are at my Granny Harriet's house in Toronto, where I usually stood by her side and licked the excess cookie dough from the bowl as she prepared her famous "Nanaimo Bars" and "Hello Dollies" for our Christmas feast. When I visit my Grandma Anne in the Rocky Mountains, we love to cook a hearty chicken stew or make our own pizzas before watching a cheesy rom-com or tv show. Even my mom—whose cooking consists of eggs, cereal, and toast (sorry, mom!)—makes a mean batch of chocolate chip cookies. She was that supermom who came to soccer games armed with boxes of homemade treats that all of my friends adored and devoured. Her food brought people together, and I met some life-long friends because of those cookies.

I was lucky to grow up in a household where we had meals that covered all of the nutritional bases every night. Our dinner staples were meatballs with brown rice and veggies, roasted chicken with root vegetables, and juicy burgers from our local butcher (fun fact: the Queen orders from the same butcher—shoutout to Lidgate!). I was also the one kid who had a packed lunch (even though I didn't have any allergies) because my parents wanted us to have proper fuel for the school day. While I was snacking on fruit, nut butter, organic salads, and sandwiches, my friends were having huge blood sugar spikes and crashes because of the sweets and simple carbohydrates that were served at school. Although the penne pasta with garlic bread looked pretty darn delicious, I am grateful that I prioritized nutrient-rich foods. This taught me from a young age that packing meals ahead of time and making food that you love will give you the longevity and energy to tackle any challenges during the day.

The women in my life have taught me that homemade cooking with fresh ingredients is the most gratifying and nourishing. As an elite ice dancer, I have learned to prioritize nutrition and treat my body as a temple that fuels me to perform at my best. Cooking fresh food each week is a game-changer in my performance. There is a pride and fulfillment that comes with knowing that you made something delicious and wholesome for yourself. Getting a personal best, first place, or feeling your strongest means having good health. The main contributor to good health is good nutrition. Fueling up on nutrient-dense foods means that you'll feel more satisfied, and therefore you're less likely to crave sugary snacks. Many athletes look for quick energy to get them through a training session. Although this might give you a boost in the short term, processed foods are nutrient-poor and provide mass without sustenance. This can cause negative health consequences, especially when training puts so much stress on the body. In order to be healthy, energized, and stay in any sport for the long run, athletes must have a varied diet that includes healthy fats, protein, complex carbohydrates, veggies, minerals, antioxidants, and vitamins.

Most people believe that eating "healthy" means eating boring, bland foods, or just a big bowl of salad. That is so not true! I have found many ways to fuel my body with whole foods while still creating delicious meals that are unrestrictive and nutritious. I hope this cookbook shows you that being elite nutritionally doesn't mean food can't be fun.

NOTE: foods affect everyone differently. Never try a new recipe or food the night before or the day of a competition. Slowly incorporate and experiment with new foods before training sessions and take note of what works and feels best for you.

~Sasha

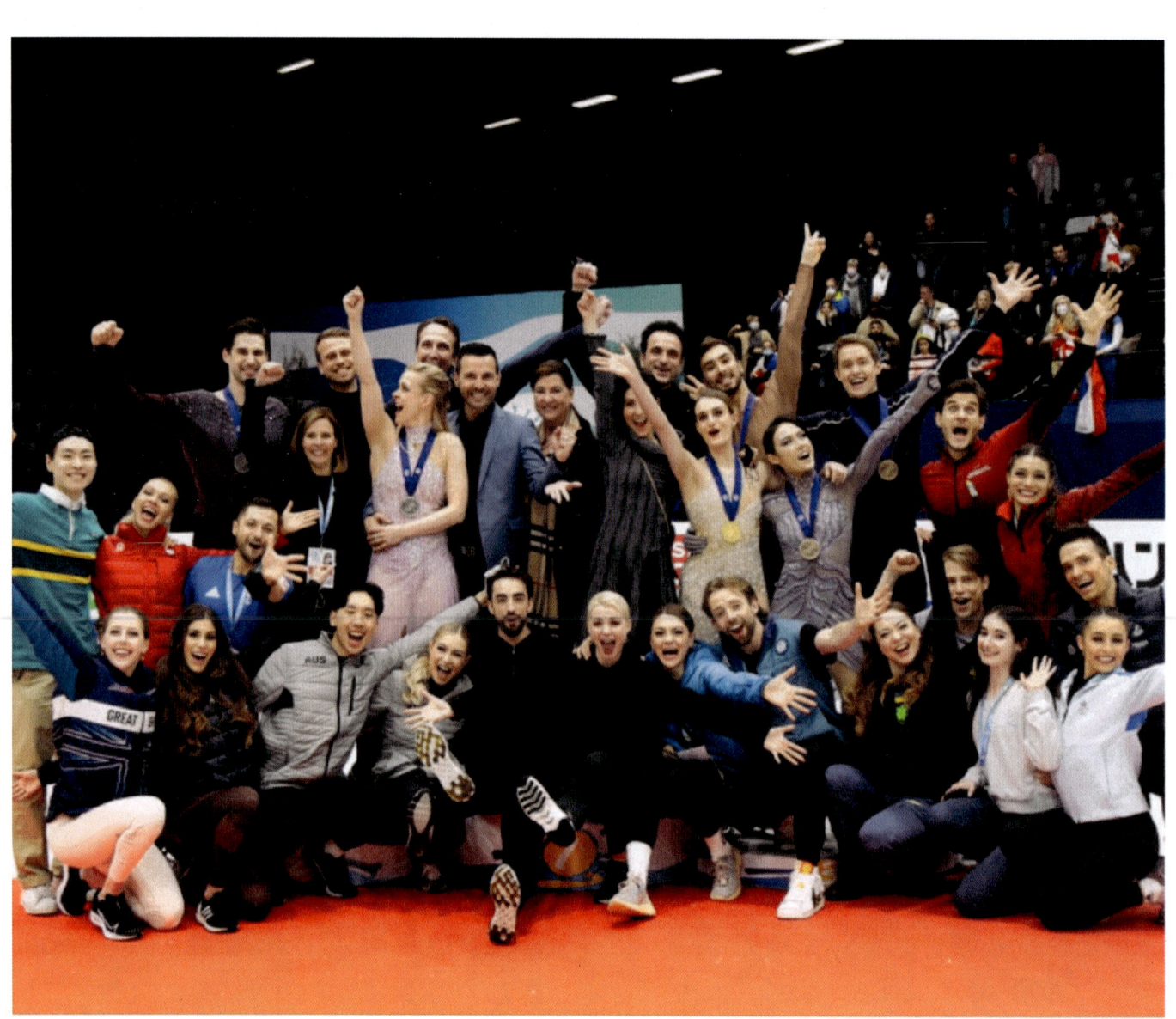

My wonderful skating family, Team I.AM, at the World Figure Skating Championships 2022 in Montpellier, France. Image by Oliver Braj.

How to use this book:

Labels to look out for:

- **gf** = gluten-free
- **v** = vegan
- **df** = dairy-free
- **nf** = nut-free
- 🕐 = time-saving tip
- 🏅 = pro nutrition tip

BONUS RECIPE = although most athletes just have one recipe each in this cookbook, some athletes had an extra recipe that was just too delicious not to include!

Each recipe will have these labels at the top right-hand corner so that you know whether they are dairy-free or vegan, for example. But don't feel restricted by the labels! Let's say you're nut-free and there is a recipe you want to try that isn't nut-free. Just substitute any of the ingredients to make it work for you!

In any recipe with oats, use gluten-free certified oats if you are sensitive to gluten. Anytime "**GF**" is written in a recipe's ingredient list, that means you can substitute the ingredient for a "Gluten-Free" alternative.

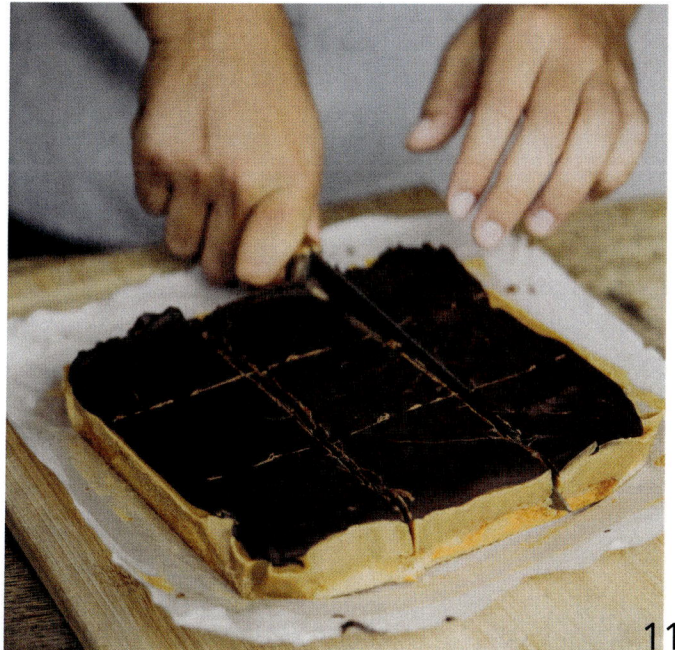

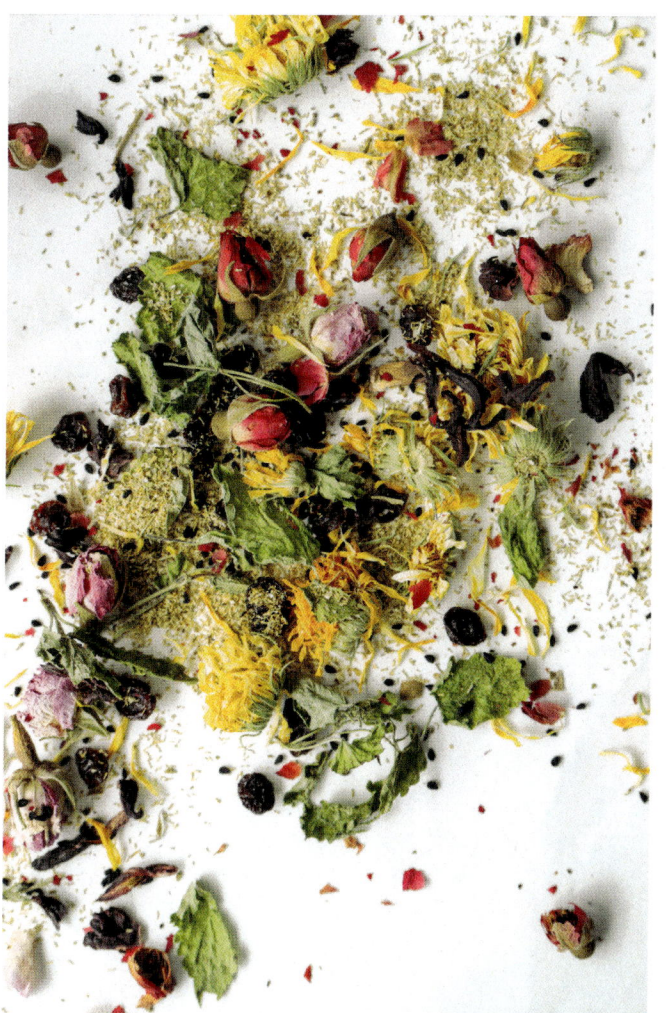

MEAL PREP LIKE A PRO

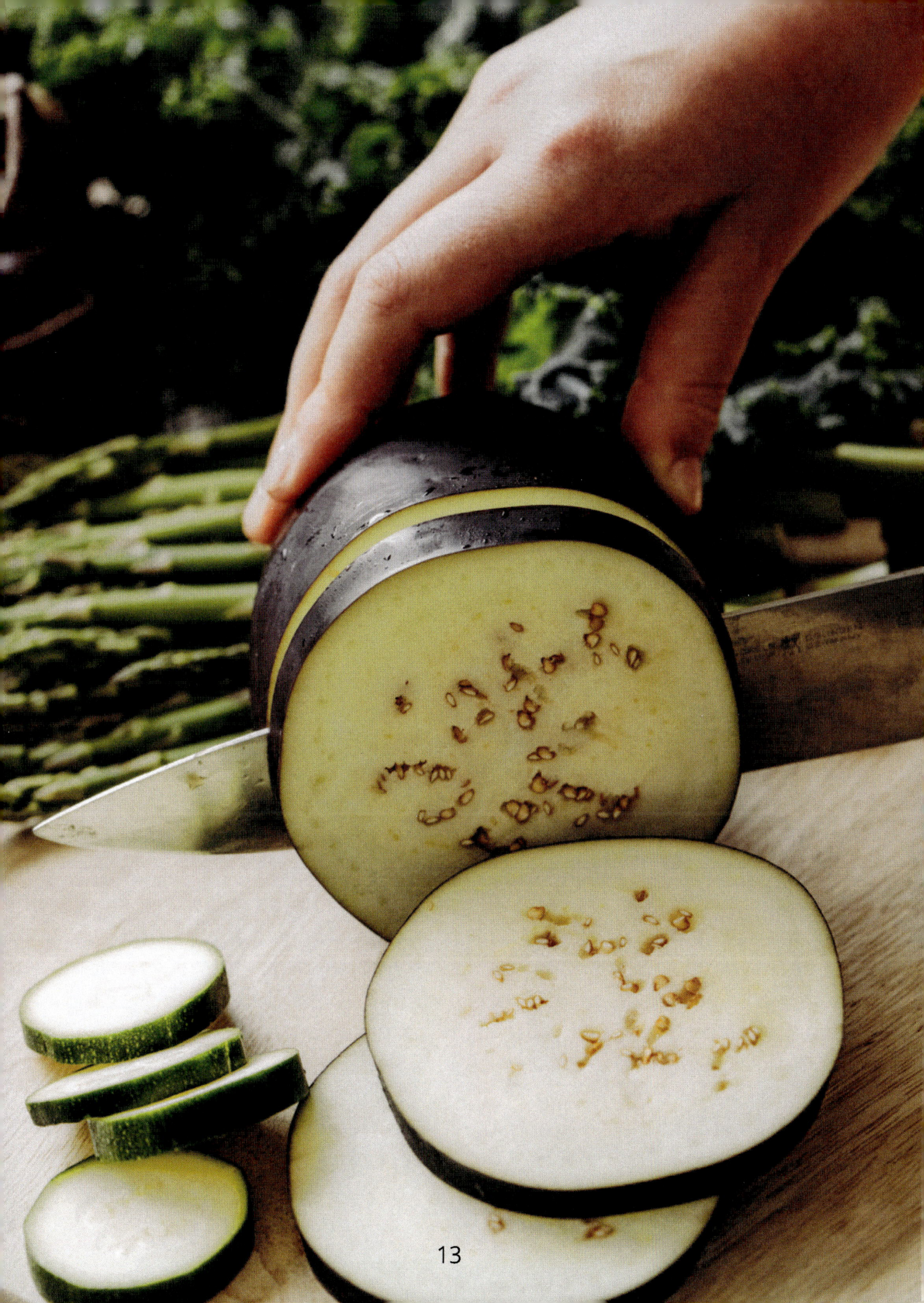

In this chapter, we talk about how preparation in the kitchen is the key to successful nutrition. I share ways to set up your environment for success; offer tips on how to save money and time, and provide lists of essential pantry staples, kitchen tools, and meal plans for every season.

Have you been hangry from long travel days, lack of sleep, tough training, or being stuck in traffic? Well, meal prepping will save the day. When you take the time to prepare meals, you'll eat healthier all week. You'll rely less on takeout and the quick-but-non-nutritive energy provided by packaged foods.

 Money-saving tips:

1. *Never grocery shop on an empty stomach:* having a snack or meal before you go will avoid any unnecessary purchases.
2. *Plan meals ahead of time* to do just one (max two) grocery runs per week to keep the food bill down.

 Time-saving tips:

1. *Your freezer is your friend:* store leftovers in airtight containers in the freezer so that you don't have to cook a full dinner every night. If your freezer and fridge are well stocked, it will be less likely that you will order takeout.
2. *Block out an afternoon for prep time in your calendar:* use an afternoon to plan out and cook the essentials for the week ahead. This will reduce any decision-making on what to eat during the week.
3. *Plan and prepare meals that use similar ingredients:* for example, roasted vegetables used on a pizza for lunch can be used as a side for a salmon dinner that night.
4. *Lay it all out:* it is important to read the recipe in its entirety and have all of the ingredients measured and set out beforehand. This will allow the cooking process to run smoothly.
5. *Want the time to fly by?* Listen to a podcast or blast some music and have fun! Cooking doesn't have to be a chore. Invite friends or family over and meal prep as a group to save time and make it social.
6. *Use high-quality ingredients:* organic, local, high-quality ingredients are naturally more flavorful and fresh, meaning there is less work required in the kitchen to make a meal delicious.

14

Time Saving Tools

High-speed blender:
For smoothies, nut milk, energy balls, protein pancake mix, nut butter, or sauces.

Glass jars and storage containers:
Mason jars and storage containers of all sizes (freezer safe) are perfect for storing smoothie ingredients.

Silicone ice cube trays:
I particularly love the brand Souper Cubes because you can easily freeze single portions of soups, stews, or any leftovers.

Sheet pans:
Have at least two rimmed baking sheets for roasting veggies, baking cookies, or baking proteins. Using parchment paper on a baking sheet reduces clean-up time.

Large mixing bowls:
Having more space to mix ingredients means less spilling when mixing, and therefore less clean-up! They are great to have in varied sizes for recipes with different components, and they can also be used as serving dishes for pasta and salads.

Utensils:
A peeler, can opener, whisk, spatula, and wooden spoons.

Large cutting board:
How else will you cut up all of those fruits and veggies for meal prep? This tool is great for big batch cooking and easy clean-up if it is dishwasher-safe. It's a no-brainer!

Quality chef knives:
Prepping veggies, meat, and fruit requires a lot of chopping. Do yourself (and your fingers!) a favor and get professionally sharpened knives to reduce the risk of any accidents. Dull knives are dangerous as they're more likely to slip when cutting. Resharpen the knives every few months.

Non-stick muffin tins and 9 x 5-inch loaf pans:
Try to get tins and pans with a non-stick surface for quick release. It's best to use paper liners for easy muffin storage and cleanup.

Measuring cups and spoons:
Sure, I usually eye-ball the measurements for a recipe, BUT sometimes it is very important to properly measure each ingredient!

Cast-iron skillet:
This bad boy can be used for pretty much anything: pancakes, veggies, pizzas, frittatas, and more.

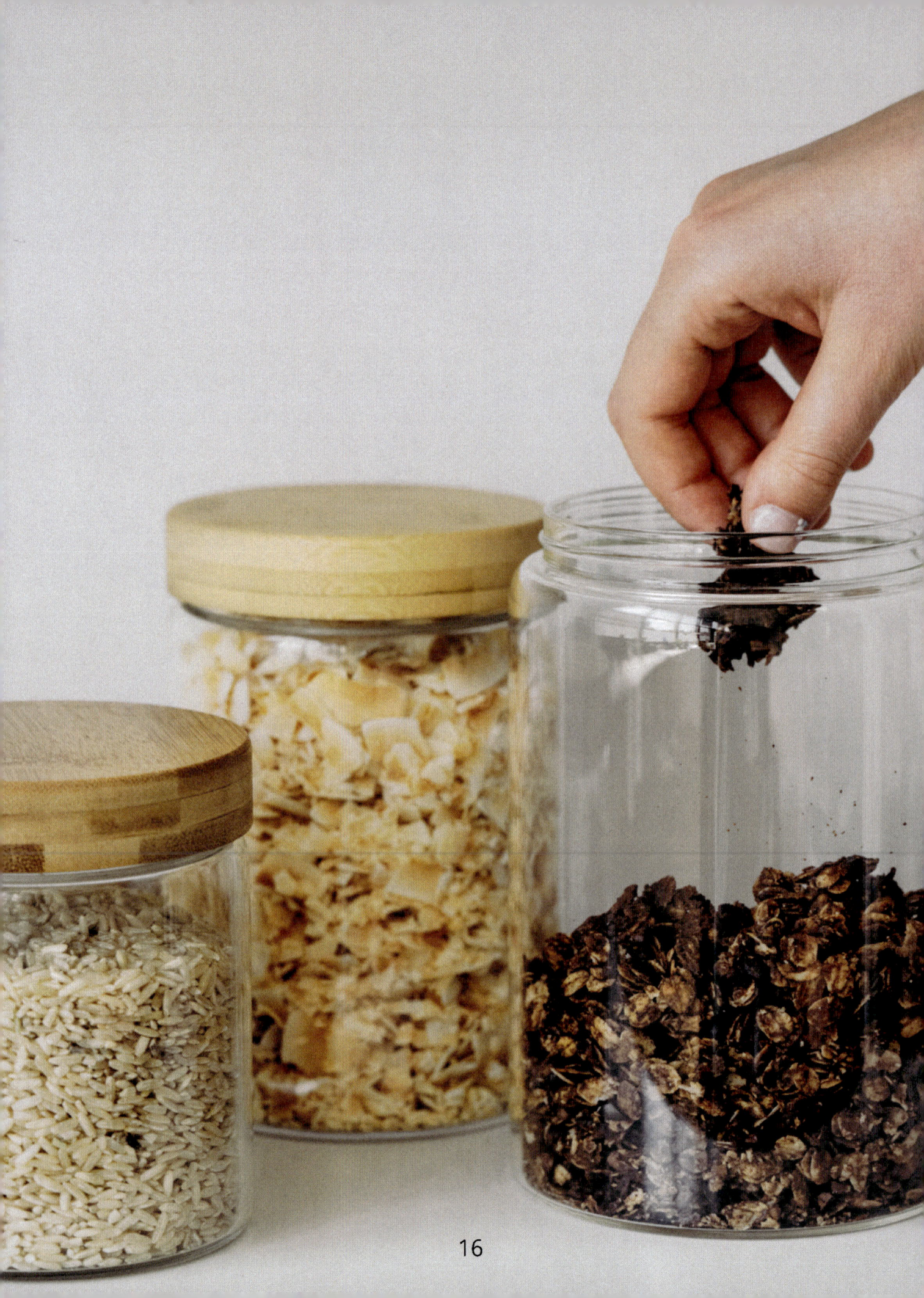

PANTRY AND FRIDGE STAPLES:

Nuts and Nut Butters: Stock up on a variety of nuts like almonds, walnuts, cashews, pecans, peanuts, and brazil nuts. Nuts have diverse uses, as they can be used to make nut milks or butters, or can be eaten raw or in a trail mix to snack on. For nut-free readers, try sunflower-seed butter and creamy tahini.
Benefits: They are a great source of fat, add flavor and texture to baked goods, and also are an amazing on-the-go snack.

Seeds and Dried Fruit: Our favorites include chia, flax, sunflower, hemp, and pumpkin seeds. Seeds are a great way to add a subtle nutrient kick into any recipe. For dried fruit, I love buying dates, unsweetened coconut flakes, cranberries, and blueberries in bulk as they have long shelf lives and can be added to granola, oatmeal, or homemade desserts for sweetness. (Note for dried fruit: check the ingredient list beforehand to avoid any unnecessary added sugar).
Benefits: Seeds are a superfood packed with omega-3 fatty acids, fiber, and protein. Dried fruit is full of antioxidants called phenols that aid digestion and blood flow.

Flours: Keep whole-wheat, sprouted spelt, and all-purpose flours handy, as well as gluten-free flours like buckwheat, corn, coconut, hazelnut, and almond flour. Almond flour is nutrient dense as it is high in fiber and protein compared to other flours, but more filling than traditional flours like all-purpose. Store opened bags of grain-free flours in the fridge to maintain freshness.

Oats and Oat Flour: Stock up on rolled oats, instant oats, or steel-cut oats as they are great for oatmeal, overnight oats, energy balls, pancakes, and more. To make your own oat flour, simply blend the oats in a food processor until they become the consistency of flour.
Benefits: They are naturally gluten-free; lower your blood sugar levels; and are loaded with important vitamins, minerals, fiber, and antioxidants. They also contain higher levels of protein and fats than other grains.

Sweeteners:

Natural sweeteners: I prefer using sweeteners that are natural and low on the glycemic index such as coconut sugar, pure maple syrup, honey, and blackstrap molasses.

Benefits:
- Coconut sugar: lower on the glycemic index than white sugar, meaning less of a sugar spike and crash.
- Pure maple syrup: jam-packed with antioxidants and minerals. Antioxidants help to protect your cells from oxidation and help with preventing disease. (Store maple syrup in the fridge).
- Honey: reduces inflammation, contains antioxidants, boosts digestion, and is a great way to treat a sore throat or cough.
- Blackstrap molasses: high in calcium, iron, magnesium, 18 amino acids, and other micronutrients that are important for athletes' performance and bone health.

Chocolate: First thing's first, I had to give chocolate its own pantry category because COME ON, it is CHOCOLATE. Don't trust anyone who says otherwise...(just kidding, kind of, not really). Stock up dark chocolate bars or chips (70% minimum) and unsweetened cocoa powder. My favorite dark chocolate chips are Hu's Baking Gems, or I chop up Hu's Sea Salt Dark Chocolate bar. If you aren't big on sugar, replace chocolate chips with cacao nibs for a less sweet but tasty alternative.

Benefits: It's a powerful source of antioxidants, may lower blood pressure, and it tastes AMAZING!

Baking essentials: Most baking recipes require baking soda, baking powder, and vanilla extract.

Whole grains: Most whole grains have a long shelf life, making them budget-friendly! The whole grains I use the most are rice (organic short-grain brown rice, jasmine, basmati rice), quinoa, farro, whole-grain teff pasta (regular brown rice or gluten-free options), and soba noodles.

Benefits: Grains are a great source of carbohydrates, which are essential for athletes to feel energized, satisfied, and fueled for training. Most whole grains are easy to prepare, so perfect for a quick noodle bowl, quinoa salad, or spaghetti bolognese.

Spices, Herbs, and Salt:
The spices and herbs I use the most include cinnamon, turmeric, ginger, cardamom,

oregano, nutmeg, garlic powder, freshly ground black pepper, chili powder, taco seasoning, and fine or Himalayan sea salt.
Benefits: Spices add extra flavor to bland-tasting meals, have antioxidants, and make meals more satisfying overall. Sea salt is great to add to homemade energy drinks to rehydrate after training and is also a fabulous addition to nourishing treats like our banana nut butter bites, granola, or cookies.

Fats and Oils: I use extra-virgin olive oil, virgin coconut oil, and avocado oil. When baking, I prefer using grass-fed butter for a lighter and more tasty result!
Benefits: Time and time again I hear athletes worry that "fats will make you fat." This could not be further from the truth. Our muscles need fatty acids as metabolic fuel for endurance exercise. Fats also fight inflammation, help build lean muscle, and are crucial for healthy brain function. Athletes should incorporate polyunsaturated fats into their diets like olive oil, coconut oil, nuts, seeds, butter, whole-milk yogurt, and fatty fish (salmon is high in Omega-3). Good fats are carriers of flavor and nutrients, so they make everything better!

Try to avoid processed foods and cooking oils like canola oil and sunflower oil as they contain hydrogenated fats that do not have any beneficial health properties.

Canned Goods: Keep stock of legumes like dried black beans, red lentils, and white beans. I also keep tomato sauce or pizza sauce as a ketchup alternative, and I store purees such as pumpkin, sweet potato, and unsweetened apple sauce.
Benefits: Legumes are a good source of protein and fiber if you are avoiding meat, and they are rich in folate, potassium, iron, and magnesium. (Warning: will definitely cause gas!)
Purees: sweet potato and pumpkin are flavorful, packed with antioxidants, and vitamins, and are a great source of carbohydrates. They are naturally sweet and add moisture to recipes, making them a perfect addition to pancakes, muffins, or breakfast cookies. (Check the labels for any unnecessary added sugar).

Fridge staples to have ready or cooked for the week:

1-2 Grains or Carbs: For example, quinoa, rice, whole-grain pasta, farro, or sweet potato.

2-3 Proteins: Wild salmon, free-range chicken, grass-fed beef, antibiotic-free turkey, tofu, tempeh, and free-range eggs are great options. You can roast a whole chicken and salmon, or prepare the beef and turkey into meatballs or burger patties ahead of time.

2-3 Breakfast or Snack Ideas: Granola (pages 44, 47), BYOYP (page 150-153), Energy Balls (pages 163, 165), or Champion Chia Overnight Oats (page 51).

3-4 Frozen and Cooked Vegetables: To save time, roast an assortment of vegetables on 1-2 large sheet trays lined with parchment paper. Store them in the fridge for the week. Keeping a bag of cauliflower in the freezer is a great way to add some vegetables into smoothies without tasting them (not to mention they make it extra creamy!). Also, it's good to have raw greens like spinach, kale, or lettuce on hand to add to any meals. Chop up fruits and raw vegetables (like cucumber, celery and carrots) and store in airtight containers in the fridge. This is perfect for when you need something quick for on-the-go nourishment.

Homemade Teas, Nut Milk, or Energy Drinks: (see pages 183-191)

One Sweet Treat: Our favorites are **Zucchini Banana Bread** (page 173), **Granola** (pages 44, 47), dark chocolate bark, and **Almond Butter Banana Bites** (page 140) to name a few!

Remember, the meals don't have to be complete and portioned during preparation, but having the base ingredients already prepared is a huge time saver during busy weekdays.

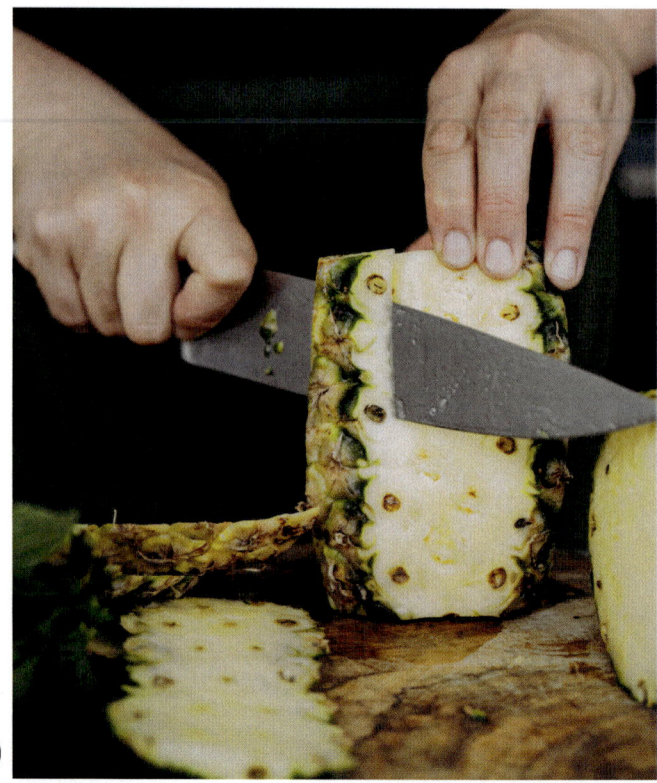

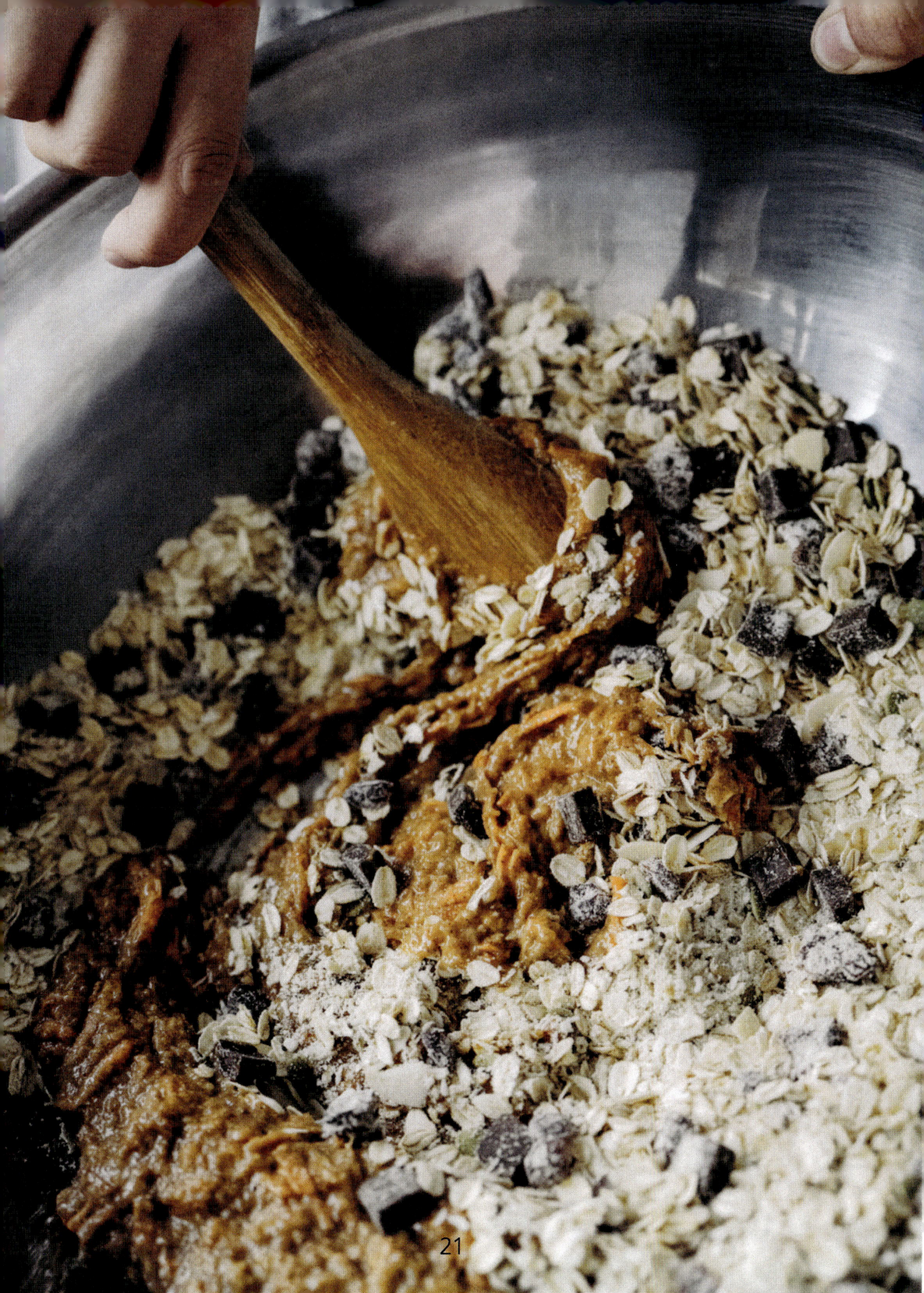

Eating Like A Pro

These are seasonal sample meal plans that include a mixture of my favorite recipes from different Olympians. These meals can be stored as leftovers and used again for lunch or dinner. Also, any snacks can be eaten before lunch or saved for the afternoon depending on your training schedule or appetite.

Remember that everyone is different! Getting adequate fuel for training depends on your unique physiology and training intensity. Some athletes eat three large meals a day, whereas others eat five-to-six smaller meals a day. This meal plan is a template of an average athlete's full day of eating, so do what works best for you.

(Note: Not every week needs to be this diverse! You can bake one or two desserts and snacks to rotate through and rely more on leftovers).

Depending on your energy output and training intensity, your portion sizes will vary, so adjust the template to fit your personal needs. On a day-to-day basis, focus on getting enough protein and fueling your body well pre-and post-training.

It is always good to have a rehydration drink like the **Electrolyte Water** (page 183) and the **Cool as a Cucumber Water** (page 193) on hand for any day of the week.

SPRING/ SUMMER	Monday	Tuesday	Wednesday
Breakfast	Matcha smoothie bowl (page 54) Cool as a Cucumber Water (page 193)	Champion Chia Overnight Oats (page 51) Immunity Booster (page 187)	Sunrise Smoothie (page 195) Cool as a Cucumber Water (page 193)
Lunch	Mediterranean Roast Salad with Chicken (page 89)	Leftover Veggies and Dip Platter with protein of choice (page 132)	Leftover Instagram Chicken Fried Rice (page 108)
Snack	Lemon Chia Energy Ball (page 163) Golden Milk Latte (page 189)	Build Your Own Yogurt Parfait (page 150-153)	Post-workout Electrolyte Lemon Limeade (page 183) The Ultimate Power Cookie (page 161)
Dinner	Veggies and Dip Platter with protein of choice (page 132)	Instagram Chicken Fried Rice (page 108)	Zucchini Tacos (page 102)
Dessert	Strawberry Nice Cream (page 143) Tranquility Tea (page 191)	Almond Butter Banana Bites (page 140) Tranquility Tea (page 191)	Mint Chip Nice Cream (page 143) Tranquility Tea (page 191)

Thursday	**Friday**	**Saturday**	**Sunday**
Slice of Honey Cinnamon PB Toast (page 65) + Slice of High Protein Toast (page 62) Cool as a Cucumber Water (page 193)	Greek yogurt with Chocolate Granola and Berries (page 47) Vanilla Nut/Seed Milk Latte (coffee/tea/matcha latte) (page 185) and water	Alkalizing Smoothie (page 178) Anti-Inflammatory Golden Milk Latte (coffee/tea/matcha latte) (page 189) and water	Chocolate Protein Pancakes (page 42) Immunity Booster (page 187) and water
Leftover Zucchini Tacos (page 102)	Leftover Pork BBQ Baby Back Ribs (page 112)	Mediterranean Roast Salad with protein of choice (page 89)	Leftover Tempeh Tabbouleh Bowl (page 121)
Vegetable and Apple slices with leftover Honey Cinnamon Peanut Butter (page 67)	Chocolate PB + Banana "Milkshake" (page 181)	Lemon Chia Energy Ball (page 163) with Greek yogurt and sliced vegetables	Sliced vegetables and rice cakes with Honey Cinnamon Peanut Butter (page 67), banana, and hemp seeds
BBQ Pork Baby Back Ribs (page 112)	Miso Salmon Nourish Bowl with Lemon Vinaigrette (page 95, 96)	Tempeh Tabbouleh Bowl (page 121)	Chicken Schnitzel (page 85)
Cookie Dough Power Ball (page 165) Tranquility Tea (page 191)	Sugar Mint Pineapple (page 156) Tranquility Tea (page 191)	Chocolate Nice Cream (page 143) Tranquility Tea (page 191)	Lemon Chia Energy Ball (page 163) Tranquility Tea (page 191)

FALL/ WINTER	Monday	Tuesday	Wednesday
Breakfast	G.O.A.T.meal (page 39) Vanilla Nut/Seed Milk Latte (page 185) and water	Avocado Toast with Poached Eggs (page 58) Cool as a Cucumber Water (page 193)	Chocolate Protein Pancakes (page 42) Anti-Inflammatory Golden Milk Latte (coffee/tea/matcha latte) (page 189)
Lunch	Cypriot Grain Salad (page 100) with protein of choice	Leftover Chill Out Chili (page 123)	Tofu Pasta (page 82)
Snack	Champion Chia Overnight Oats (page 51) and sliced vegetables	Ultimate Power Cookie (page 161) and sliced vegetables	Leftover Veggie and Dip Platter (page 132)
Dinner	Chill Out Chili (page 123)	Veggie and Dip Platter (page 132) with protein of choice	Winner Winner Chicken Dinner (page 124)
Dessert	Caramelized Pears (page 159) Tranquility Tea (page 191)	Apple and Blackberry Crumble (page 167) Tranquility Tea (page 191)	Zucchini Banana Bread (page 173) Tranquility Tea (page 191)

Thursday	Friday	Saturday	Sunday
Breakfast Sandwich (page 36) Cool as a Cucumber Water (page 193)	Build Your Own Yogurt Parfait (page 150-153) Ultimate Power Cookie (page 161) and water	G.O.A.T.meal (page 39) Immunity Booster (page 187) and water	Chocolate Protein Pancakes (page 42) Immunity Booster (page 187) and water
Leftover Winner Winner Chicken Dinner (page 124)	Leftover Lasting Lentil Soup and a Crispy Salad Burrito (page 79, 76)	Leftover Turkey Bacon Bowl (page 92)	Leftover Shrimp Stir Fry (page 118)
Electrolyte Lemon Limeade (page 183) and Build Your Own Yogurt Parfait (page 150-153)	Zucchini Banana Bread (page 173) with Greek yogurt	Microwave apple and cinnamon with Honey Cinnamon Peanut Butter (page 67) and sliced veggies	Cookie dough Power Ball (page 165) with Greek yogurt and sliced veggies
Lasting Lentil Soup (page 79) with crackers and hummus	Turkey Bacon Bowl (page 92)	Shrimp Stir Fry (page 118)	Uncle Johnny's Meatballs (page 115)
Race Ready Rice Pudding (page 169) Tranquility Tea (page 191)	Apple and Blackberry Crumble (page 167) Tranquility Tea (page 191)	Walnut Brownie (page 147) Tranquility Tea (page 191)	Millionaire Square (page 171) Tranquility Tea (page 191)

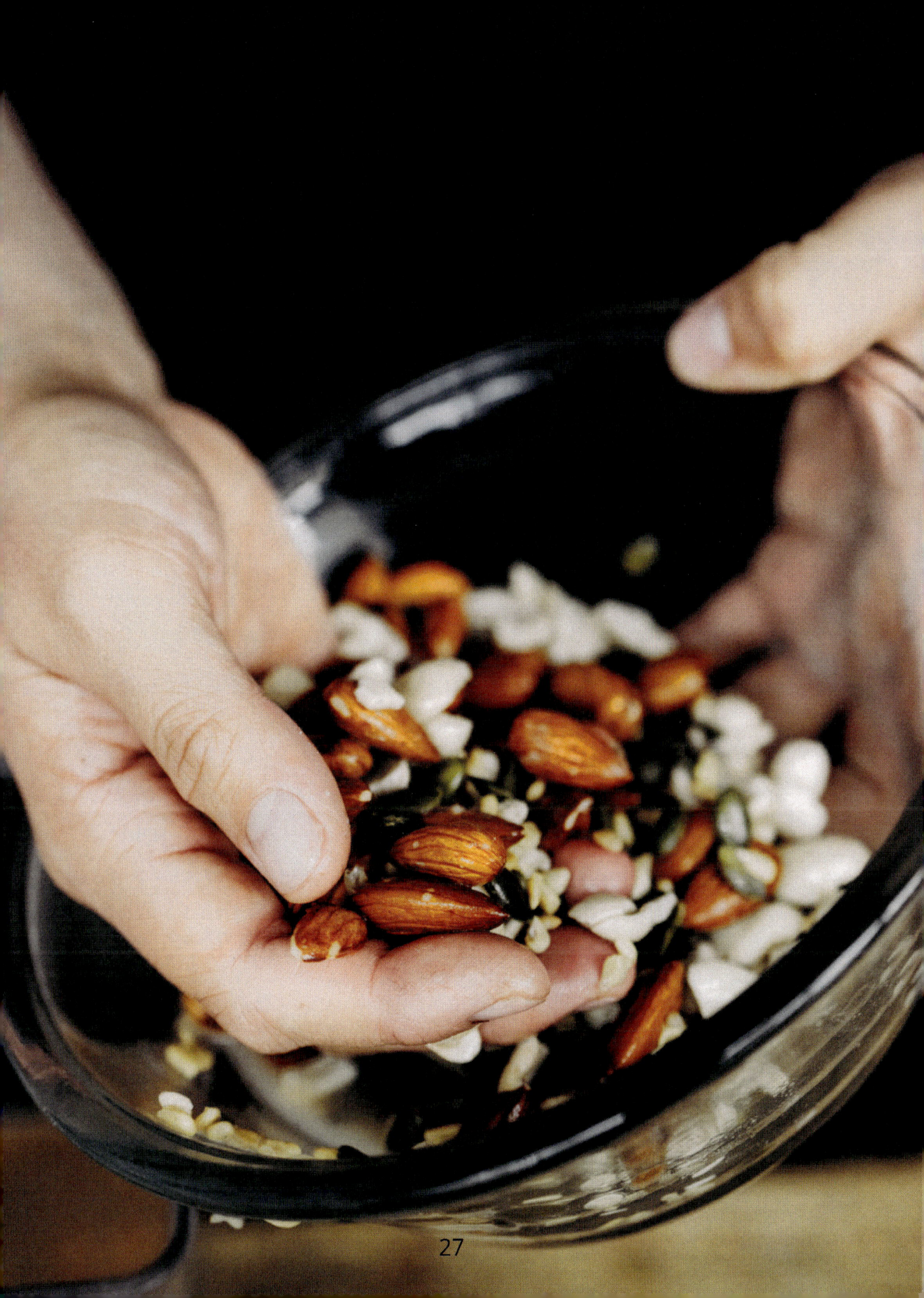

Interview with Nutritionist and Trainer, Kristine Williams:

On setting up your environment for success, nutrition tips before competition and travel, and the importance of sleep.

Q: Most common mistakes young athletes make with their nutrition?
The biggest mistake I find young athletes make with their nutrition is not having a plan for food prep and what they are going to eat on a daily basis. Schedule it in!

Q: What are some tips to set up your environment for success?
Make sure that your kitchen is set up efficiently. Appropriate storage containers, cooking utensils, pots and pans and general organization in your cooking space. Also if you have some foods that are not as nutritionally optimal (like sugary snacks), keep them out of sight, plan them into your schedule, or don't have them in the house at all so that you eliminate any temptation.

Q: What are some ways to sneak in vegetables for those who don't love them?
Throw extra vegetables like spinach, for example, in soups or a smoothie. I also find having chopped fresh vegetables prepared can be so helpful in getting in a bit more each day.

Q: Do you have any meal prepping hacks?
Create a consistent schedule of the days of the week that you will prepare food and meals. Cook big batches so you have some emergency go-to meals for busy days. Stick to 3-5 recipes that you consistently use per meal and change it up when you are needing variety. Keep things as simple as possible, you do not have to get fancy!

Q: Explain the importance of hydration
Hydration is so important for performance and taking care of your body. Not being hydrated is especially noticeable as an athlete as it can reduce both your strength and endurance performance.

Q: Explain the 80/20 rule and 90/10 rule

As a Precision Nutrition L1 coach, I really encourage the 80/20 rule. This means that 80% of the time you eat the most optimal nutrition choices and 20% of the time would be any other option you enjoy fitting in. If you are performing at a high level, are close to a competition, or your sport has an aesthetic aspect, then you may have to spend a period of time being in the 90/10 range. This will mean making a small adjustment to your 80/20 guideline before competing.

Q: How should athletes approach nutrition before travel and competition?

I believe the best approach for an athlete going into a competition or travel is to stay as close to the nutrition intake they have already been consuming so as not to eat any food that may cause an upset stomach or may not make them feel their best. Staying well hydrated before and during travel is of high importance so that the body is not dehydrated for competition. Having a plan, such as where you will buy your food or groceries before you go, can be helpful so you are organized once you arrive.

Q: How does sleep impact cravings and nutrition?

Lack of sleep or poor sleep patterns can throw off your appetite regulation and also cause you to feel hungrier. Rest and recovery are so important!

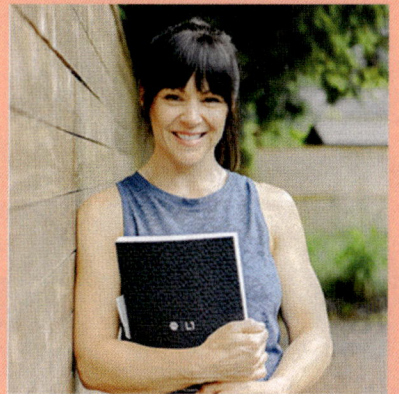

Pure Strength + Nutrition is a full-service personal fitness and nutritional guidance program that gives the gift of whole health.

Visit Kristine's website **purestrengthnutrition.com** for more.

 **WARNING:** Before we get into the recipes, note that some recipes use protein powders. Make sure to check the brand, labels, and ingredients of the protein powders to see if they are safe and doping-approved for your sport.

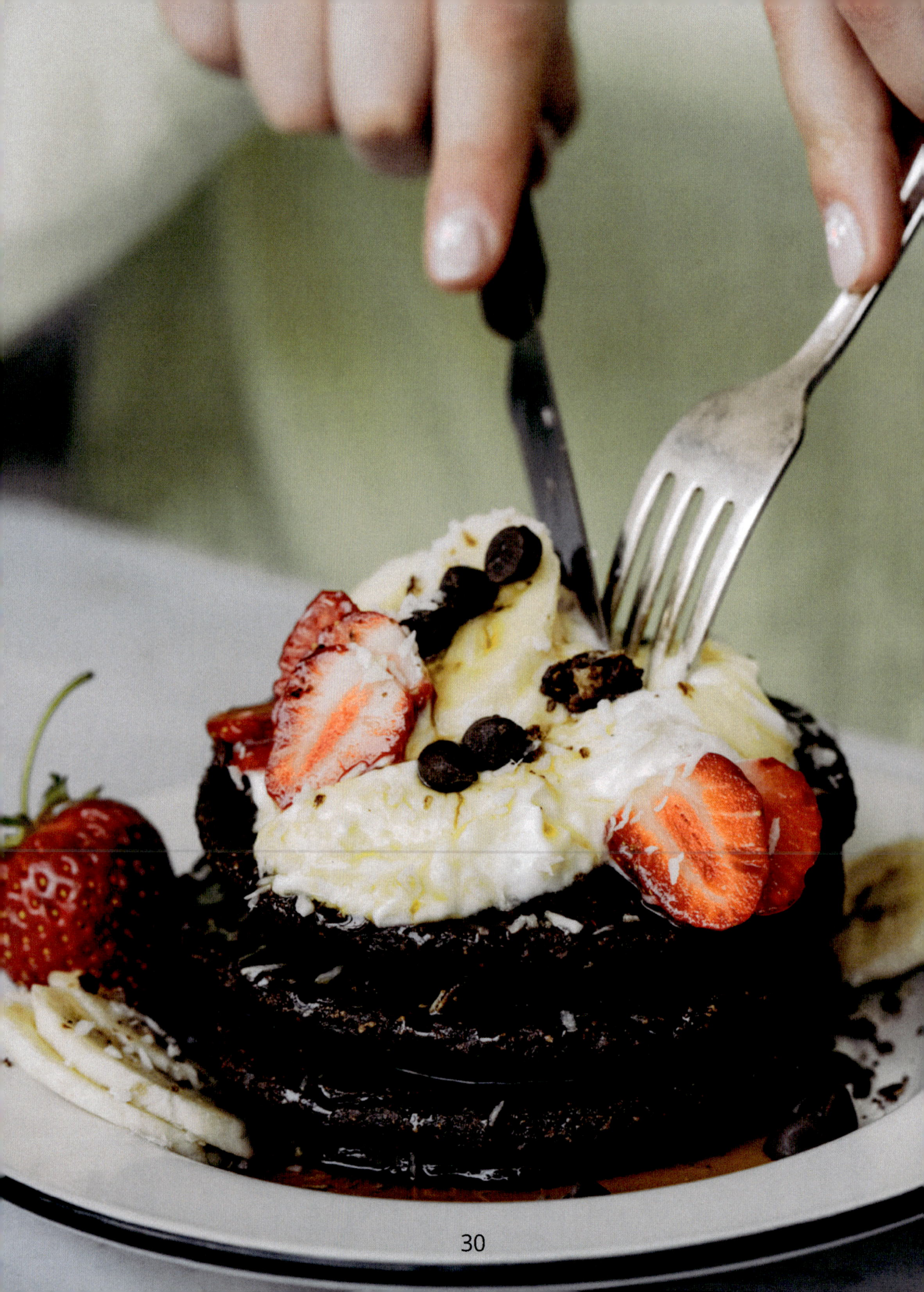

THE BREAKFAST OF CHAMPIONS

Breakfast Sandwich   34

G.O.A.T.meal   37

Chocolate Protein Pancakes   40

Maple Coconut Granola   43

Chocolate Sea Salt Granola   46

Champion Chia Overnight Oats   49

Matcha Smoothie Bowl   52

TOASTS: because toast deserves its own section

- Avocado Toast with Poached Eggs   56
- High Protein Toast   60
- Cinnamon Raisin Bread   63
- Honey Cinnamon Peanut Butter Toast   66

Mornings are special. They represent a blank slate—a fresh start where you can design your day and how you want to show up for yourself. Establishing a consistent morning routine is important in setting yourself up for success and reducing scheduling overwhelm.

An alarming number of young athletes skip breakfast without realizing the negative impact this has on their training. Without sufficient energy, your muscles will not respond as well, your focus and energy will drop, and your overall performance will decrease. Getting a nutritious, energy-dense breakfast will prepare your body to burn more energy, kick-starting your metabolism so that you can train harder and better. Breakfast really *is* what makes champions!

Here are 7 ways to boost your mornings and increase productivity:

Set an intention for the day:
What energy do you want to bring, and how do you want to show up to work, family time, or downtime? This could be something like "Today, I intend to eat mindfully" or "Today, I intend to be the best partner I can be."

Face the sun:
Direct sunlight first thing in the morning activates your circadian rhythm. This brings your melatonin production down so you feel more awake in the morning and boosts it in the evening to improve the quality of your sleep.

Movement is key:
Movement of any form wakes up the body and metabolism, releases tension, and energizes you for the day. BONUS: try to get outside and in nature to feel extra energized and calm.

Get grateful:
Start the day by writing down 3 things you're grateful for. This simple practice focuses on the positives, encouraging you to live a life of abundance rather than focusing on lack.

Don't hate, just meditate:
Taking just 5 minutes in the morning to be still and connect with your body and your breath is a powerful practice. Athletes love meditation because it preps and calms their bodies mentally so they can perform physically.
Tip: Start small to build consistent, long-term results. Set a timer for just 1 minute per day. Once that is comfortable, increase the time gradually until you're a pro!

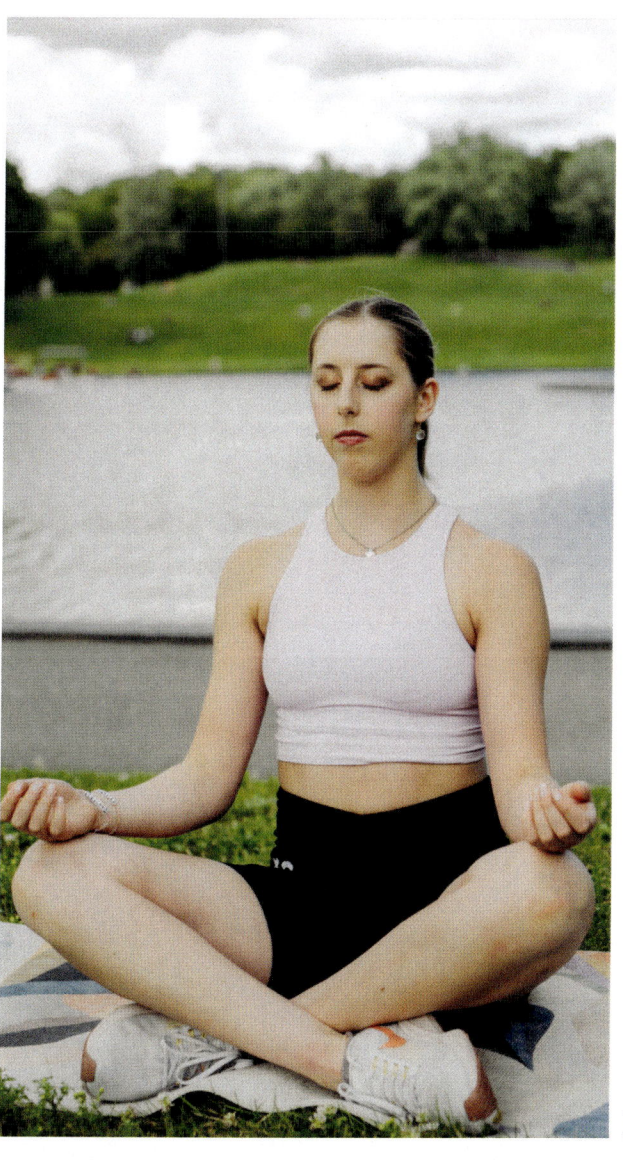

Create before you consume:
Each day our brains have a limited supply of fuel which is replenished each morning. That means that doing low-energy tasks like chores, scrolling through emails, social media, or messages first thing in the morning will drain your precious brain power and prime the brain for distractions (not to mention, this increases stress). Choosing to work on a project, get a workout done, meditate, or do something creative before turning to screens will boost your productivity and maximize your morning peak-focus hours. Are you someone who rushes out the door? Try setting your alarm 30 minutes earlier (and going to bed 30 minutes earlier) to have just a few extra minutes to set an inspiring tone for the day.

Review your success plan:
Each night write down your schedule for the next day. Find blocks of time to dedicate to projects, family, self-care, workouts, screen time, breaks, etc. Don't overstuff the day, but in those focused blocks of time be 100% present for the tasks or people you're with.

GUILLAUME CIZERON

Ice Dance

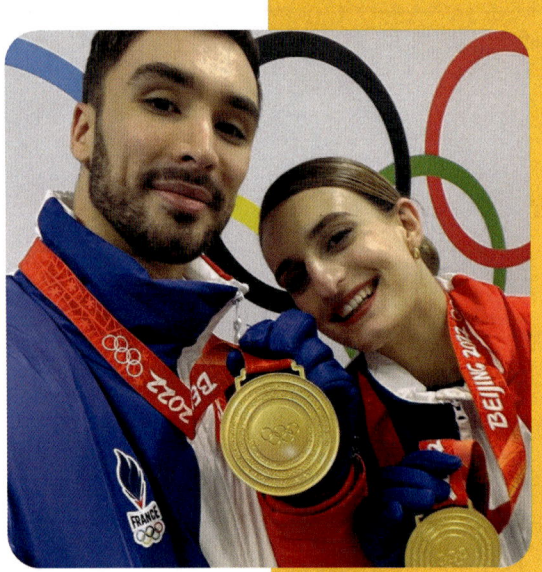

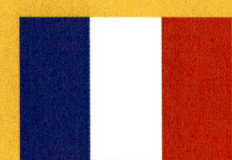

Morning Routine

"Wake up, coffee, big glass of water. Then I take my dog out. I usually make an oatmeal breakfast if I'm in a rush. If I have time, I make avocado toast, eggs, and labneh. Then shower, prepare, and go to the rink."

Mental Prep Tip

"I like breathing exercises. I also do a lot of visualization with different goals or focuses for each one. It can be breath, emotion, technique, or energy management."

Recovery Tip

"Taking my dog out for a walk, watching tv, or going out for dinner with friends!"

Olympic Memory

"My favorite moment was in the 'Kiss and Cry' when we had just won and all of our friends came and hugged us!"

Image by Guillaume Cizeron

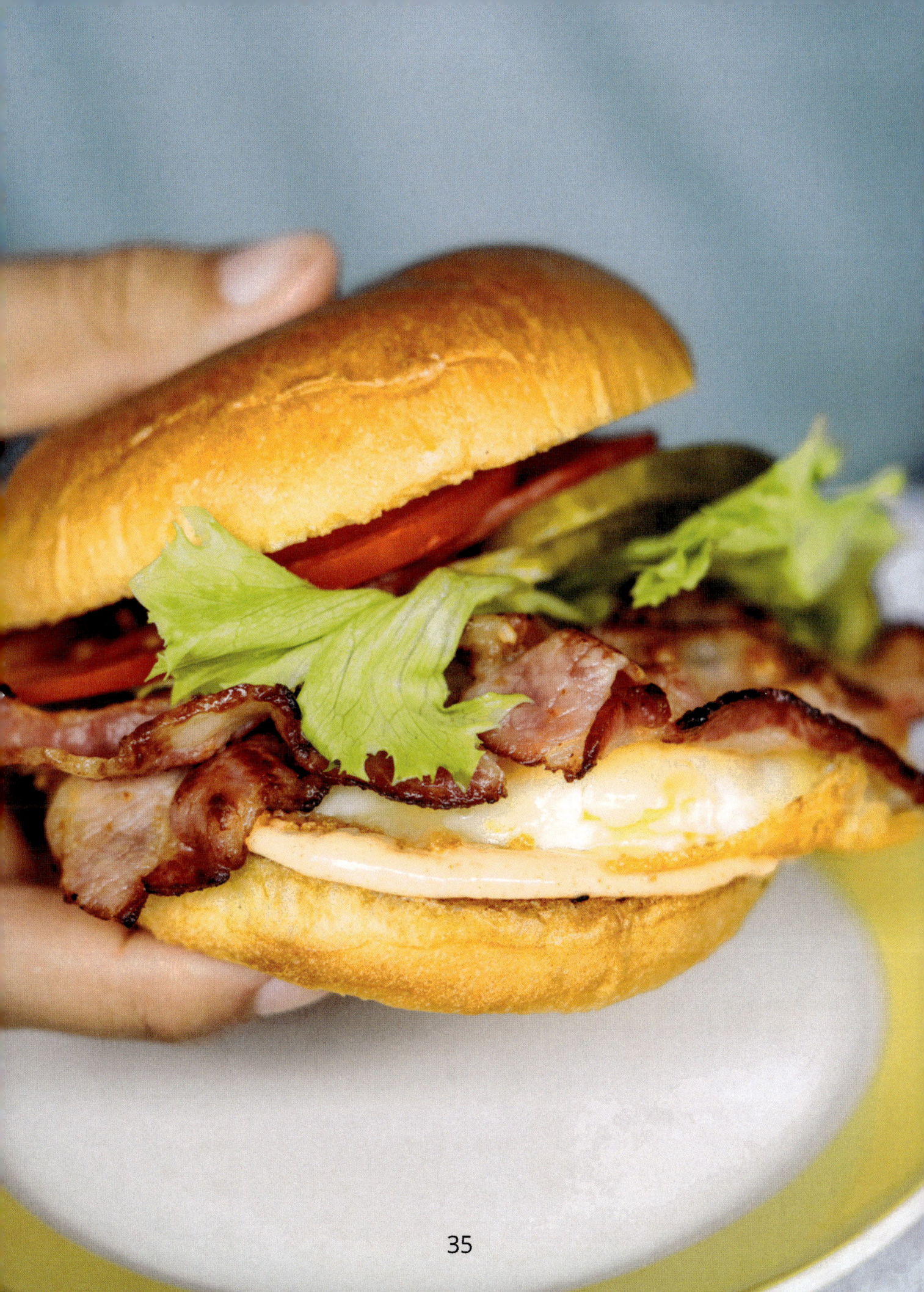

Breakfast Sandwich
for a savory start

nf

Guillaume Cizeron is a French ice dancer who won Silver in Pyeongchang 2018 and Gold in Beijing 2022 alongside his partner Gabriella Papadakis. Not only is he an Olympic Champion, but he is also a 5x World Champion, a 5x consecutive European Champion, a 7x National Champion, and he has broken world records 28 times. Guillaume and Gabriella are known for their lyrical and modern movements, and the quality of their skating skills is unparalleled. It's a privilege to train with G&G, and they are some of the best ice dancers of all time. Check out Guillame's beautiful book *Ma Plus Belle Victoire* where he opens up about his homosexuality and becoming his truest self.

Makes 1 serving

2 tablespoons mayo
1 teaspoon sriracha
1/2 teaspoon smoked paprika
1 tablespoon salted butter
1 egg
1 tablespoon cheddar cheese, shredded
2 strips of bacon
1 brioche bun
1 small head iceberg lettuce
1/2 large dill pickle, thinly sliced
1/2 medium tomato, thinly sliced

> This recipe is inspired by Guillaume's favorite breakfast sandwich in Montréal. It is so delicious because of the different textures and layers like the crunchy lettuce, salty bacon, and the soft brioche bun. The spicy mayo melts in your mouth and adds an extra kick of flavor!

1. Mix mayo, sriracha, and smoked paprika in a bowl. Set aside.
2. Crack the egg in a small ramekin to avoid eggshell pieces falling in. Then, melt the butter in a non-stick pan. Add the egg. Cook one side, flip, then add the cheese on top of the egg. Cook for 1 minute to allow the yolk to firm.
3. Add bacon to the pan and cook until both sides are crispy brown.
4. If needed, add more butter to the pan and place each half of the brioche bun face down and cook until toasted.
5. Assemble the sandwich by spreading mayo on each bun, then add the egg, bacon, lettuce, pickles, and tomato.

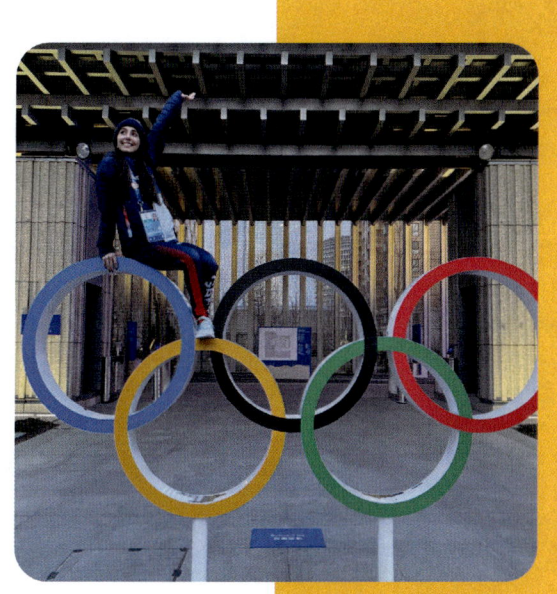

LILAH FEAR
Ice Dance

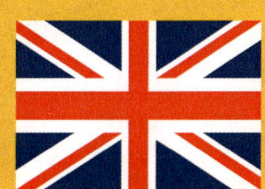

Mental Prep Tip

"Breath work is very powerful, as well as intentional self talk to empower oneself." (See more page 211)

Morning Routine

"Wake up at 5:45am, journal, and get ready while listening to a podcast. Then sit down for a mindful, relaxed breakfast and coffee. Warm up for skating at home, then drive to the rink at 6:45am."

Olympic Memory

"The sense of community, friendship, and encouragement. It was an honor to connect with so many miraculous humans and share their experiences."

Sleep Habits

"Wind down with a generous amount of time before bed. Limit technology, switch to a book, and drain lactic acid from my legs by lying on my back and putting my legs up the wall. I dim the lights and like to use lavender oil to relax."

Recovery Tip

"I like to have an Epsom salt bath with a hot cup of tea, some dark chocolate, and a soothing face mask!"

Image by Lilah Fear

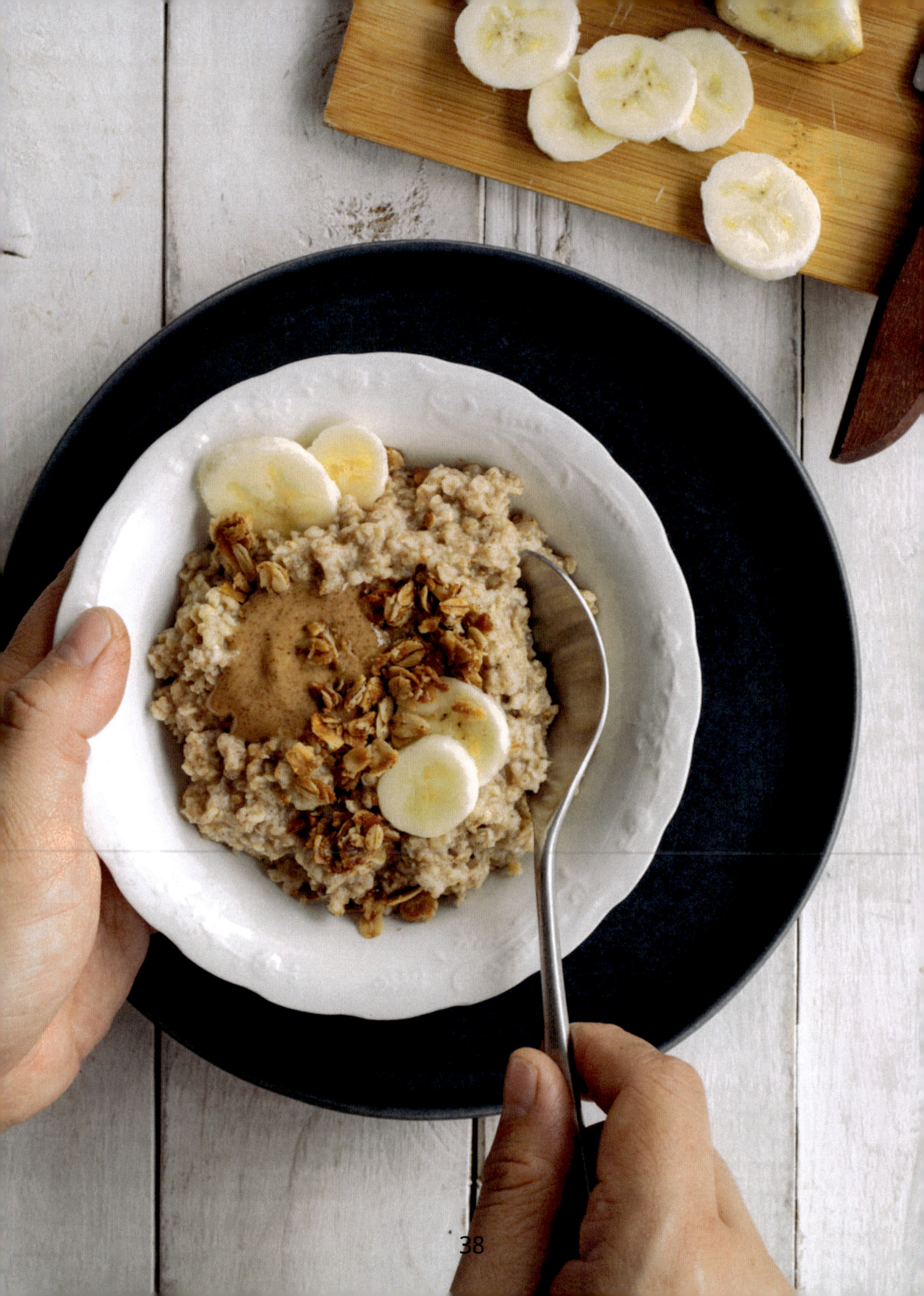

G.O.A.T.meal
for a cozy but quick pre-training breakfast

gf v df

Lilah Fear is an ice dancer representing Great Britain alongside her partner Lewis Gibson. The pair competed in Beijing 2022 at their first Olympic Games and placed 10th. (In case you didn't notice, YES, we are SISTERS!) They most recently finished 2nd at the European Championships and 4th at the World Championships 2023.

This warm bowl of cinnamon oatmeal is Lilah's go-to breakfast before intense on-ice training. Using hot water from the kettle to make the oats is a great time saver for rushed mornings. She insists on eating two heaping spoonfuls of nut butter. Period. End of story. Non-negotiable. (I mean, twist my arm!)

Serves 1
1/2 cup quick oats (or GF if sensitive)
1/2 teaspoon ground cinnamon
Pinch of sea salt
3/4 cup of boiling water
1/2 banana sliced
1-2 tablespoons nut butter of choice (Lilah loves using both almond butter and crunchy peanut butter)
1/4 cup maple coconut granola (see recipe on next page)

1. Combine the oats, cinnamon, and salt in a cereal bowl. Add 3/4 cup boiling water from an electric tea kettle and stir.
2. Cover the bowl with a plate, pot lid, or towel for 3 minutes or until the oats have thickened.
3. Top with banana slices, nut butter of choice, and granola!

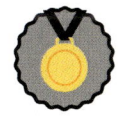

🕒 For slower mornings, use steel-cut or rolled oats and cook over the stovetop with 1 cup of water until thickened. For a banana bread taste, add the banana slices into the pan and cook them with the oats.

🏅 For extra protein add 1/2 cup plain whole milk greek yogurt, or stir in 2 tbsp hemp seeds.

Other topping ideas:
- Fresh berries or raisins
- Dark chocolate chips
- Honey

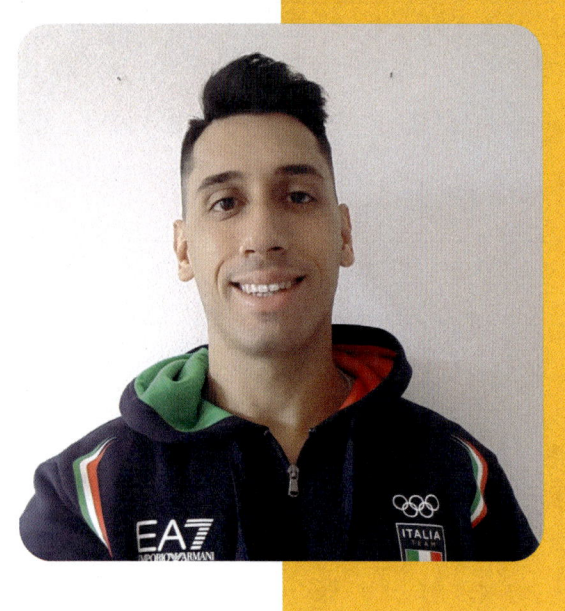

FRANCESCO COSTA

Bobsled

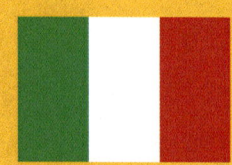

🇮🇹

Sleep Habits

"I get 8-9 hours of sleep. I use a ZMA supplement to sleep well."

Mental Prep Tip

"I prepare for competitions by listening to music, focusing on the goal, and imagining the action to do. I want to feel good." (See more page 212).

Recovery Tip

"I like to sit in the garden and chill in the sun, or play with my PlayStation."

Olympic Memory

"The first Winter Olympics in Russia was a dream—a dream that came true. Representing my country has been fantastic. I have a good memory of my team, and my opponents, and sharing those moments with them was unique."

Image by Francesco Costa

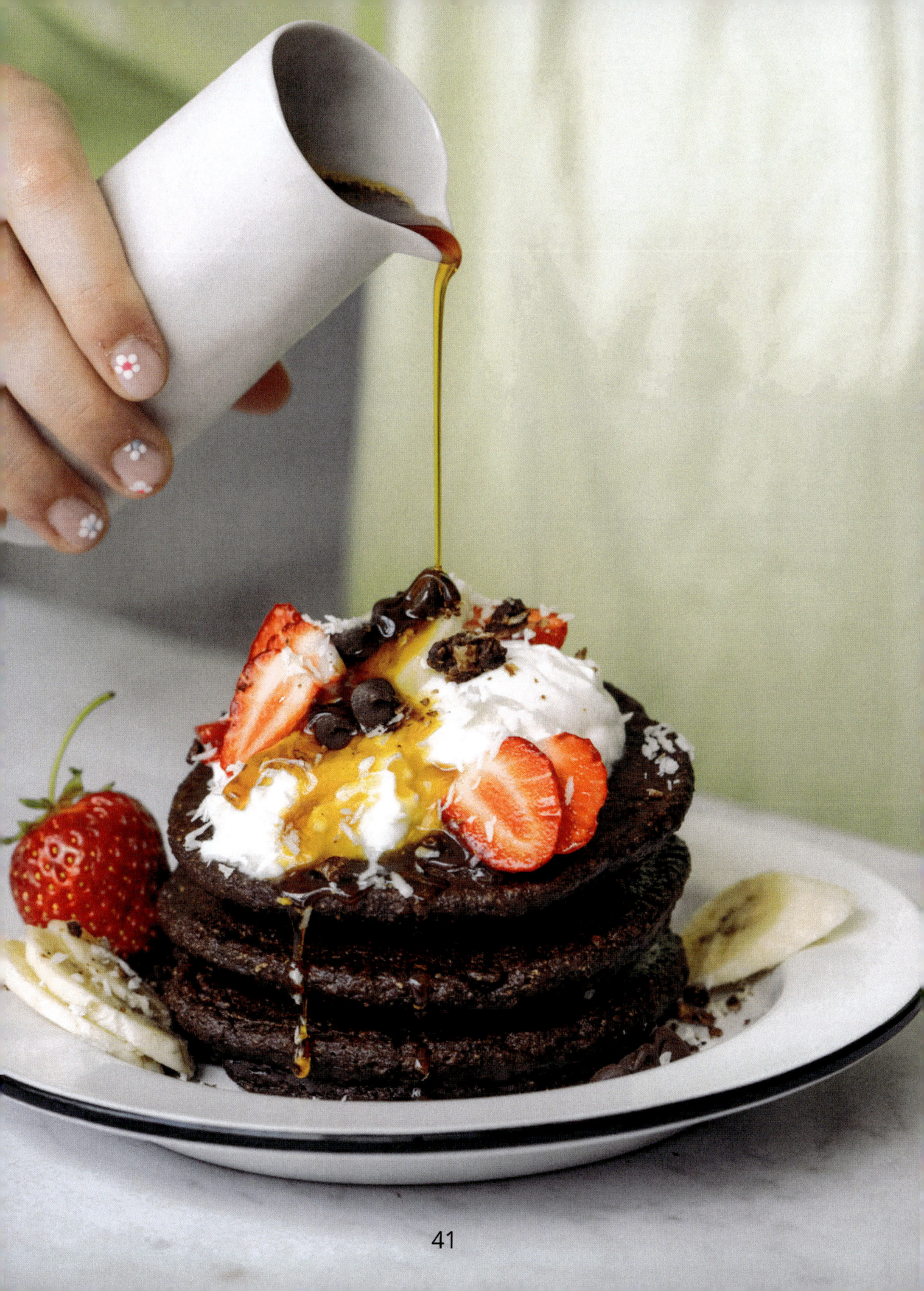

Chocolate Protein Pancakes
for sustenance and power

df gf nf

Francesco Costa is a bobsledder who represented Italy at the Sochi 2014 and Pyeongchang 2018 Olympics in the four-man event. He is also a 3x Europa Cup winner and 3x Italian Champion, and he now is focused on his career as a gym trainer.

Here, Francesco shares his protein pancake recipe which is made with only 3 ingredients! Egg whites are naturally packed with protein, and the oats provide energy and keep you sustained. This recipe is perfect for meal prep because you make a big batch and freeze the pancakes, then simply pop each one in the toaster or microwave to reheat!

Makes 2 Servings

Pancakes:
1 cup egg whites
1 cup oats
1/2-1 tablespoon cacao powder
1 tablespoon coconut oil or butter for frying

Topping ideas:
Drizzle honey or maple syrup
Chocolate chips
Shredded coconut
Sliced fruit (strawberries and bananas are Francesco's favorite!)
Nut or seed butter
Sprinkle of granola
Greek yogurt for extra protein

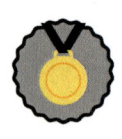

Add 1 banana and chocolate chips into the pancake batter with the egg and oats for a chocolatey banana bread taste!

1. In a high-speed blender, add the egg whites, oats, and cacao powder until smooth.
2. Heat a tablespoon of coconut oil or butter on a non-stick skillet on medium-low heat. Add 2-3 tablespoons of pancake batter for each pancake and cook until the edges of the pancake harden, then flip.
3. Remove once both sides are hardened or golden brown.
4. Serve with as many toppings as you like!

Want to switch it up?
Use **1/2 tablespoon of ground cinnamon** and **1 teaspoon of vanilla extract** instead of cacao powder for a cinnamon bun flavor.

42

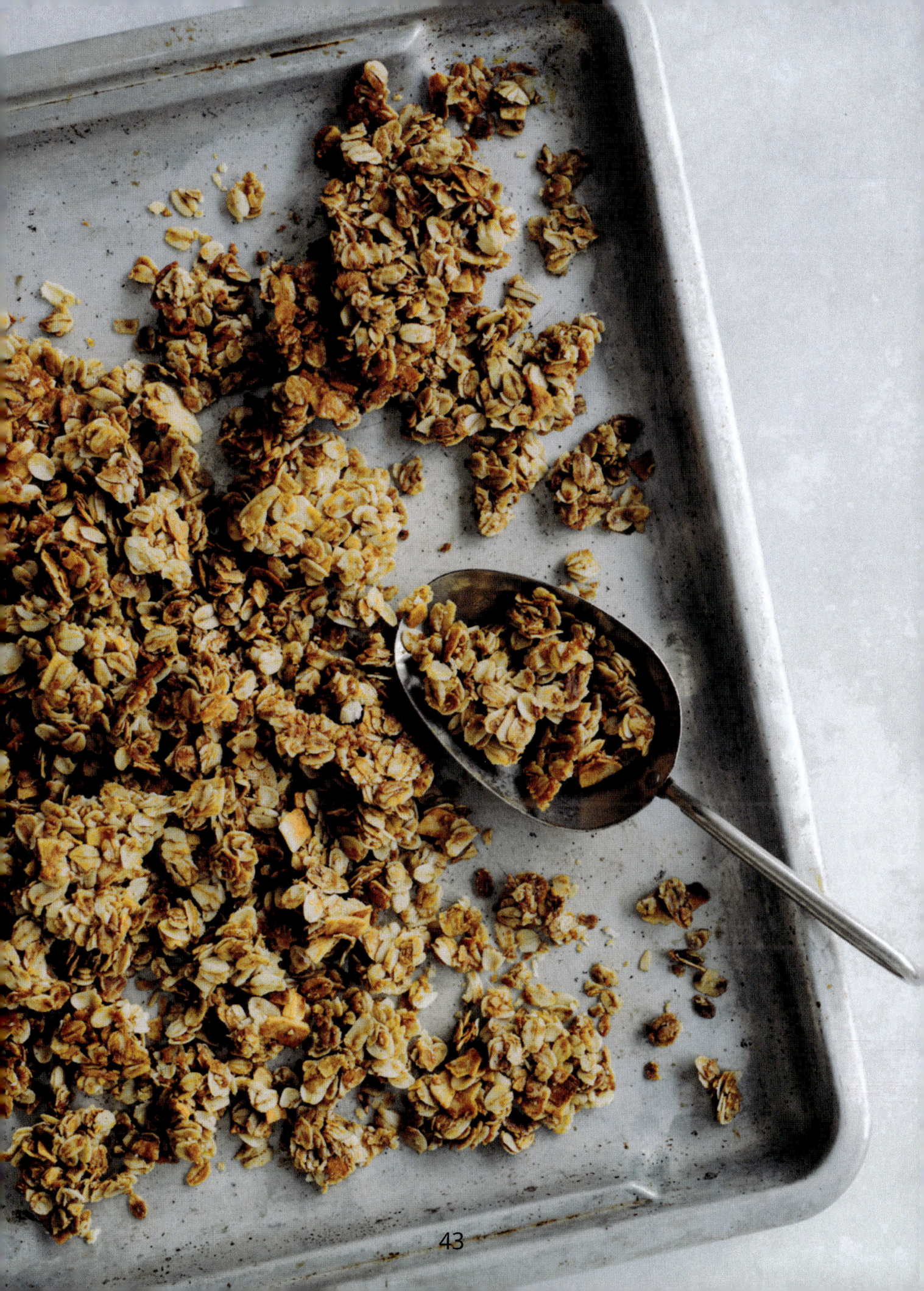

Maple Coconut Granola

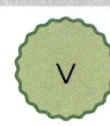

for a crunchy burst of energy

nf gf v df

The story about this granola is pretty special. At the beginning of the pandemic, I had a granola business, and came up with this delicious chunky granola recipe. Since Lilah lives just down the hall, she stopped by frequently to be my "taste tester" when I was in the process of developing the recipe. Let's just say she became addicted!

Athletes need carbs as energy for training and competition. This chunky granola is great because it uses natural sweeteners such as coconut sugar and maple syrup, which are low on the glycemic index. This means that you won't get a huge sugar spike or crash. It is also the perfect addition to oatmeal, yogurt, and smoothies. Or, you can just eat it straight out of the bag (that's my preference!). Allow it to cool completely before storing so that it's extra chunky!

Makes 10 servings

Dry ingredients:
1 1/2 cups rolled oats (or GF if sensitive)
1/4 cup unsweetened coconut flakes
1 teaspoon coconut sugar
1/4 teaspoon sea salt
1/4 teaspoon ground cinnamon

Wet ingredients:
4 tablespoons coconut oil
1/4 cup maple syrup
1 teaspoon pure vanilla extract

1. Preheat oven 325°F and line a large baking tray with parchment paper.
2. In a large bowl, combine the oats, coconut flakes, coconut sugar, sea salt, and cinnamon.
3. In a saucepan on the stovetop, combine the wet ingredients: coconut oil, maple syrup, and vanilla. Let simmer, and stir continuously on low heat. Remove from the stovetop once the mixture starts to bubble.
4. Pour wet ingredients onto dry ingredients. Mix well to evenly coat.

5. Transfer the mixture onto the baking tray and press down so the ingredients stick together as one layer.
6. Bake for 20 minutes, then turn the pan around so the other end goes into the oven first (so that it bakes evenly).
7. Bake 5-7 minutes more, watching carefully so that it doesn't burn. Remove once the granola is golden brown.
8. Let cool, then break the large cluster into smaller pieces. Store in an airtight container at room temperature for several weeks.

Memories from my granola business. I brought the Maple Coconut Granola packs with me everywhere as an easy snack!

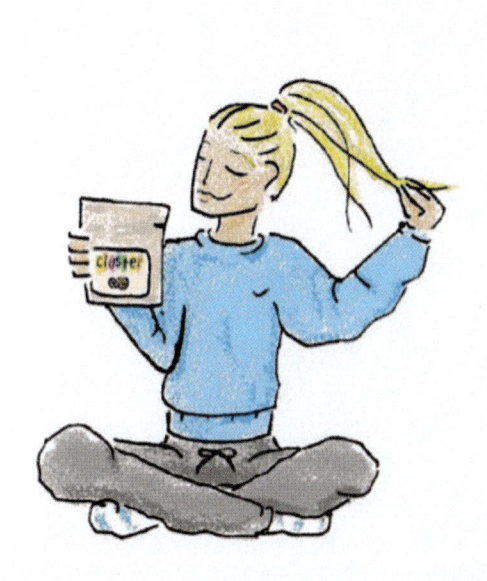

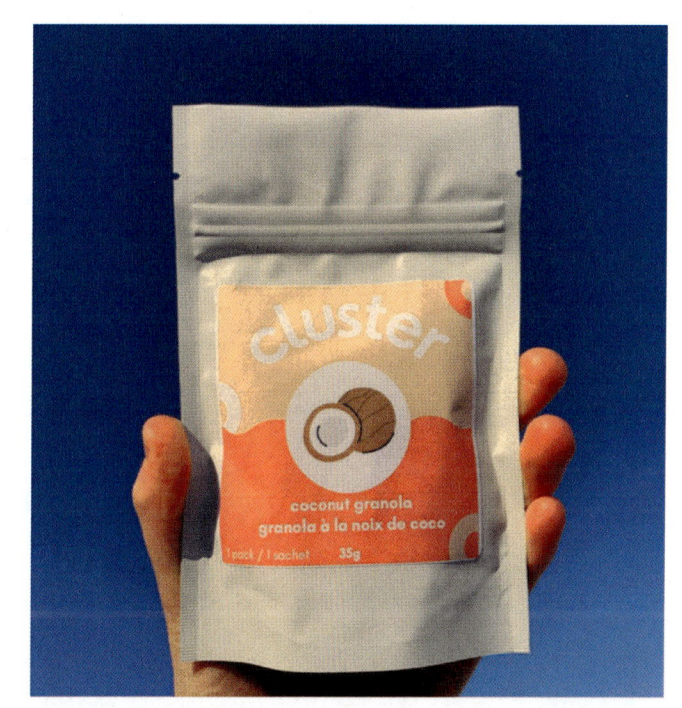

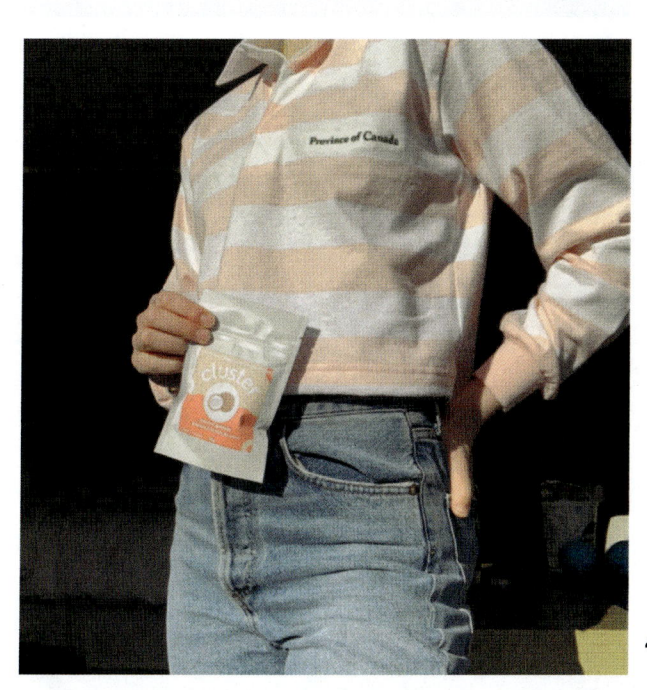

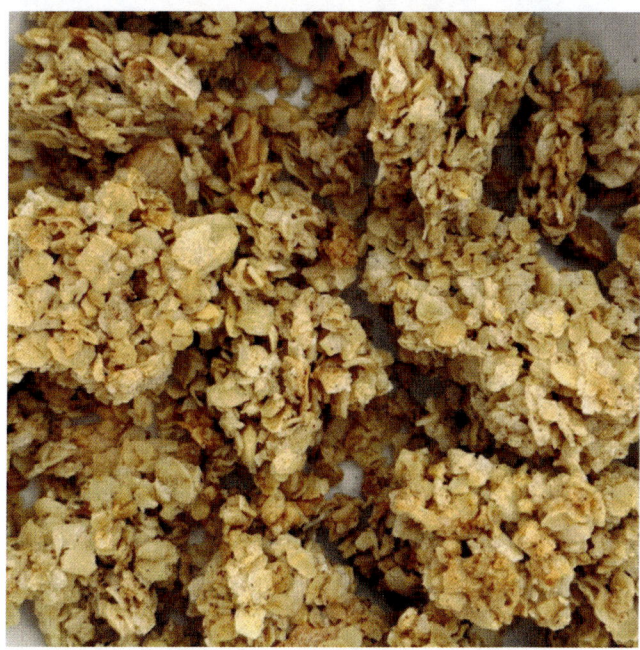

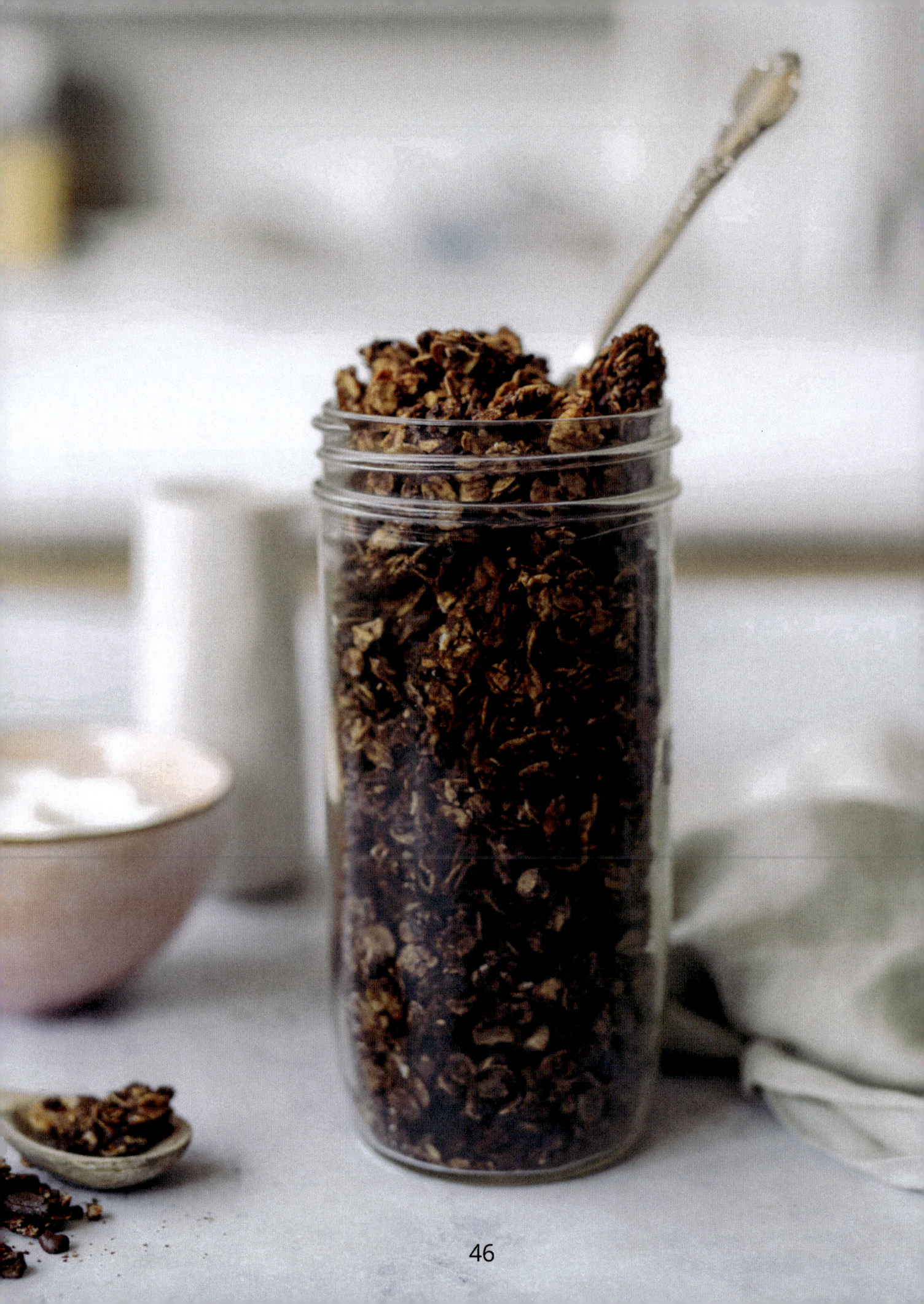

Chocolate Sea Salt Granola

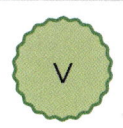

for a sweet start to the day

nf gf v df

The chocolate granola was the second granola flavor that my business released, and it has to be my favorite! The cocoa powder and maple syrup combined make sweet chocolate syrup, and the cacao nibs are a crunchy surprise in every bite (and packed with antioxidants and heart-healthy flavonoids!)

I had to test so many recipes to find the perfect combination of sweet, salty, and chunky, and, let me tell you, this granola ticks all the boxes. It is lightly sweetened with maple syrup and coconut sugar, and the sprinkle of salt balances the rich cocoa powder. Allow the granola to cool completely before storing so that it's extra chunky!
Warning: you will definitely want to lick the bowl, and your kitchen will smell like freshly baked brownies.

Makes 10 servings

Dry ingredients:
1 1/2 cups rolled oats (or GF if sensitive)
1/4 cup cocoa powder
1 teaspoon coconut sugar
1/4 cup cacao nibs
1/4 teaspoon sea salt

Wet ingredients:
4 tablespoons coconut oil
1/4 cup maple syrup
1 teaspoon pure vanilla extract

1. Preheat oven 325°F and line a large baking tray with parchment paper.
2. In a large bowl, combine the oats, cocoa powder, coconut sugar, cacao nibs, and sea salt.
3. In a saucepan on the stovetop, combine the wet ingredients: coconut oil, maple syrup, and vanilla. Let simmer and stir continuously on a low heat. Remove from the stovetop once the mixture starts to bubble.
4. Pour the wet ingredients onto the dry ingredients and mix well to evenly coat.

5. Transfer the mixture onto the baking tray, and press down so the ingredients stick together as one layer.

6. Bake for 20 minutes, then turn the pan around so the other end goes into the oven first (so that it bakes evenly).

7. Bake 5-7 minutes more, watching carefully so that it doesn't burn since the mixture is already chocolatey brown.

8. Let cool, then break the large cluster into smaller pieces. Store in an airtight container at room temperature for several weeks.

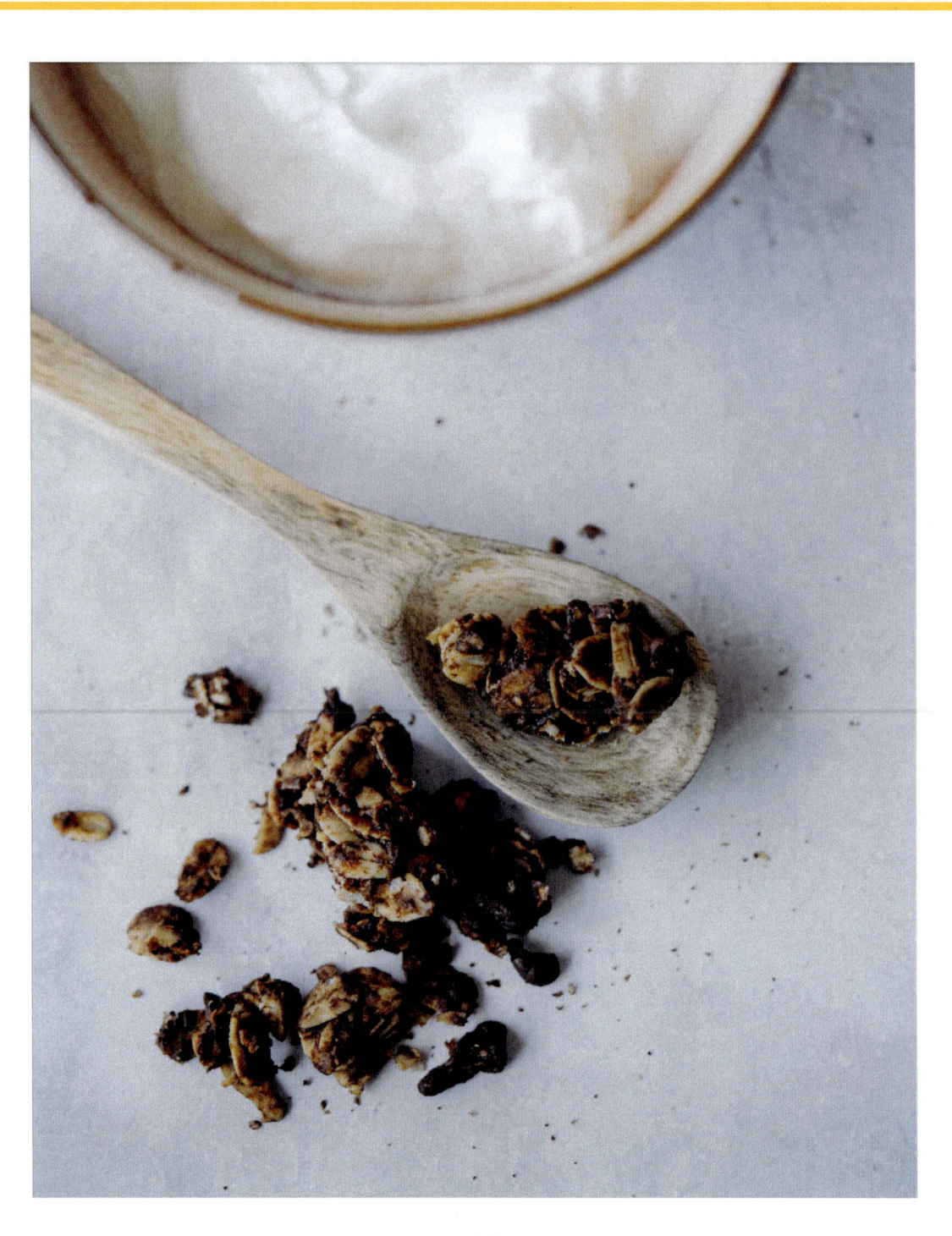

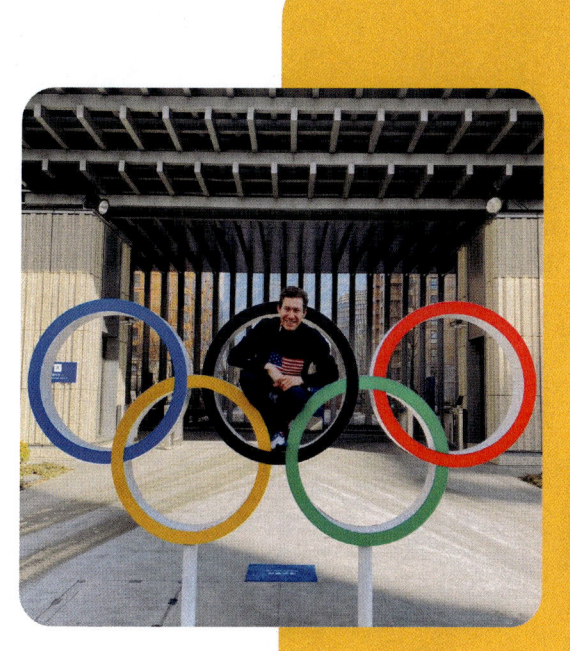

JASON BROWN

Figure Skating

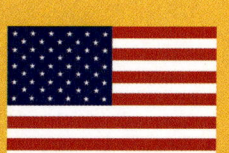

Mental Prep Tip

"Mental preparation is so crucial prior to competitions. On competition days, I always try to take an hour nap or even just set aside 10 mins (depending on how tight the schedule is) to breathe, slow down my heart rate, and calm my mind. I remind myself that I am prepared, repeating the mantra "preparation beats fear". Before I step onto the ice, I clear my head as best as possible, telling myself how lucky I am to have this opportunity to perform and get to show people what I have been working so hard on...and then I take one big, deep breath right before the music starts to ground myself in the present moment." (See more page 211).

Recovery Tip

"I always spend about 1 hour a day cooling down after training. This is where I will stretch and roll out. On top of this, I usually end the night with a good book, some ice, and my Normatec pants.`'

Olympic Memory

"I have to say the interactions with other athletes and getting to cheer on my teammates are probably my favorite memories from the Olympics. We all knew how hard we worked for this moment, so to get to share it and be there to support one another was really special. Plus, it's beyond surreal to be surrounded by the best athletes in their fields from all over the world!"

Image by Jason Brown

50

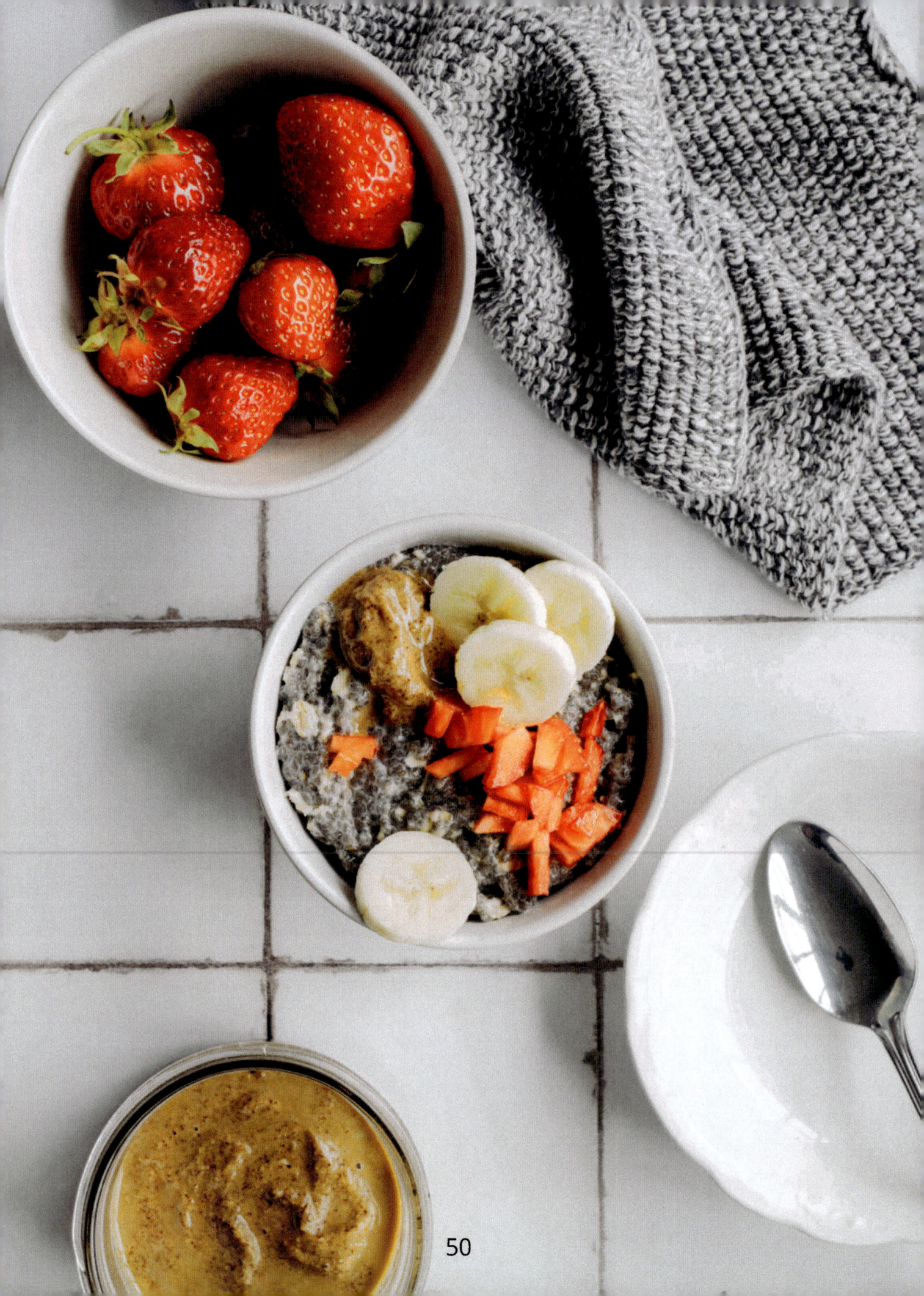

Champion Chia Overnight Oats
for a light breakfast

gf

Jason Brown is a figure skater who represented the USA at the Sochi 2014 and Beijing 2022 Olympic Games. He is a 9x Grand Prix Medalist, a 2x Four Continents Champion, and the 2015 USA National Champion. His incredible artistry, flexibility, and interpretation on the ice set him apart, and he has been a true asset to Team USA throughout his career.

Jason LOVES chia overnight oats with a passion: "It travels well and sits well in my stomach no matter what I am doing. I eat it prior to competing at events. Satisfying, hearty, and settling."

Makes 1 serving

1/3 cup chia seeds
1/4 cup rolled oats (or GF if sensitive)
1 cup unsweetened vanilla almond milk
1/4 teaspoon ground cinnamon
1 tablespoon almond butter (or any other nut butter)
1/2 cup fruit of choice (recommend frozen berries and sliced banana)

1. In a glass jar or airtight container, mix the chia seeds, oats, milk, and cinnamon until fully combined.
2. Let it set and thicken in the fridge for 4-12 hours (overnight is best).
3. After it's thickened, top with nut butter and fruit of choice.

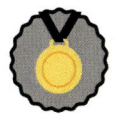

Use our Anti-Inflammatory Golden Milk (see page 189) instead of almond milk for an extra nutrient boost, or add 1 teaspoon of cocoa powder to give it a chocolatey taste.

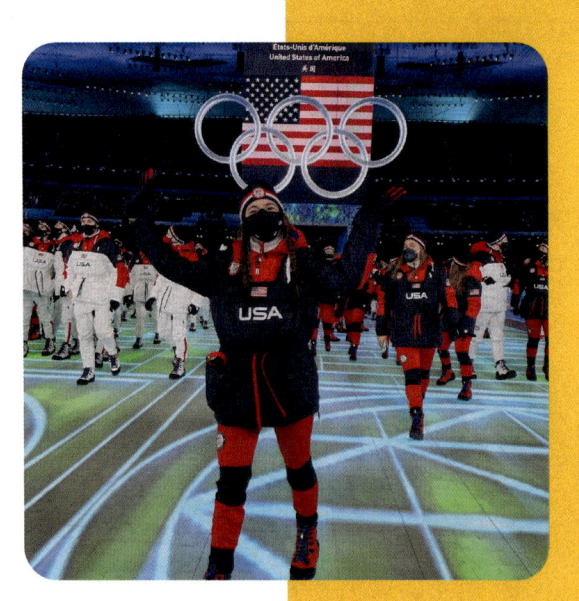

JAELIN KAUF

Freestyle Skier

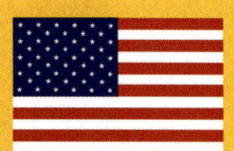

🇺🇸

Olympic Memory:

"My favorite moment from the Olympics was standing at the top of the course for my final run. In my last Olympics, I'd missed out on that final round of 6 and finished in 7th. This time, I made it; I felt so relieved and excited to finally get that chance to ski for gold. I knew my teammates, my coaches, and everyone back home were proud of me, and I was excited to give it everything I had this time around."

Recovery Tip:

"Some yoga and stretching are the best ways for me to wind down. If there is a sauna, you will definitely find me there every day after training."

Mental Prep Tip:

"I have recently gotten into writing down positive moments from every day. Before competing, I reflect on the most positive things I've been doing in training to feel best when going out for my competition." (See more page 212).

Sleep Habits:

"I sleep 9 hours at least most nights. Putting my phone away and not allowing myself to look at it until my alarm goes off in the morning is the best way to fight jet lag and optimize my sleep."

Image by Jaelin Kauf

53

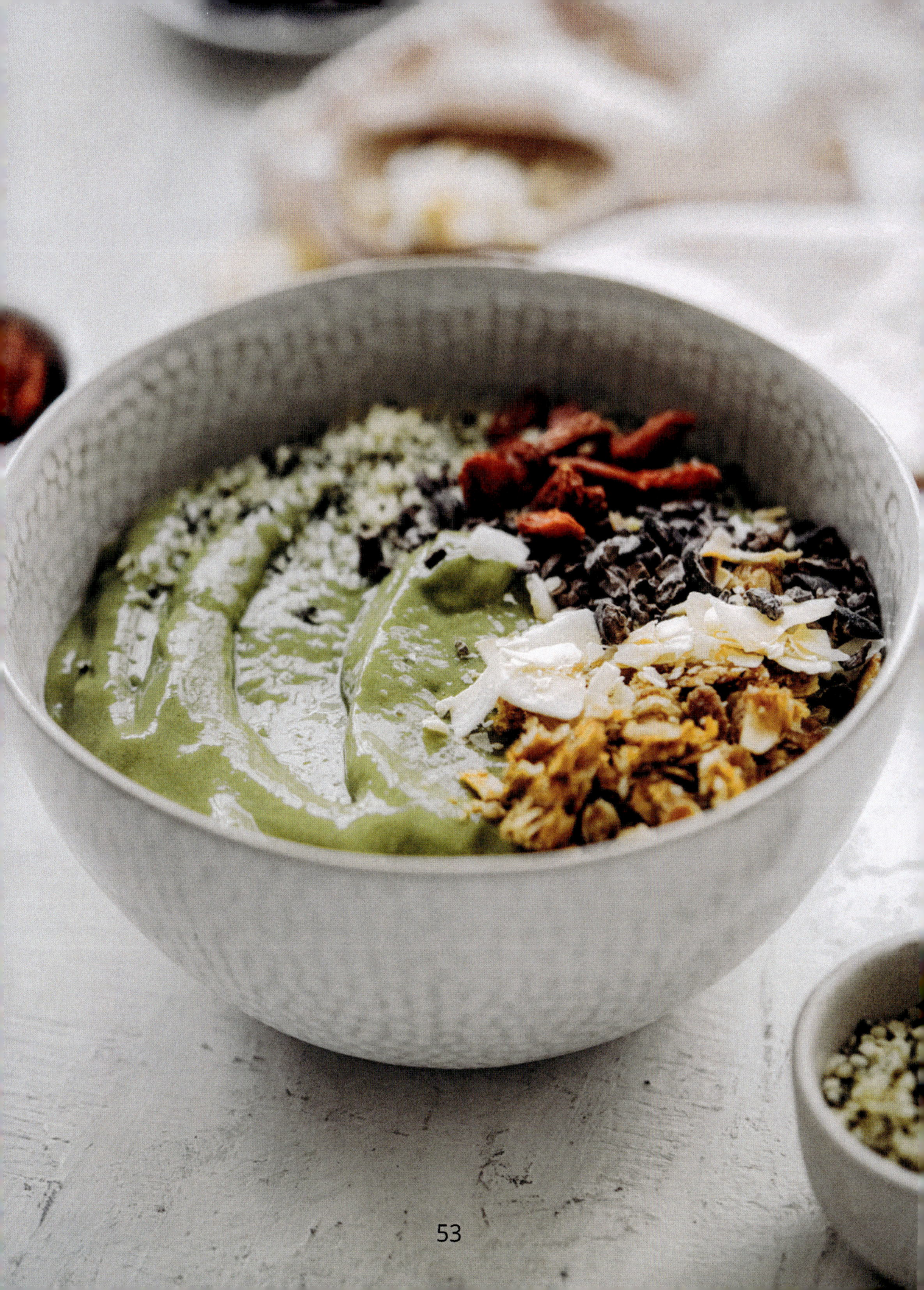

Matcha Smoothie Bowl
to energize and detoxify

v | df | nf | gf

Jaelin Kauf is a freestyle skier who represented the USA at the Pyeongchang 2018 and Beijing 2022 Winter Olympic Games. She won Silver in Beijing in the freestyle moguls and is also a 2x World Championship Medalist. You go, girl!!

Here, Jaelin shares her matcha smoothie bowl recipe, which is packed with antioxidants from the matcha and fruit, and is sustaining due to the healthy fat and protein (from the avocado and protein powder). Get creative with this recipe; add extra toppings like cacao nibs, frozen berries, hemp seeds, or nut and seed butter to make this bowl even more delicious!

Makes 1 Serving

3 tablespoons of matcha powder
1 frozen banana
1/4 cup frozen pineapple
1/2 avocado (frozen for a creamier texture)
1 scoop of vanilla protein powder
1 cup milk of choice

Topping ideas:
- Granola (see pages 44, 47)
- Nut/seed butter (see page 67)
- Cacao nibs
- Coconut flakes
- Goji berries
- Hemp seeds (for extra protein)

1. In a high-speed blender, blend the matcha powder, banana, pineapple, avocado, protein powder, and milk until fully combined.
2. Transfer the smoothie into a serving bowl. Top with granola or anything you desire and enjoy!

NOTE: Use less milk to make it thicker and more milk for a thinner consistency.

TOASTS

Because toast deserves its own chapter

Savory:

Avocado Toast with Poached Eggs   56

High Protein Toast   60

Sweet:

Cinnamon Raisin Bread   63

Honey Cinnamon Peanut Butter Toast   66

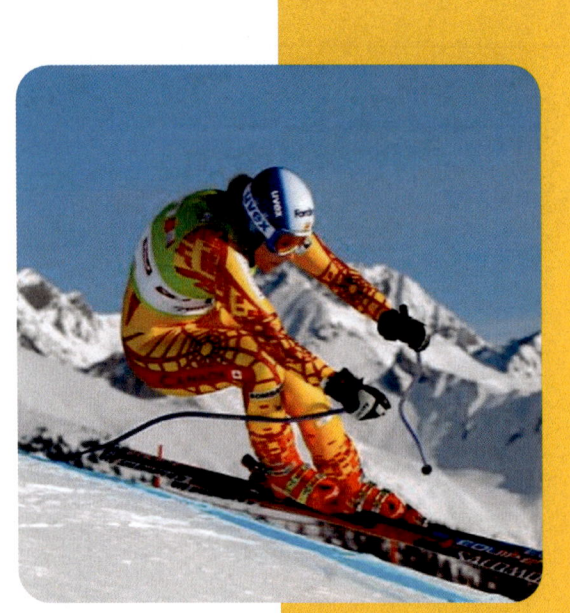

EMILY BRYDON

Alpine Skiing

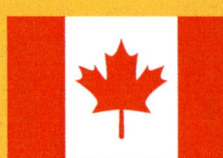

Mental Prep Tip

"I spend a lot of time focused on mental preparation, especially post injuries. Given that my sport involves a lot of fear, you need to be in the right headspace on race day to really charge. I spend hours visualizing racecourses, techniques, and ideal performance states. I also know that when I am in a good place mentally, my performance self is going to be in a stronger position, so I spend time taking care of myself and my state-of-mind. At the top of a racecourse, most of my mental prep is dedicated to running through the racecourse, feeling the turns, and visualizing how I execute the tough sections. But when I get into the actual start gate, I clear my mind and let my body, intuition, and trust lead the way."

Sleep Habits

"When I'm training, I need at least 8 hours to sleep. I try to stay away from electronic devices before sleep. Reading is something I enjoy, and when I was competing, I always had a book to pick up if I wasn't quite ready to sleep and my roommate was. Give yourself time to wind down at the end of the day, it is really hard to go from hero to zero on a consistent basis. I would also recommend setting healthy sleep boundary conditions—like "don't stay up past x o'clock" or "don't eat right before bed," for example. Figure out what is best for you."

Olympic Memory:

"Standing in the start gate, feeling the energy of the people lining the course, and wearing the Canadian downhill suit."

Image by Jed Jacobsohn

57

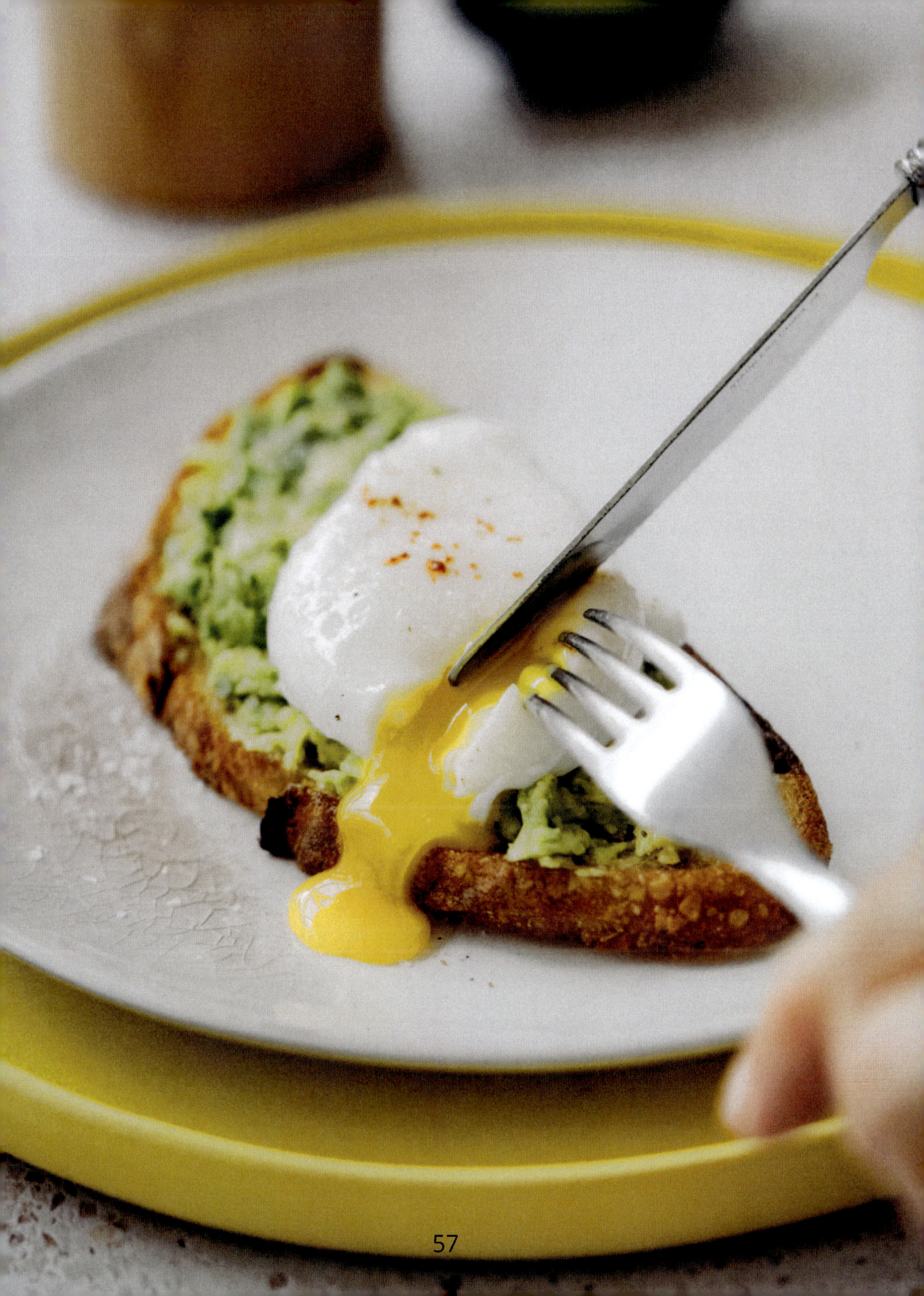

Avocado Toast with Poached Eggs
for a savory breakfast

gf nf

Emily Brydon is a 3x Olympic Alpine Skier who represented Canada at the Salt Lake 2002, Turin 2006, and Vancouver 2010 Olympic Games. She also competed in multiple World Championships, is a 9x World Cup Medalist, and was a member of the Canadian National Team for 13 years. In 2006, Emily started The Emily Brydon Youth Foundation as a way to give funding to children in the Elk Valley so that they could pursue their dreams, whether they were in sport, education, or the arts. Emily was born and raised in Fernie, BC (which is where my mom is from!) and is a true inspiration and legend in our town. She is also fearless, funny, and definitely knows how to make a mean avocado toast.

Here, Emily will share her classic avocado toast recipe, which is a breakfast staple when she has training mornings off. Emily loves to use sourdough bread, and, if you have time, she recommends making it yourself for extra freshness. Avocado is a superfood because it is nutrient-dense and a great source of healthy fats, vitamin K, B, potassium, and magnesium. Eggs are high in protein and iron and are important for brain health. All in all, this meal will give you energy, sustenance, and is packed with nutrients to fuel your day.

Makes 1 serving

1/2 avocado, mashed
Pinch of salt and pepper to taste
1 poached egg (see page x)
1 slice of sourdough bread
Squeeze of lemon
Paprika to taste (optional)

1. Slice an avocado in half, scoop out the filling, and mash it up with a pinch of salt and pepper.
2. Poach the egg in an individual silicon egg poacher (best thing ever, according to Emily!).
3. Put the toast in the toaster around the same time you start poaching. It doesn't take too long if you like a soft poached egg.

4. To assemble, spread the chunky avocado mixture on the toasted sourdough slice, squeeze a bit of lemon on top, and put the poached in the middle of the toast. Sprinkle some paprika and salt on top for added flavor.

How to poach an egg:
step-by-step guide to making the perfect poached eggs

1. Get a teacup (ideally one with a rounded base).
2. Pour in 1cm of water, and a pinch of salt and stir.
3. Carefully crack 1 egg into the cup
4. Cover with a moist piece of paper towel, and microwave for 90 seconds.
5. Check the firmness of the yolk (if you want a firmer yolk, put it in for another 30 seconds).
6. Use a slotted spoon to scoop out the poached egg and drain it. Season with a pinch of salt and pepper if desired.

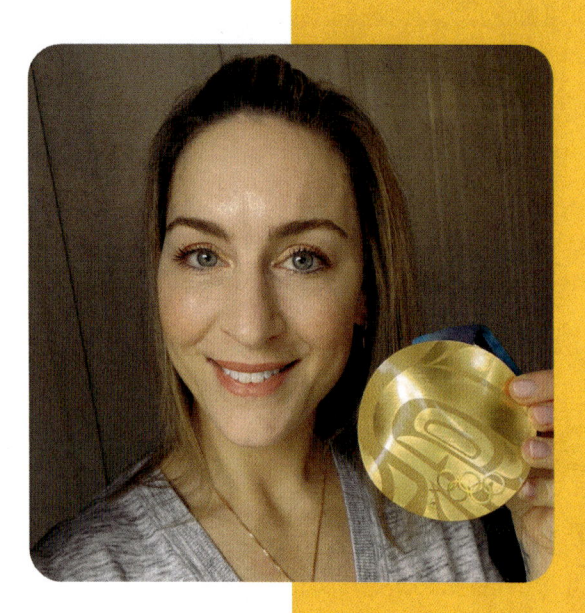

AMY WILLIAMS MBE

Skeleton

Mental Prep Tip

"Focus only on YOU. You are the only one who can make your performance better. Be consistent in your training routines and then competition day so you are prepared and have a plan for all eventualities. Smile and enjoy yourself, you are prepared, excited and ready to see what performance you can achieve."

Recovery Tip

"Olympic Amy used to get about 8-9 hours a night during summer training. Now as a mummy to 2 boys, I've got used to having as little as 4-6 hours sleep. My top tips are, when traveling to bring your own pillow, read a book before sleep, and have a "sleep time" tea. Deep box breathing can help switch off the mind too."

Image by Amy Williams MBE

Morning Routine

Summer training:
"Wake up 7am, do back stretches, and glute activations. Cuppa tea, coffee, and breakfast at 7:30am. Drive to the gym at 8-9am, warm-up and stability work 9:30am. Weights/strength session. Protein Shake/snack. 11am post-workout stretch. 11:30/12pm Lunch."

Winter Training:
"Walk to the ice track if we had morning training times to look at the ice and corners. Watch other athletes slide before my session started."

Sleep Habits:

"Always a stretching session of about 30 minutes. Then food to recover, getting in good quality protein and nutrients. Once back at home, I watched movies, and I used to go to the cinema a lot to switch off my brain and turn my focus to something else."

61

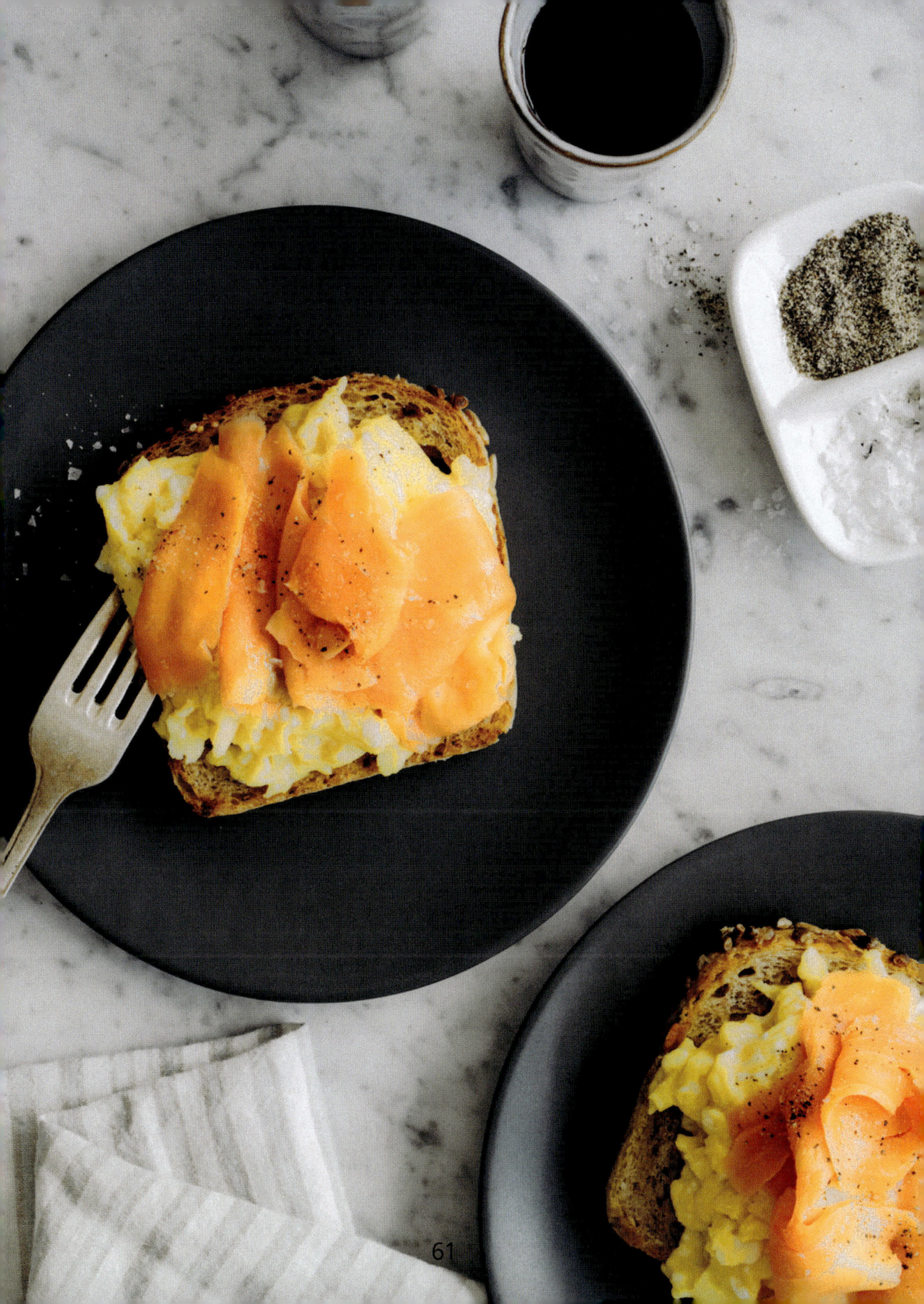

High Protein Toast
for a filling breakfast

df nf gf

Amy Williams, MBE (Member of the Order of the British Empire) is a skeleton racer who represented Great Britain at the Vancouver 2010 Olympics. She was the first British individual gold medalist at a Winter Olympics for 30 years and was the only British medalist at that Games! Amy is also a World silver medalist and a European bronze medalist; she now commentates and presents for high-level sporting events.

Here, Amy shares her high-protein toast breakfast recipe. This recipe has over 30g of protein, as the smoked salmon provides 15g of protein, and the eggs provide 15-18g of protein! This meal sustains you for high-intensity training days, but is also a great post-workout meal as your body needs protein to repair and build muscle.

Makes 1 serving

3 eggs
Pinch of salt and pepper
1 tablespoon butter
2 slices of seeded whole grain bread (or GF if sensitive)
3 ounces smoked salmon

1. In a small bowl, whisk the eggs and salt and pepper. In a non-stick skillet, melt the butter on medium heat.
2. Pour the egg mixture into the skillet, and reduce the heat to low. As the eggs set, gently move a spatula across the bottom and the side of the eggs until large, soft curds form. Cook until no liquid egg is remaining, but the eggs should not be dry.
3. Toast the bread in a toaster, spread butter on each slice, then add the smoked salmon, and finally top with the scrambled eggs. Season with more salt and pepper if desired.

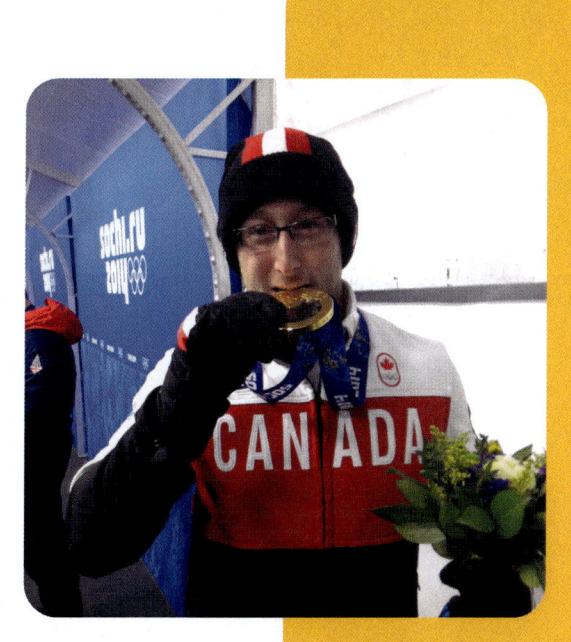

RYAN HARNDEN

Curling

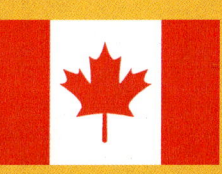

Mental Prep Tip

"Our team has a sports psychologist; I meet with him before every event, and our chats are roughly 2 hours along. We talk about sport, everyday life, the team, the event coming up, how I'm feeling mentally and physically, my job, family etc."

Recovery Tip

"After an event, which is typically a week long, I relax for the first couple days after I arrive home. I don't touch a weight, if anything, I will stretch because my body is sore from the event and also from the travel home."

Olympic Memory

"Winning the gold medal was an amazing moment, especially because my brother and first cousin were on the team, so that was special. I'd also say being in attendance for the Women's hockey final was one of my favorite moments: seeing the puck hit the post, Canada tying it up, then winning in overtime. The atmosphere was incredible. I remember all of us Canadian athletes in attendance going wild and high five-ing."

Sleep Habits:

"I generally try for 7-8 hours of sleep. If we have an early morning game, it's less, but for the most part, I hit my sleep goal. I use CBD at night as I've found this has helped my sleep scores increase."

Image by Ryan Harnden

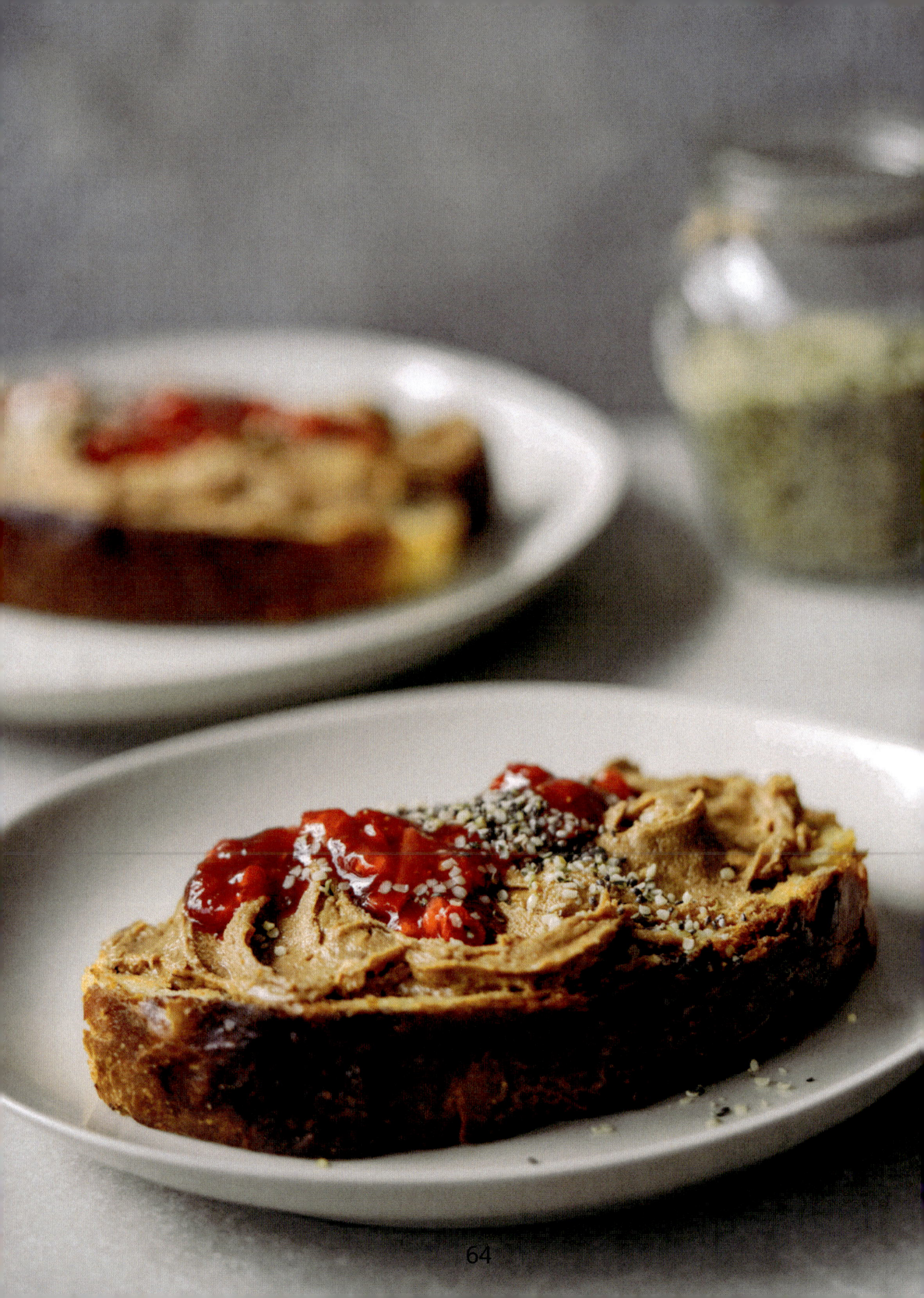

Honey Cinnamon PB Toast

for simple but effective fuel

gf df

Ryan Harnden is a curler who represented Canada at the Sochi 2014 Olympics where his team won the gold medal. He is the former lead for the Brad Jacobs rink, is the 2013 World Silver Medalist, and is the son of three-time Northern Ontario Champion Eric Harnden. I guess pro curling runs in the family!

When not in the gym or on the ice, Ryan is a Real Estate Agent and Real Estate Appraiser. He admits that he doesn't cook much, but loves peanut butter on toast for breakfast. This meal is so simple, but sometimes the most simple of recipes are the most delicious! The peanuts provide healthy fats, fiber, a some protein and will keep you sustained for longer periods of time. The spice of the cinnamon and sweetness of the honey elevate the peanut butter to create a tasty and gooey spread.

Serves 1

1 tablespoon smooth or crunchy peanut butter
1 tablespoon honey
1 teaspoon ground cinnamon
1 slice of whole-grain toast (or try Gabriella Papadakis's Cinnamon Raisin Bread page 70)
Unsalted butter (optional)

Extra topping ideas:
- Banana slices
- Berries or berry jam
- Hemp seeds
- Chia seeds
- Coconut flakes

1. In a bowl, mix the peanut butter, honey, and cinnamon until combined.
2. Toast the bread in the toaster.
3. Spread a layer of unsalted butter on the toast (optional).
4. Spread the peanut butter mixture on the toast, add any extra toppings if desired, and enjoy!

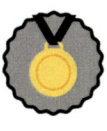

Want to make your own Honey Cinnamon Peanut Butter (with a special secret ingredient)? Check out page 67 for more.

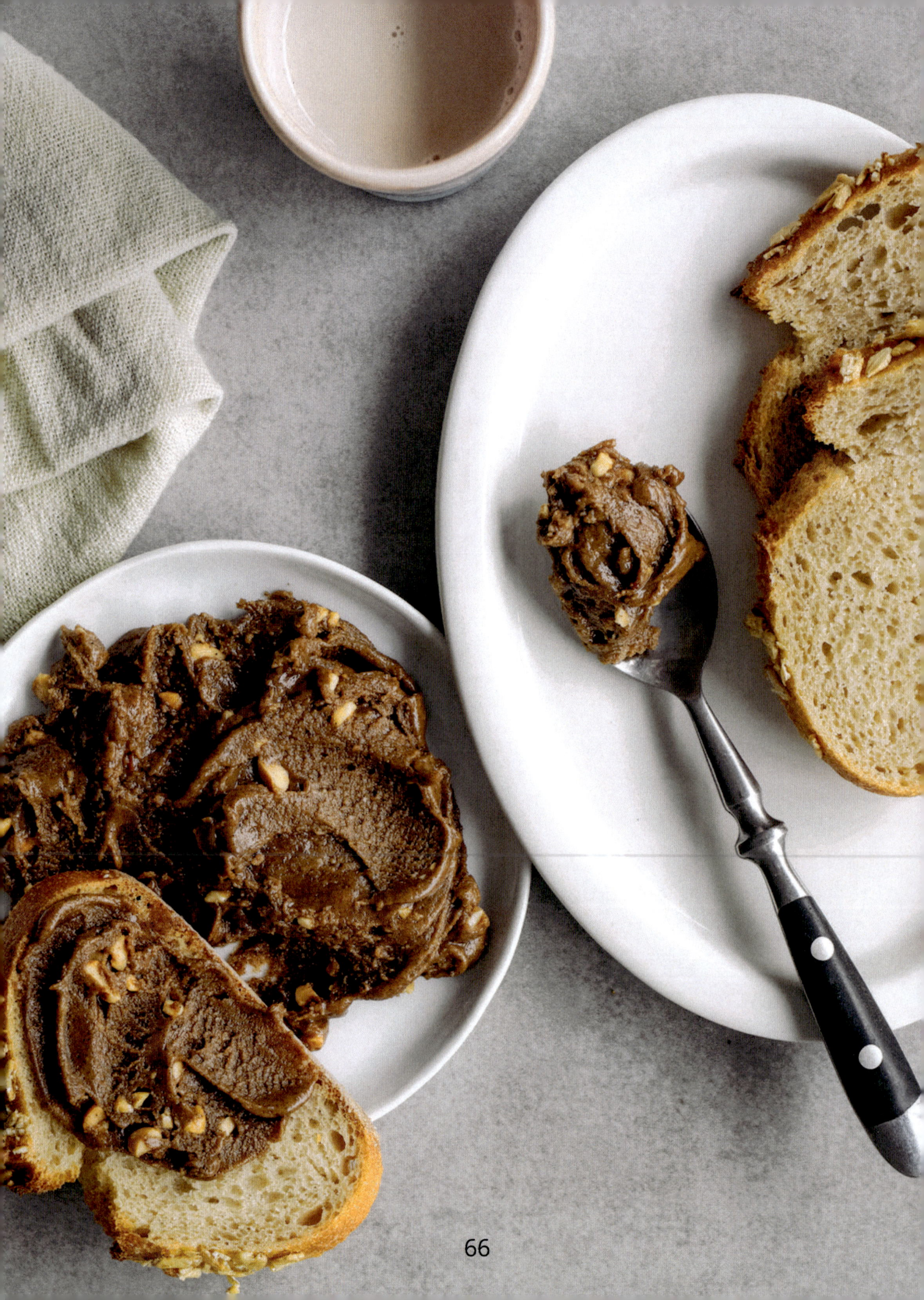

Honey Cinnamon Peanut Butter

for a sweet and salty addition to any meal

gf df

Anyone who knows me knows that I LOVE PEANUT BUTTER. This honey cinnamon peanut butter is the glue that holds my life together.

This peanut butter is great on toast (Cinnamon Raisin Bread page 70), in smoothies (see pages 178, 195), and by the spoon. Or just dunk your head in it and call it a day.

Makes 1-1 1/2 cups

2 cups cocktail peanuts
2 Medjool dates
2 teaspoons ground cinnamon
2 tablespoons honey
1/4 teaspoon sea salt
3 tablespoons coconut oil

1. In a high-speed blender or food processor, blend the peanuts down to a paste. Scrape the sides of the blender/food processor or use the tamper on a Vitamix to ensure they are all mixed.
2. Add the dates, cinnamon, honey and salt. The mixture will thicken.
3. Add the coconut oil one tablespoon at a time, and blend everything until a smooth and creamy peanut butter forms.
4. Store in an airtight glass jar or container in the fridge for up to a month.

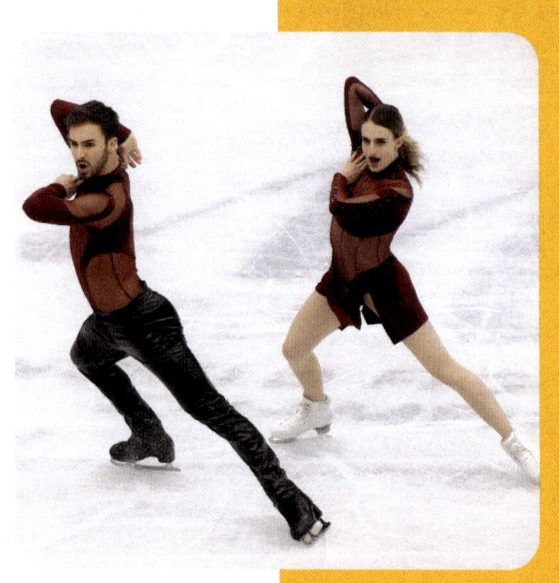

GABRIELLA PAPADAKIS

Ice Dance

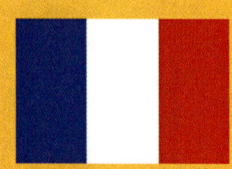

🇫🇷

Mental Prep Tip

"I like to remind myself that I'm just a person dancing on frozen water, wearing boots with knives attached to them, and that I shouldn't take it too seriously... this takes the pressure off and reminds me that I love this absurd sport."

Recovery Tip

"After spending a whole day in a cold ice rink, I love taking a long bath with soft music and candles (and sometimes Nutella by the spoon, but that's a secret)"

Olympic Memory

"Winning the Olympics was insane, obviously, but my close second favorite moment was hugging all of my competitors and teammates right after. Loved these moments of friendship."

Sleep Habits:

"I try to sleep about 8 hours, but I tend to become hyperactive around 9pm and struggle to go to bed early enough. To fight that, I usually have dinner before 7pm, then dim the lights, and generally turn my brain off (not the time to try and figure out what the meaning of life is)."

Morning Routine:

"I wake up, boil some water to make tea, eat a lot, and then start moving. I am useless on an empty stomach and don't like having to eat so much during the day. So breakfast is my favorite and most important meal, and the one I make the most time for."

Image by Oliver Braj

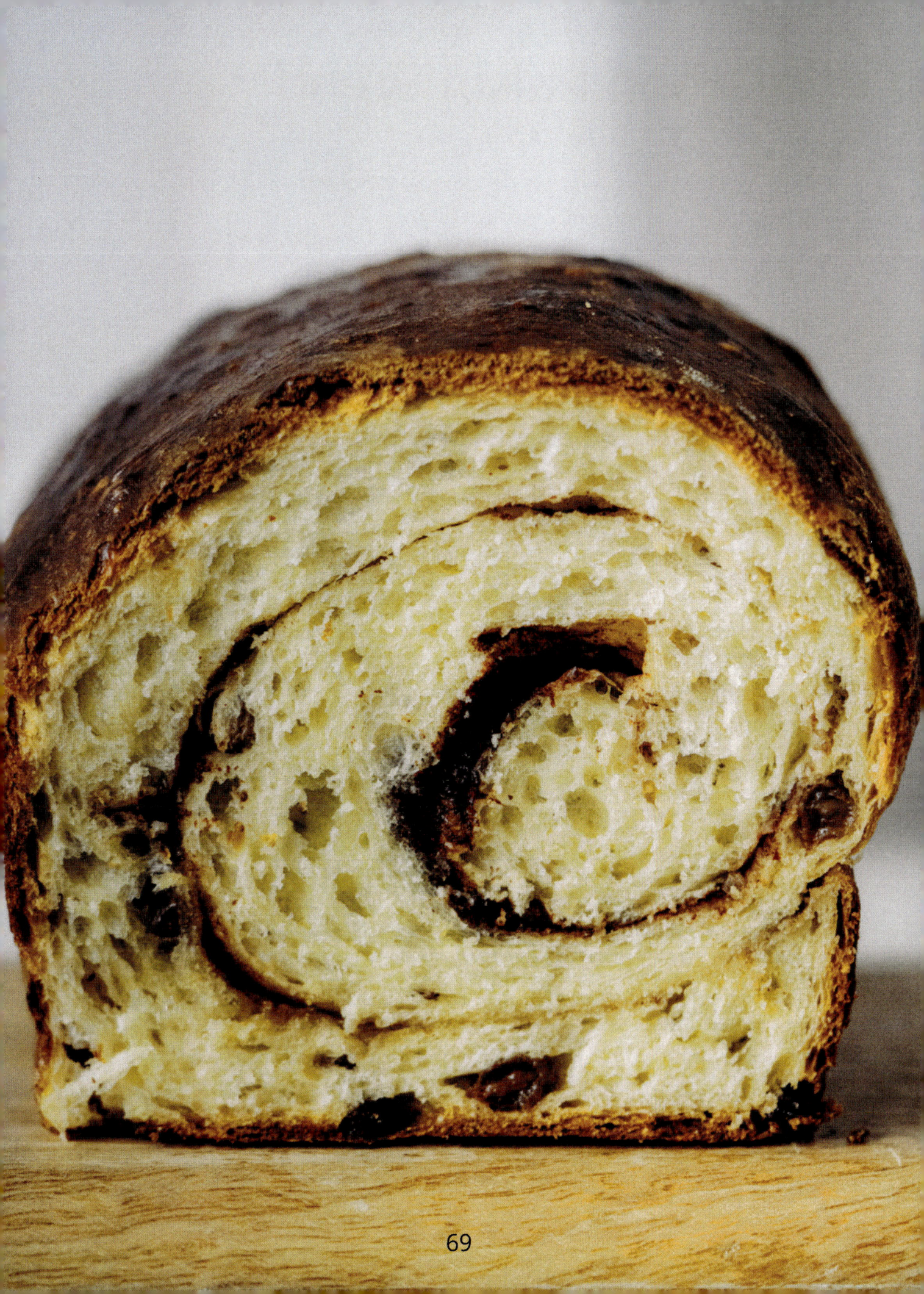

Cinnamon Raisin Bread
for cinnamon bun lovers

nf gf

Gabriella Papadakis is a French ice dancer who won silver in Pyeongchang 2018 and gold in Beijing 2022 alongside his partner Guillame Cizeron. Not only is she Olympic Champion, but she is also 5x World Champion, 5x consecutive European Champion, 7x National Champion, and she has broken world records 28 times. Guillaume and Gabriella have been skating together since they were 9 and 10 years old; they are known for their lyrical and modern movements, and the quality of their skating skills is unparalleled. Gabriella recently released her own clothing line of sportswear, knitwear, and loungewear that she designed herself over the last year. The colors and comfort of each piece is amazing, and I particularly love the red raspberry leggings set with orange trim. Elles sont très jolies!

Gabby likes to start her mornings with honey, nut, and cinnamon toast from her local bakery, Première Moisson, topped with sunflower seed butter and avocado for healthy fats, cottage cheese for protein, and flax seeds for fiber. If she is feeling extra hungry, Gabby adds a sunny side-up egg. "It sounds strange, but it is delicious and gives me energy for the whole day!"

Makes 2 loaves or 28 slices

- 1 cup raisins
- 2 cups milk
- 10 tablespoons unsalted butter, divided
- 1/4 cup honey
- 1 tablespoon yeast
- 7-8 cups all-purpose flour (or GF if sensitive)
- 5 eggs, divided
- 1/2 cup brown sugar
- 3 tablespoons ground cinnamon

1. Put the raisins in a small saucepan and cover with water, let them simmer on low heat for 10-15 minutes. Drain, then pat dry and leave them to plump.
2. In another saucepan heat the milk, and 8 tablespoons of butter on low heat until the butter is nearly melted. Add the honey and stir.
3. Pour mixture into the bowl of a standing mixer. Mix in the yeast and 2 cups of flour until mostly combined.

4. Add 4 eggs (save the last egg), mix, then add the remaining flour.
5. Knead dough by hand for 15 minutes or use a dough hook for 7-10 minutes until smooth and elastic. Add the plump, dry raisins, and knead until evenly combined.
6. Cover the dough with cling film or a damp kitchen towel, and let it rise for 1-2 hours so it doubles in size.
7. Add flour to a flat surface to prevent sticking, and cut the dough into 2 even pieces. Roll the dough into a long, thin strip.
8. Melt the extra 2 tablespoons of butter in a bowl. Use a brush to spread it across the dough strip. Leave an inch untouched at the top.
9. Mix the cinnamon and sugar, sprinkle it over the butter, then roll up the dough edge to edge. Repeat with the other strip of dough. Place into a greased loaf pan. Cover the loaves with a damp kitchen towel and let rise for another hour.
10. Preheat the oven to 375°F. Place an empty pan at the base of the oven and add 1 cup of water to the hot pan (for moisture).
11. Mix the last egg with 1 tablespoon of water and brush the egg wash on the top of the loaves. Bake for 40-50 minutes or until golden and it sounds hollow when thumped.
12. Let cool before serving. Store in the freezer for up to 6 months.

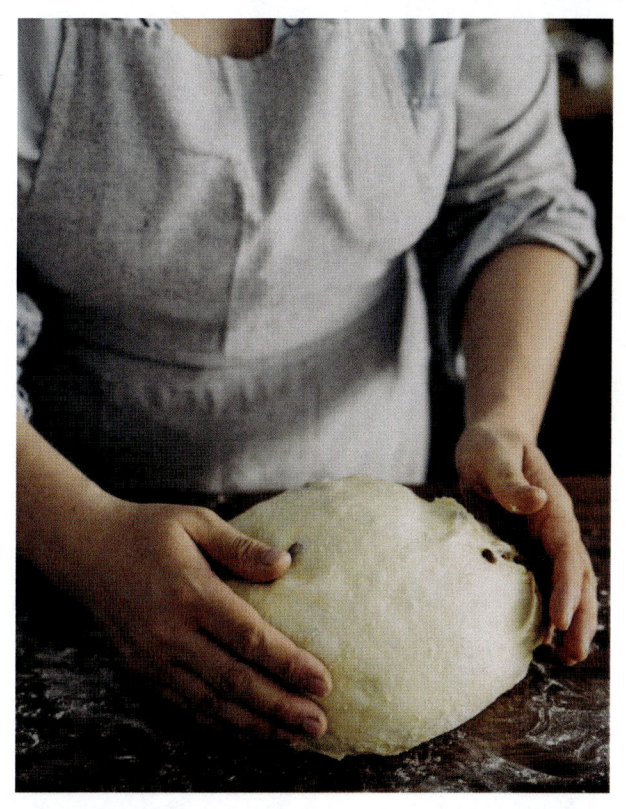

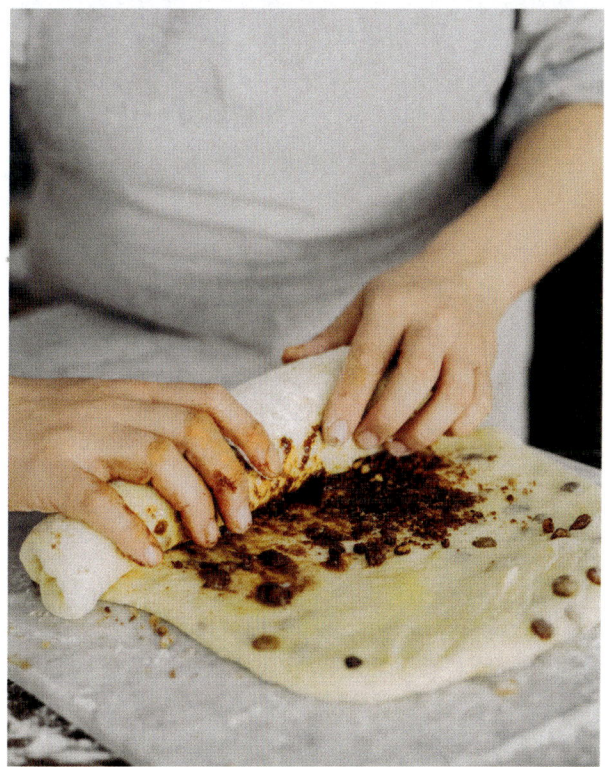

Gabby's favorite toppings:
1 tablespoon of sunflower seed butter, with 2 tablespoons of cottage cheese, 1/4 sliced avocado, a drizzle of honey, and a sprinkle of flax seeds.

72

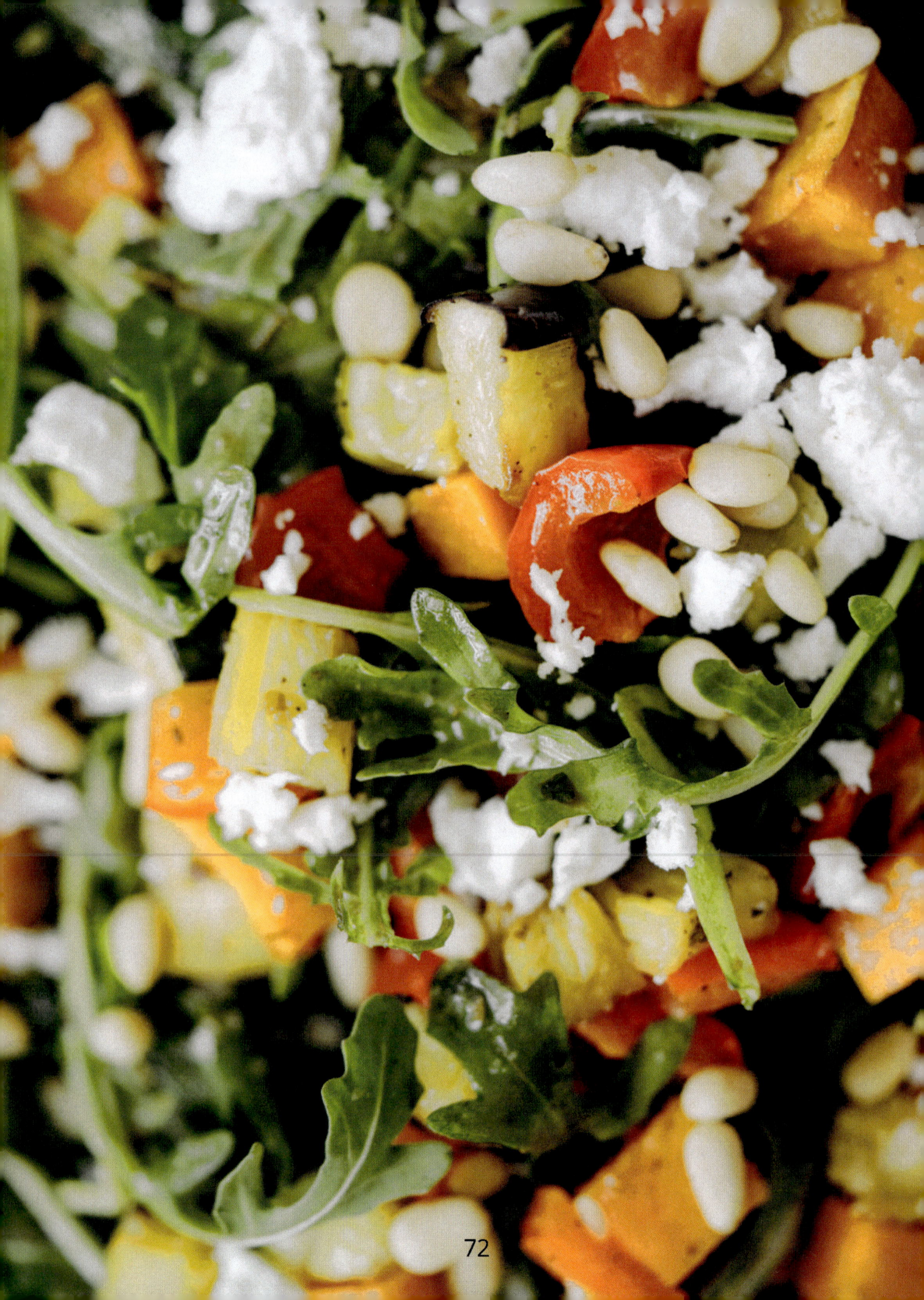

LUNCH TIME CRUNCH TIME

Crispy Salad Burritos   74

Lasting Lentil Soup   77

Tofu Pasta   80

Chicken Schnitzel   83

Mediterranean Roast Salad   87

Turkey Bacon Bowl   90

Miso Salmon Nourish Bowl   93

Lemon Vinaigrette   97

Cypriot Grain Salad   98

BONUS RECIPE: Zucchini Tacos   101

LEWIS GIBSON

Ice Dance

🇬🇧

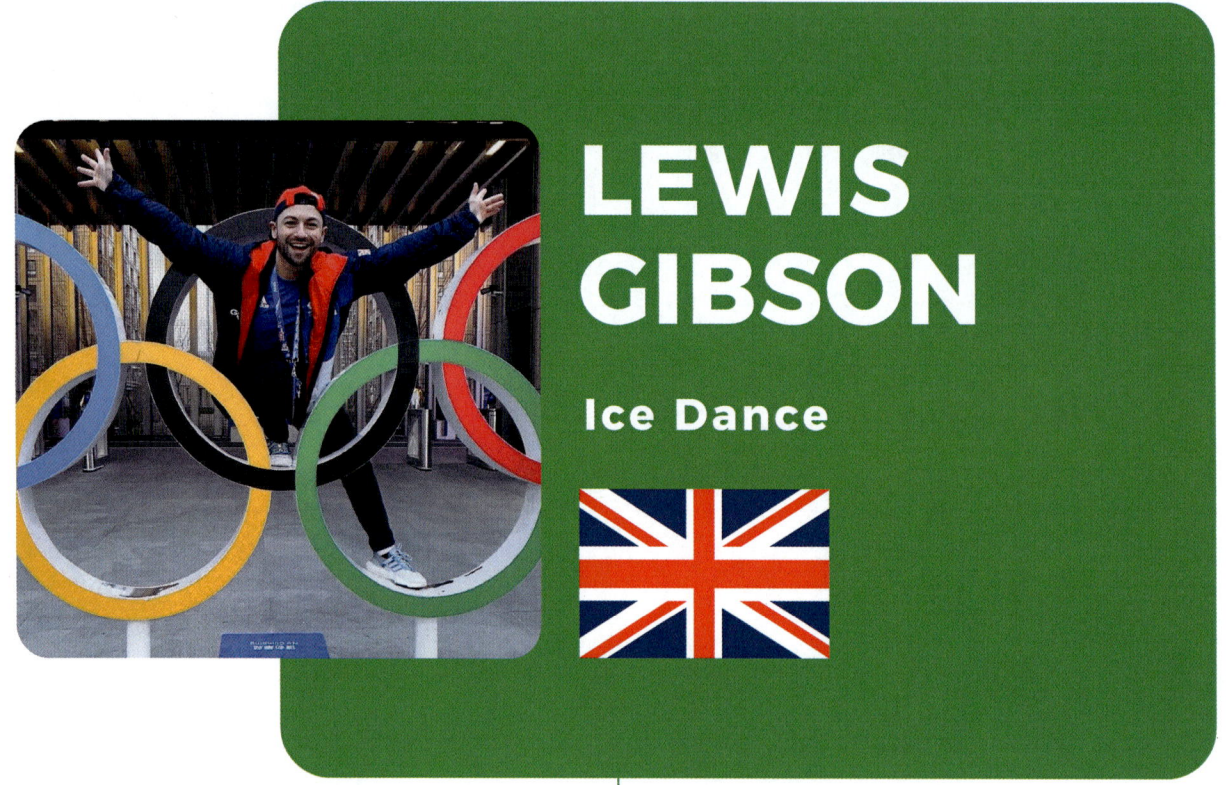

Morning Routine:

"Wake up and the first thing I do is drink a large glass of water. Then, I shower and get dressed. The night before I prepare my training clothes for the next day just to save time in the morning. Next, I make breakfast, coffee, and lunch/snacks for the day ahead. I have breakfast on the sofa and do a quick five-minute morning meditation. I feel like this allows me the chance to check in and remind myself of the dream that I'm living."

Olympic Memory:

"My favorite memory was the fun I had at the whole event. I was told by many former Olympians to just embrace the whole occasion, and I'm so glad I really took that on board. I remember specifically reminding myself to just ENJOY. I kept repeating that to myself as I was skating the free dance. And enjoy is what I did."

Recovery Tip:

"Watching a comedy, whether it's a show or stand-up, is a great way to boost my mood and just laugh. At the same time, I can wind down and take my mind away from my sport."

Sleep Habits:

"I sleep roughly 8 hours. My number 1 tip (which is more of a wake-up tip) is to get yourself a sunrise alarm clock. I travel everywhere with this; the light starts to turn on 20 minutes before the alarm sound so I find myself already out of my deep sleep and less jolted awake by the dreaded alarm noise."

Mental Prep Tip:

"I always start by forming a great playlist to get me in the right character to perform and I listen to this on my way to the competition venue. Just before I compete I do a short mediation/visualization of my performance."

Image by Lewis Gibson

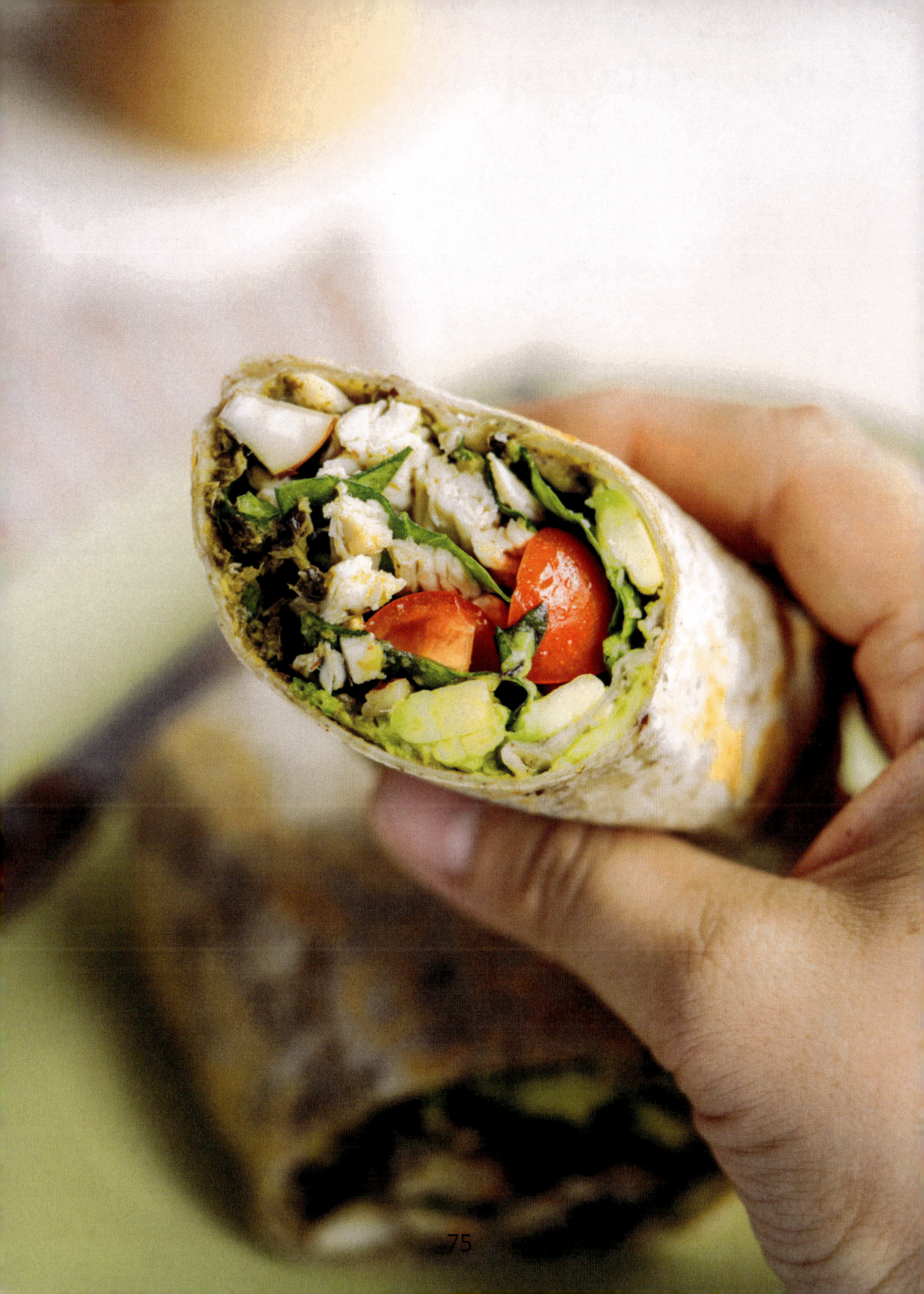

Crispy Salad Burritos
for a crunchy lunch

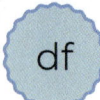

df gf v

Lewis Gibson is an ice dancer who represented Great Britain at the Bejing 2022 Olympics alongside my sister, Lilah. The pair placed 10th in Beijing and most recently finished 2nd at the European Championships and 4th at the World Championships in 2023. Lewis is like the big brother I never had (no offense Georgia and Lilah), a fellow cookie addict, and a home decor aficionado.

Here, Lewis shares his easy burrito recipe. Using the air fryer or oven will crisp up the wrap and warm up the inside to create a crunchy salad burrito. This simple extra step makes any old wrap or sandwich SO much tastier! Feel free to add any other ingredients and toppings to the salad and make it your own.

Makes 1 serving

1 chicken breast, shredded
1 cup baby spinach or mixed greens
1/2 cup cherry tomatoes, chopped
1/2 an avocado, sliced
1 tablespoon sunflower seeds
2 tablespoons almonds
A drizzle of olive oil
A squeeze of lemon juice
Pinch of salt
1 tortilla-style whole wheat wrap (GF if sensitive)
1 tablespoon pesto (optional)

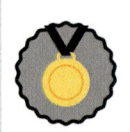

Not a fan of pesto?
Use hummus (extra protein yay!) or any other spread.

Want to make it vegan?
Sub the chicken for tofu, tempeh, edamame, beans, or hummus.

1. Preheat an air fryer to 400°F (Lewis's favorite thing) or the oven to 425°F.
2. On a cutting board shred the cooked chicken breast by using your hands to tear it into pieces or by using two forks.
3. In a mixing bowl, make the salad by tossing together the chicken, spinach, cherry tomatoes, avocado, sunflower seeds, almonds, olive oil, lemon juice, and salt.
4. Take a tortilla and spread 1 tablespoon of pesto down the center of the wrap (optional). Add the salad contents on top of the pesto, and roll up the wrap tightly into a burrito.
5. Bake the burrito for 8 minutes in the air fryer or oven until crispy and golden brown.

BRUCE MOUAT

Curling

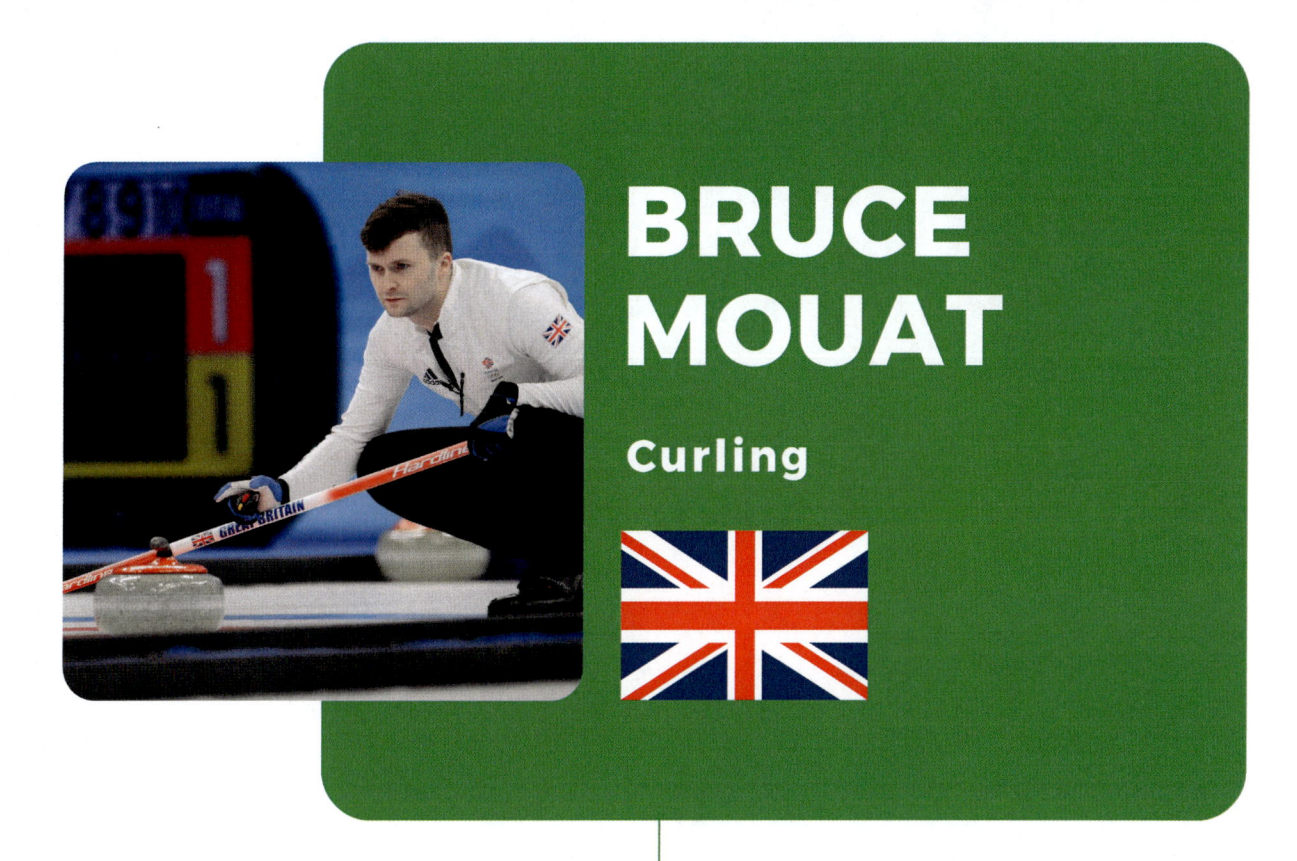

Morning Routine:

Bruce's nutrition tip for morning training:
"Try to get some protein in at least 30 minutes before training."

This increases muscle protein synthesis before a workout and improves muscle performance and recovery.

Olympic Memory:

"Winning the semi-final against the USA to guarantee Team GB their first medal at the 2022 Olympics."

Recovery Tip:

"I'm a big movie buff, so I like to find a good one to watch in the evenings."

Sleep Habits:

"I always get about 6/7 hours a night but recommend 8. I like to listen to audio books while I try and get to sleep, often it'll be Harry Potter!"

Mental Prep Tip:

"Walking always clears my mind before a big event. Try it with a good coffee and focus on the task ahead."

Image by David Pearce

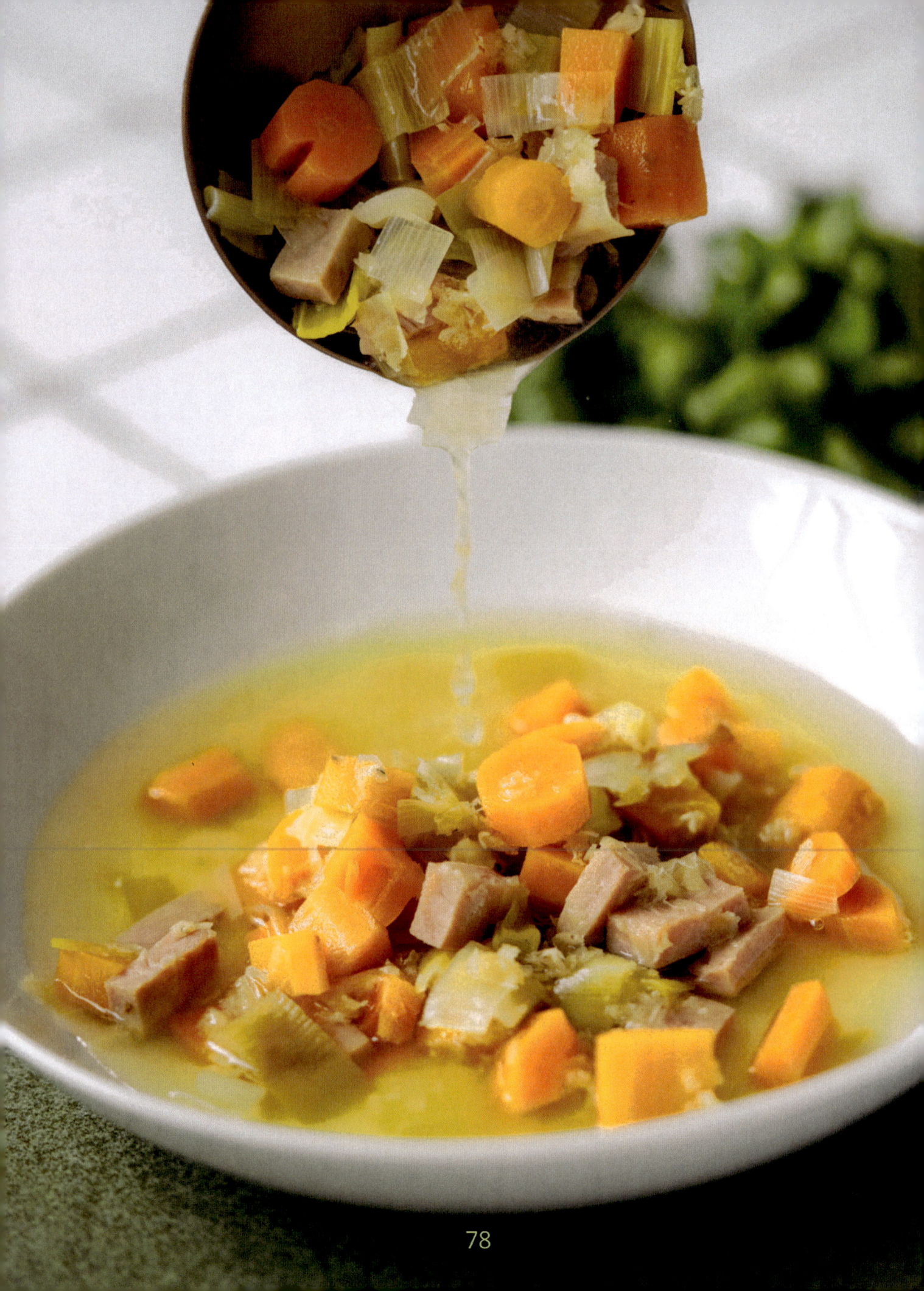

Lasting Lentil Soup

for a soup that sustains

nf gf df

Bruce Mouat is a Scottish curler who represented Great Britain at the Beijing 2022 Olympic Games. Not only did he carry the team to an Olympic Silver Medal, but he is also a 3x World Championship Medalist!

Here, Bruce shares his go-to lentil soup recipe, which he makes for lunch on training days. This rich, veggie-and-bean-packed soup is full of flavor and warms the soul on cold winter days or after an intense practice.

Makes 4-6 servings

6 ounces red lentils, rinsed
6 carrots, peeled and diced
2 medium-sized leeks, diced
6 1/4 cups of chicken broth
7 ounces ham, diced
Freshly ground pepper to taste
Sprinkle of chopped parsley to taste

⏱ Meal prep this soup on a Sunday for quick and easy lunches or dinners throughout the week.

V **Want to make it vegan and vegetarian?** Sub veggie broth for chicken stock broth and scrap the ham.

1. In a large slow cooker, add the rinsed red lentils, diced carrots, leeks, chicken broth, and ham.
2. Cover and cook on low for 8-10 hours or on high for 4-5 hours (the longer the better).
3. Serve in a cereal bowl and top with freshly ground pepper and a sprinkle of chopped parsley.
4. Remove from slow cooker and store in an airtight container in the fridge for up to 5 days, or 3 months in the freezer.

> **Bruce's tips:**
> 1. "I don't add salt as the chicken stock is enough, but feel free to add salt if you feel it's needed."
> 2. If you don't like chunky soup, blend it in a blender to make it smooth

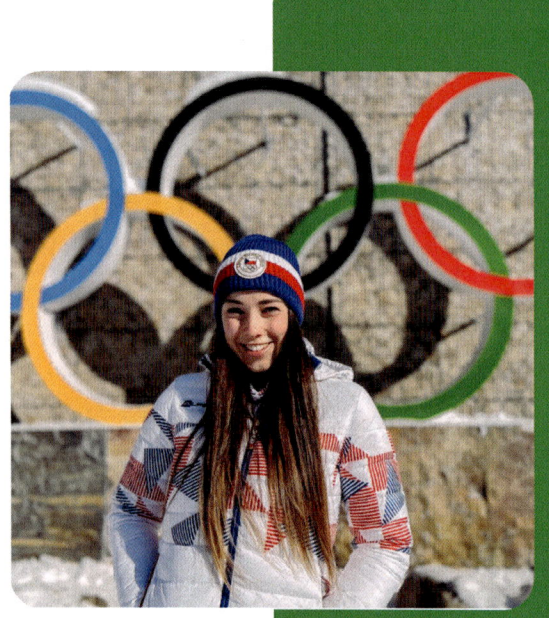

ANNA FERNSTÄDT

Skeleton

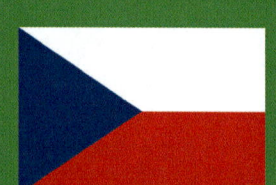

Morning Routine:
"Wake up, take a cold shower, and do a 10-15 minute 'workout' (some exercises focused on what I need to activate for training and prevent injuries). Then drink a glass of warm water with a squeezed lemon, do a 5-10 min meditation, and then I have breakfast and start my day."

Recovery Tip:
"Good, high-quality food, stable blood glucose levels, good diabetes/insulin management, and good sleep is my priority for my recovery. After training, I normally go home and eat, nap if I can (who doesn't love a good nap?), and then go for a coffee with friends or do something not sport-related (if I don't have a double session that day, otherwise it's just food, nap, go again). I also do physio, take a sauna, or go for little walks (or swims in summer) for active recovery."

Olympic Memory:
"I remember going to the start line and while waiting for the green light I said to myself: "I did it. I'm here. WE did it. I'm so proud. Now enjoy." To give a little bit of background, I got diagnosed with Type 1 Diabetes 10 days before my flight to China, so until the very last moment I didn't know if I would make it to China, through training, or to that start line. So that was a big moment for me."

Sleep Habits:
"I get 7.5-9 hours. I have alarms but I mostly wake up before it. I sleep the best when I read at night, when it is really dark in my room, and when it is cold in my room, so I always open all windows for a couple of minutes before going to bed. I try to avoid overhead lights at night because that signals your brain it's still day because of 'sunlight.'"

Image by Anna Fernsädt

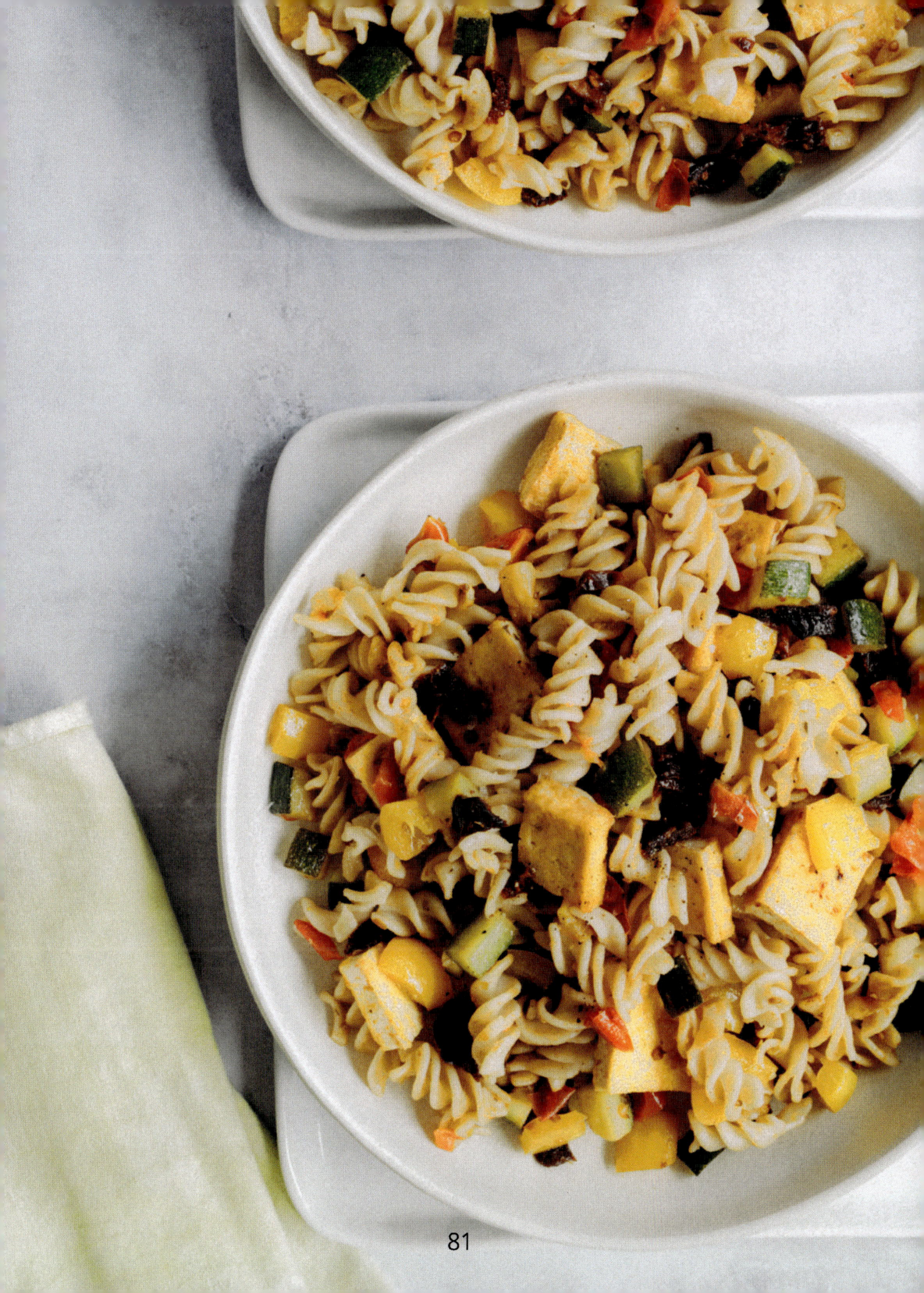

Tofu Pasta
for lunch or leftovers

df nf gf v

Anna Fernstädt is a Czech-German Skeleton racer who competed at the Pyeongchang 2018 Olympics representing Germany, and the Beijing 2022 Olympics representing the Czech Republic. After switching to Team Czech Republic, she needed to compete at lower levels to earn her World Cup quota spot, so she dominated the field by becoming the 2018, 2019, and 2020 Junior World Champion, as well as the World Mixed Team Bronze Medalist in 2017.

Czech out this recipe!! (Sorry Anna, I had to). Here, Anna shares her tofu pasta recipe which is full of flavor, easy to make, and keeps you satiated on long training days. The tofu can be replaced by any protein, so this meal is versatile when you are stuck in a recipe rut and want to try something new!

Makes 2 Servings

3/4 cup uncooked brown rice pasta
1 tablespoon olive oil for grilling
1 cup of tofu, sliced
1/2 teaspoon of salt
1 yellow bell pepper, diced
15 mini cocktail tomatoes, diced
1 cup sun-dried tomatoes
1 zucchini, diced
1/2 tablespoon dried oregano
Spicy olive oil to taste

1. Cook the pasta according to package instructions.
2. Add a tablespoon of olive oil to a skillet, and add 1/4 teaspoon of salt to each side of the tofu. Grill the tofu on a medium-high heat for 2-3 minutes each side, or until it is golden.
3. Add the bell pepper, cocktail tomatoes, dried tomatoes, zucchini, and oregano to the pan. Stir and cook until the vegetables soften.
4. Turn the heat off and stir in the cooked pasta until everything is combined.
5. Serve with a drizzle of spicy olive oil (optional).

MEGHAN TIERNEY

Snowboarding

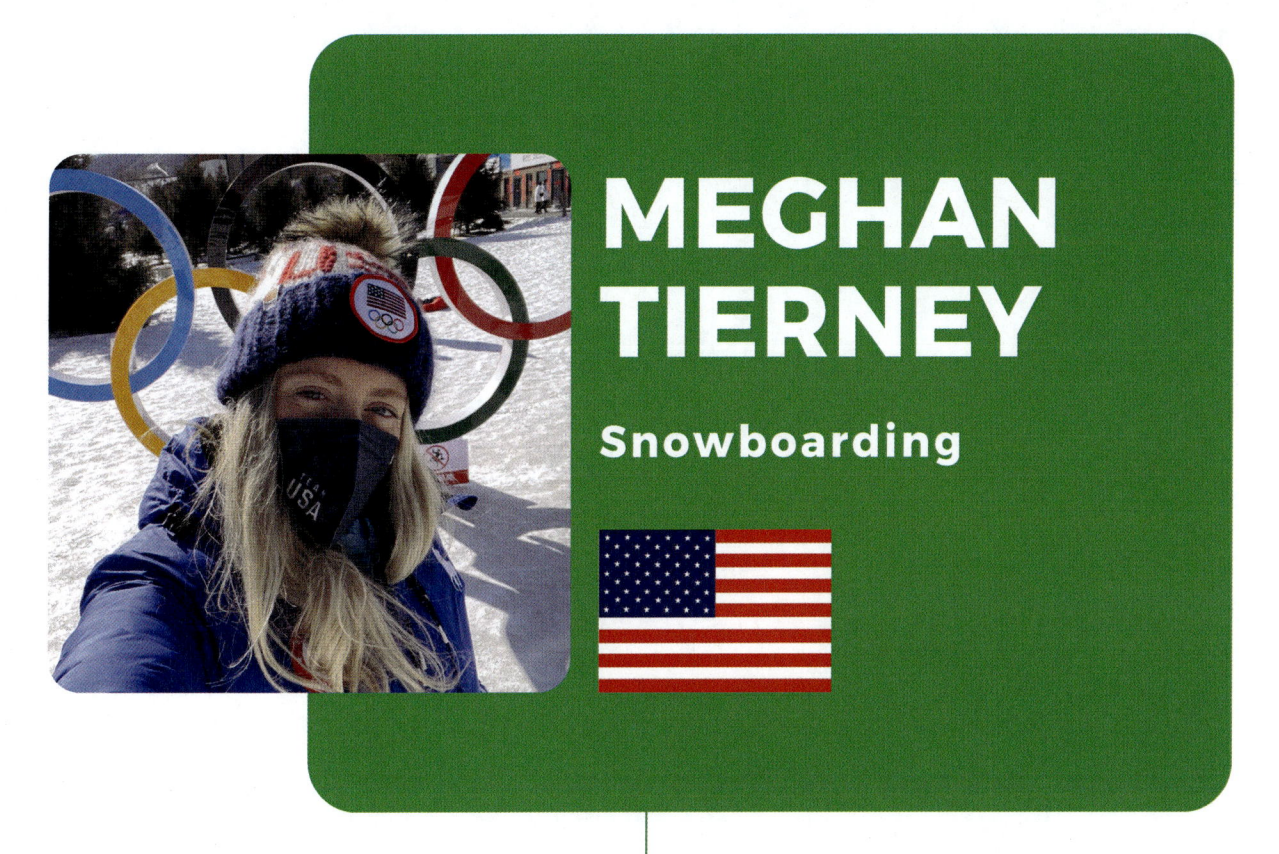

Sleep Habits:

"I try to sleep 8 hours usually. I would say try to get into a pattern of going to sleep around the same time every night. Also what has helped is making sure it's very cold in my room and taking a hot shower before bed."

Olympic Memory:

"Walking into the opening ceremonies was so incredible. It was so different both times, but an experience I will never forget."

Mental Prep Tip:

"I just try to remember that I am prepared and that I've trained hard for this. I also go over the course in my head to feel ready mentally."

Morning Routine:

"Wake up, stretch, eat some breakfast (either oatmeal, eggs and potatoes, or sometimes steak and potatoes)."

Recovery Tip:

"Go on a slow walk and drink a protein shake."

Image by Meghan Tierney

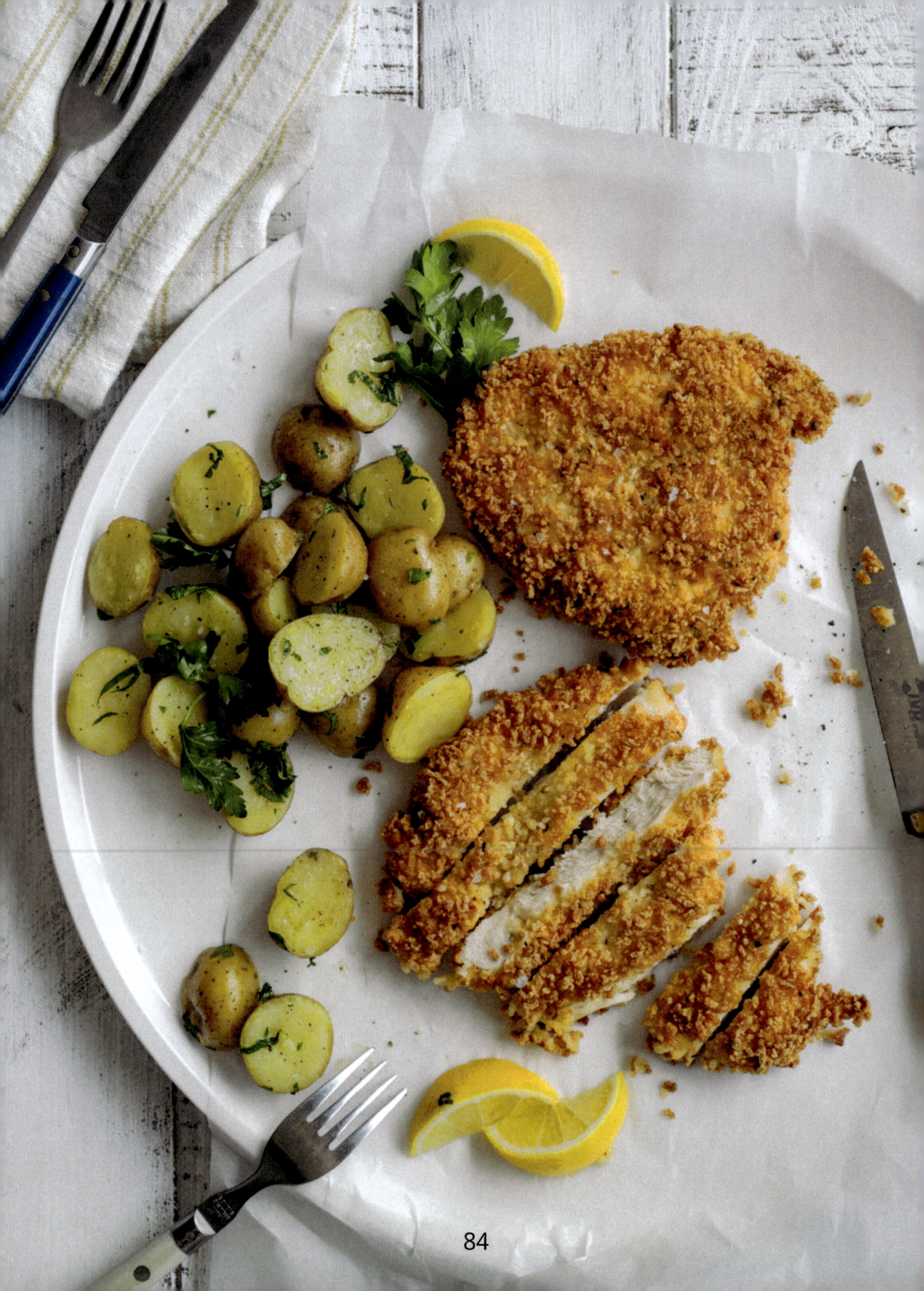

Chicken Schnitzel

for comfort after a long training day

gf nf

Meghan Tierney is a snowboarder who represented the USA at the Pyeongchang 2018 and the Beijing 2022 Olympics in the snowboard cross. She is the first-ever USA athlete to win both the NORAM and the Europa Cup Championships.

Here, Meghan shares her chicken schnitzel recipe that she learned to make while living in Austria. Traditionally it's made with veal, but she prefers using chicken. Serve this mouthwatering dish with buttered boiled potatoes and parsley to take it to the next level of tastiness!

Makes 2 Servings

2 large boneless, skinless chicken breasts
1/3 cup all purpose flour (or GF)
2 eggs
1/2 teaspoon kosher salt
1/2 teaspoon paprika
1 cup panko breadcrumbs (GF if sensitive)
1/2 teaspoon basil
1/2 teaspoon garlic powder
1/2 teaspoon black pepper
1 teaspoon dried oregano
A squeeze of lemon juice to serve

Sides:
18 ounces fingerling potatoes
1 tablespoon unsalted butter, melted
1 tablespoon extra virgin olive oil
1 teaspoon kosher salt
1/2 teaspoon black pepper
1 tablespoon parsley, finely chopped

Recommendation: add vegetables like asparagus or broccoli to serve.

1. Preheat the oven to 400°F. Place each chicken breast between two sheets of cling film. Use a rolling pin or meat mallet to pound the breasts to 1/8 inch thickness. Coat both sides of the chicken breasts in flour. Tap off any excess.
2. In a small bowl, beat the eggs and dip both sides of each chicken breast into the egg.
3. On a plate, mix the salt, paprika, breadcrumbs, basil, garlic powder, black pepper, and oregano.
4. Firmly press both sides of each chicken breast into the breadcrumb mixture 2-3 times until fully coated.
5. Bake chicken for 10-15 minutes or until golden brown.
6. Place potatoes in a large pot and cover in 1 inch of water. Add the salt. Bring to a boil. Reduce heat and simmer for 10-15 minutes. Use a fork to check

when they are tender, and remove them from heat.
7. Drain potatoes. In a bowl, mix the potatoes, melted butter, olive oil, extra salt, pepper, and parsley.

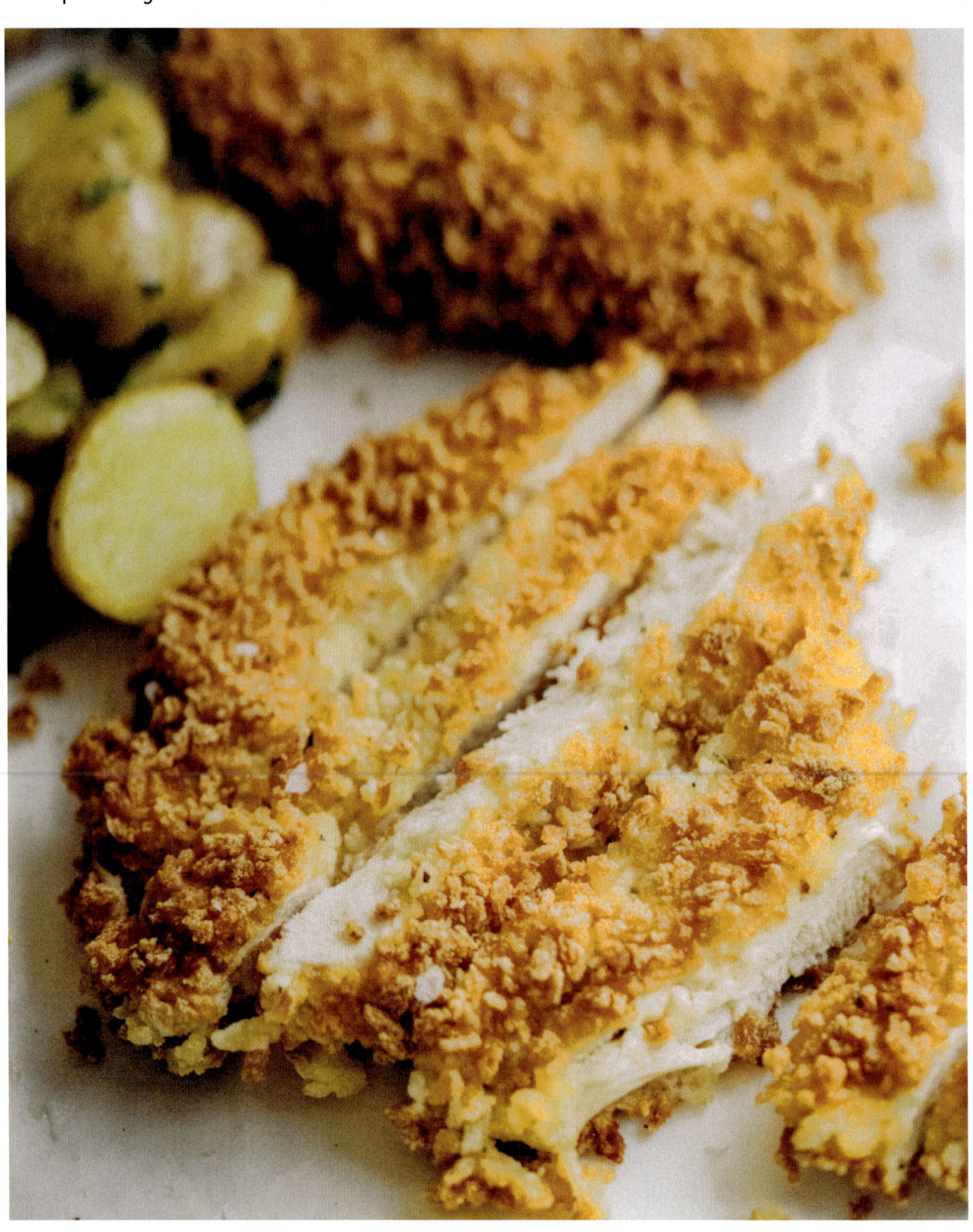

BREE WALKER

Bobsled

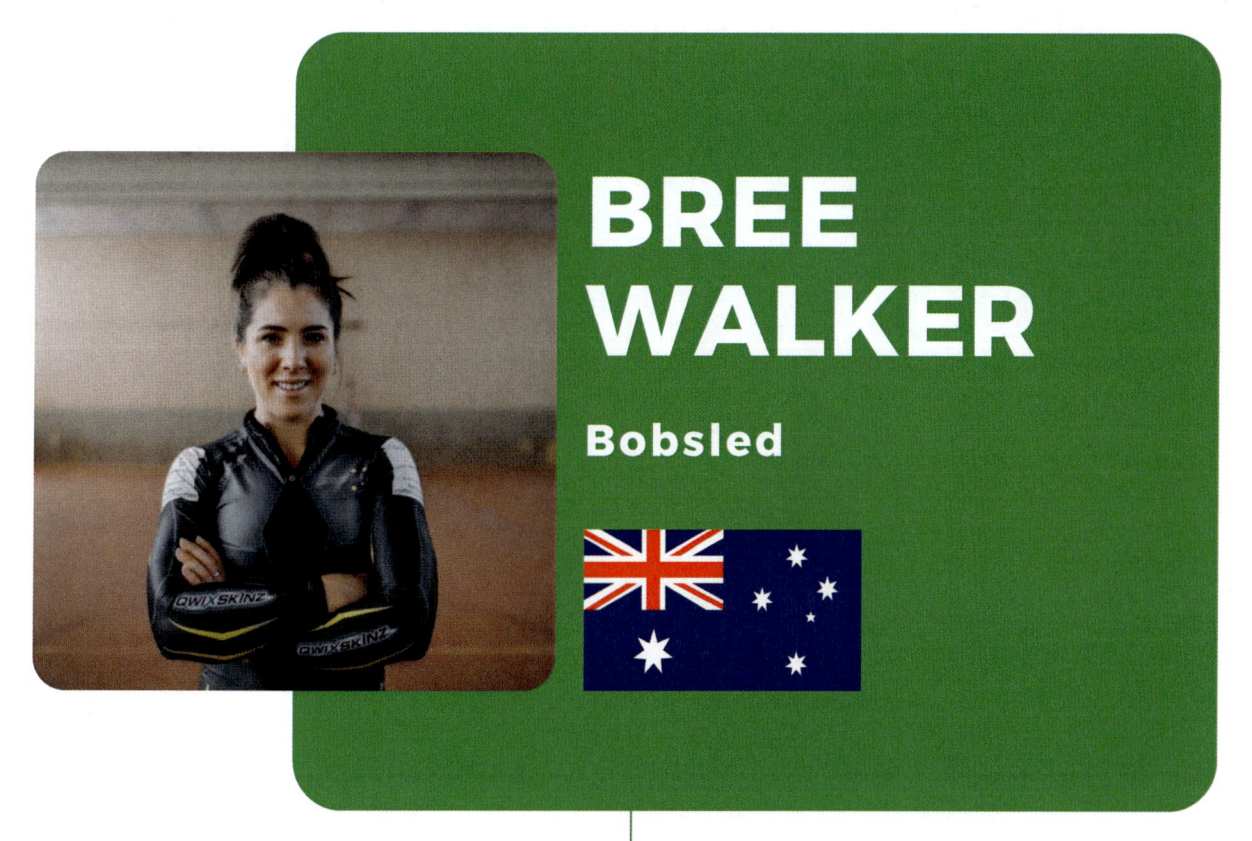

Sleep Habits:
"I sleep 7-8 hrs per night. If you are having trouble sleeping have a drink of water and put on some Biaurnal sounds to help you calm your mind"

Olympic Memory:
"It's hard to think of just one, but I think walking into the Opening Ceremony was a huge moment and I felt like I had finally achieved my lifelong goal of representing Australia at the Olympics. Also, my three-run on my second day of competition because I executed the run that I wanted to do the day before, and that allowed me to fight back from 10th place back to 5th place. That feeling will be the fire that burns in me for the next four years towards the next Winter Olympics. "

Mental Prep Tip:
"If my mind starts to wander before a competition, I bring myself back to where I am and become very present. I do this by asking myself 'where am I?,' looking around for all the details in my environment, being grateful for where I am and what I'm doing, and asking myself 'ok, what am I going to do to execute?' This brings me back to the present and always gets me to refocus."

Daily Routine:
"Wake up, breakfast and, of course, coffee! Check my emails, respond to emails, and tick a few things off my "To-Do List." Lunch. Prepare for training—rest, stretch, yoga, and pack food for during training. Physio (2-3 times a week usually before or after training). Training for about 3 hours. Dinner and bedtime routine—shower, skincare routine, chill."

Image by Bree Walker

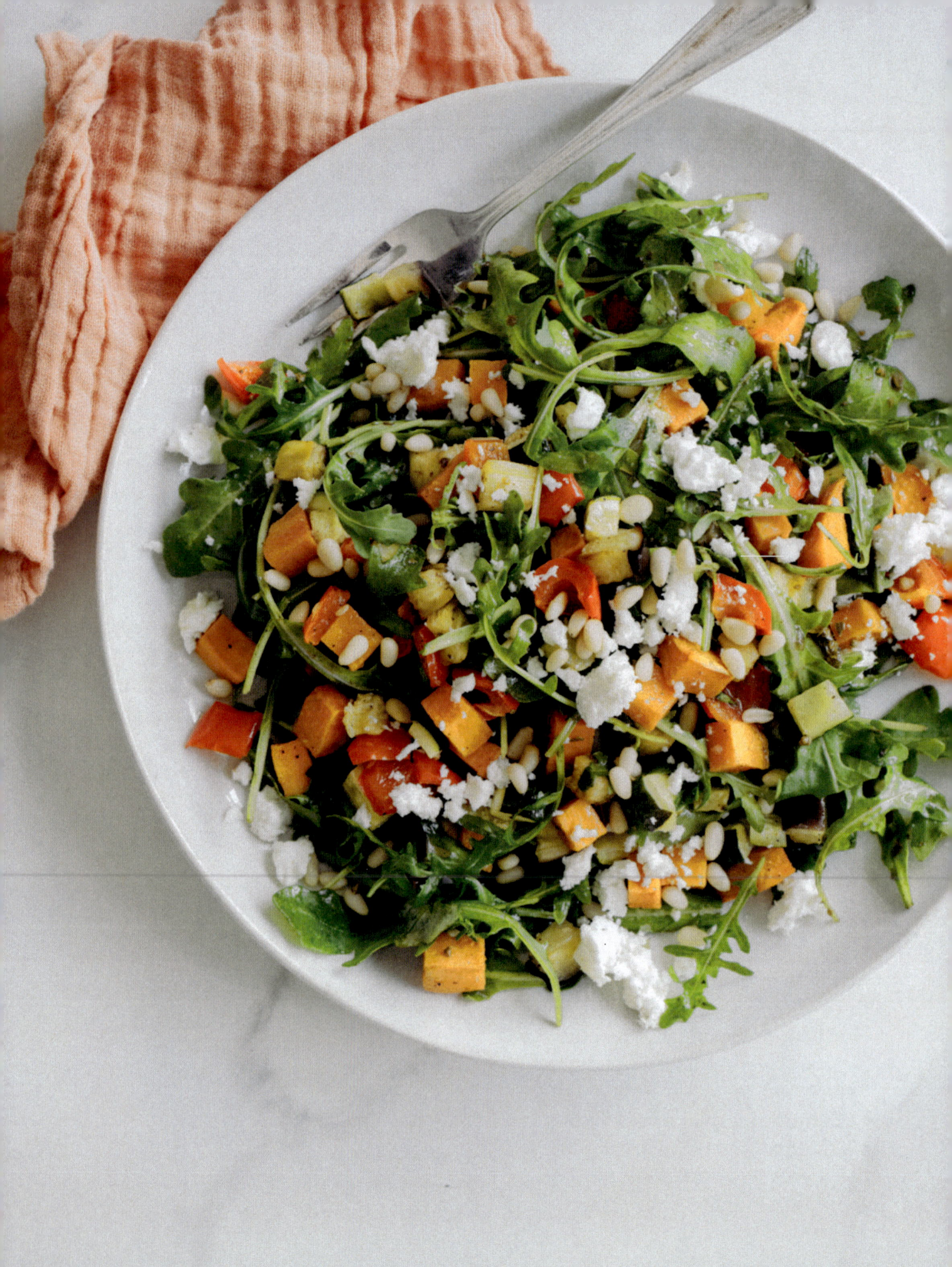

Mediterranean Roast Salad
for a fresh and easy meal

gf

Bree Walker is a bobsledder who represented Australia at the Bejing 2022 Olympics, is a top 10 World Cup Finisher, and has her sights set on the Milano Cortino 2026 Olympics. Originally a talented hurdler, Bree became Victoria's Champion in 2013, but in 2016 decided to switch from athletics to bobsledding because she saw more potential in reaching her goal of becoming an Olympian.

Here, Bree shares her Mediterranean Roast Salad recipe, which is full of colorful vegetables for fiber and has a tangy burst of flavor from the feta. The lemon dijon honey dressing is the perfect addition for a sweet and sour zing!

Makes 3 Servings

1 large red pepper, cubed
1 large sweet potato or pumpkin, cubed
1 large eggplant, cubed
1 large zucchini, cubed
2 tablespoons extra virgin olive oil
2 cups of arugula
3/4 cup feta
1/4 cup pine nuts (roasted or raw)

Dressing
2 tablespoons lemon juice
3/4 cup extra virgin olive oil
1/4 cup balsamic vinegar
1 tablespoon dijon mustard
1/2 teaspoon salt
1/2 teaspoon pepper
2 tablespoons honey
2 tablespoons oregano (fresh or dried)

1. Preheat the oven to 350°F. In a bowl, coat the pepper, sweet potato (or pumpkin), and eggplant with olive oil. On a baking tray with parchment paper, spread out the vegetables and roast them for 20-30 minutes. **NOTE:** some vegetables cook faster than others so keep an eye on the oven!
2. Remove vegetables from the oven. Let them cool completely.
3. Make the dressing by adding lemon juice, olive oil, mustard, and oregano into a glass jar. Close the lid and shake until the contents are fully combined.
4. In a salad bowl, add the rocket, feta, pine nuts, roasted vegetables, and dressing. Toss until mixed evenly. Add a protein to make it a complete meal.

NEVILLE WRIGHT

Bobsled

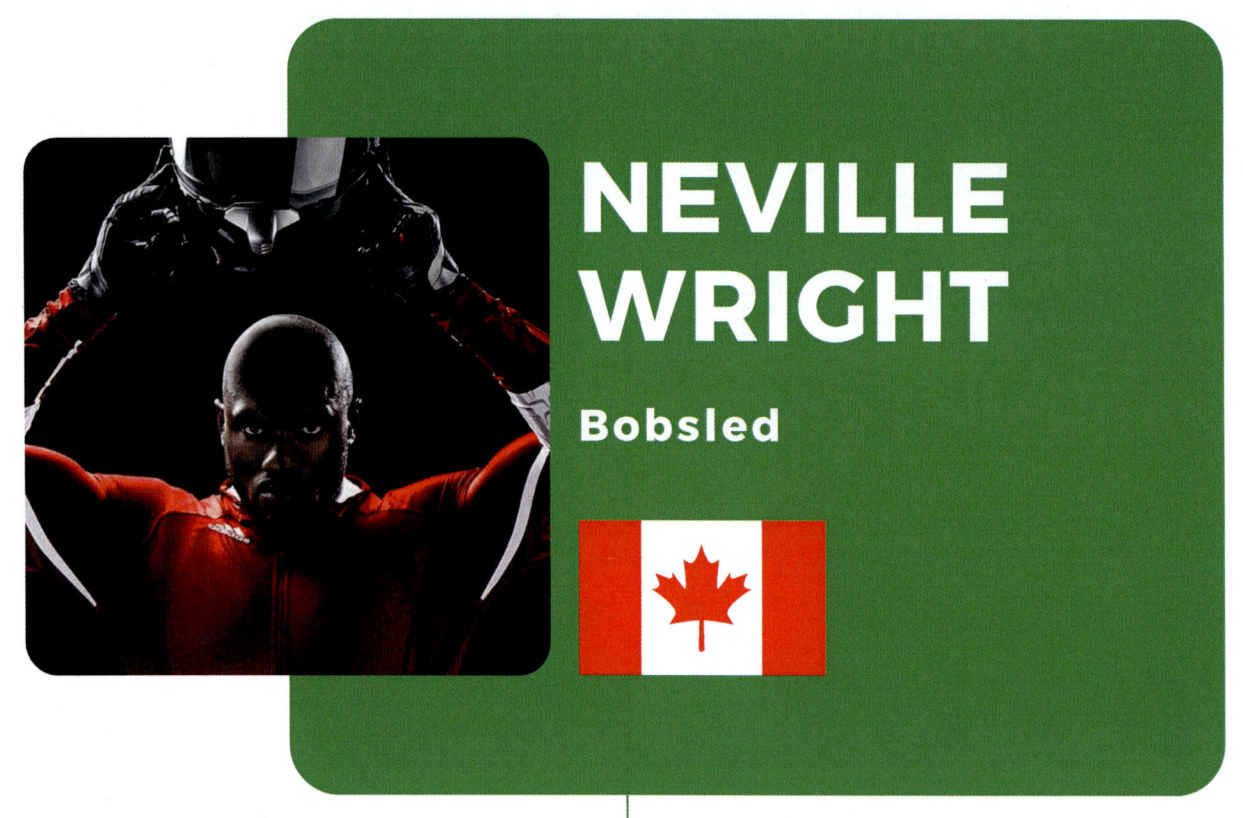

Sleep Habits:

"I'm not the best sleeper, maybe 5-7 hours a night. My best tip would be to sleep in the optimum temperature that is most comfortable for you, listen to soothing sounds with noise-canceling headphones, and/or put your phone out of arm's reach."

Morning Routine:

- Up at least 2 hours before my workout
- Sometimes pop on some music, unless I want complete silence
- Have breakfast
- Based on how I feel and the intensity of the workout, I may do a hot/cold contrast shower
- Training gear is already laid out and training bag is packed from the night before
- Head to the track and sit for about 5 minutes
- Begin training

Mental Prep Tip:

- Make sure everything is laid out the night before so I'm not panicking the day of the competition
- Try and maximize the best sleep possible
- Avoid thinking too much about the competition by having distractions like music (soft) and maybe some mellow conversation
- Do a few mental rehearsal reps in my head, but don't overthink
- Remind myself that I did the work, I don't have to try anything different. Just go out there and perform to the best of my ability and let the result be the result

Olympic Memory:

"Walking into opening ceremonies on home soil."

Image by Neville Wright

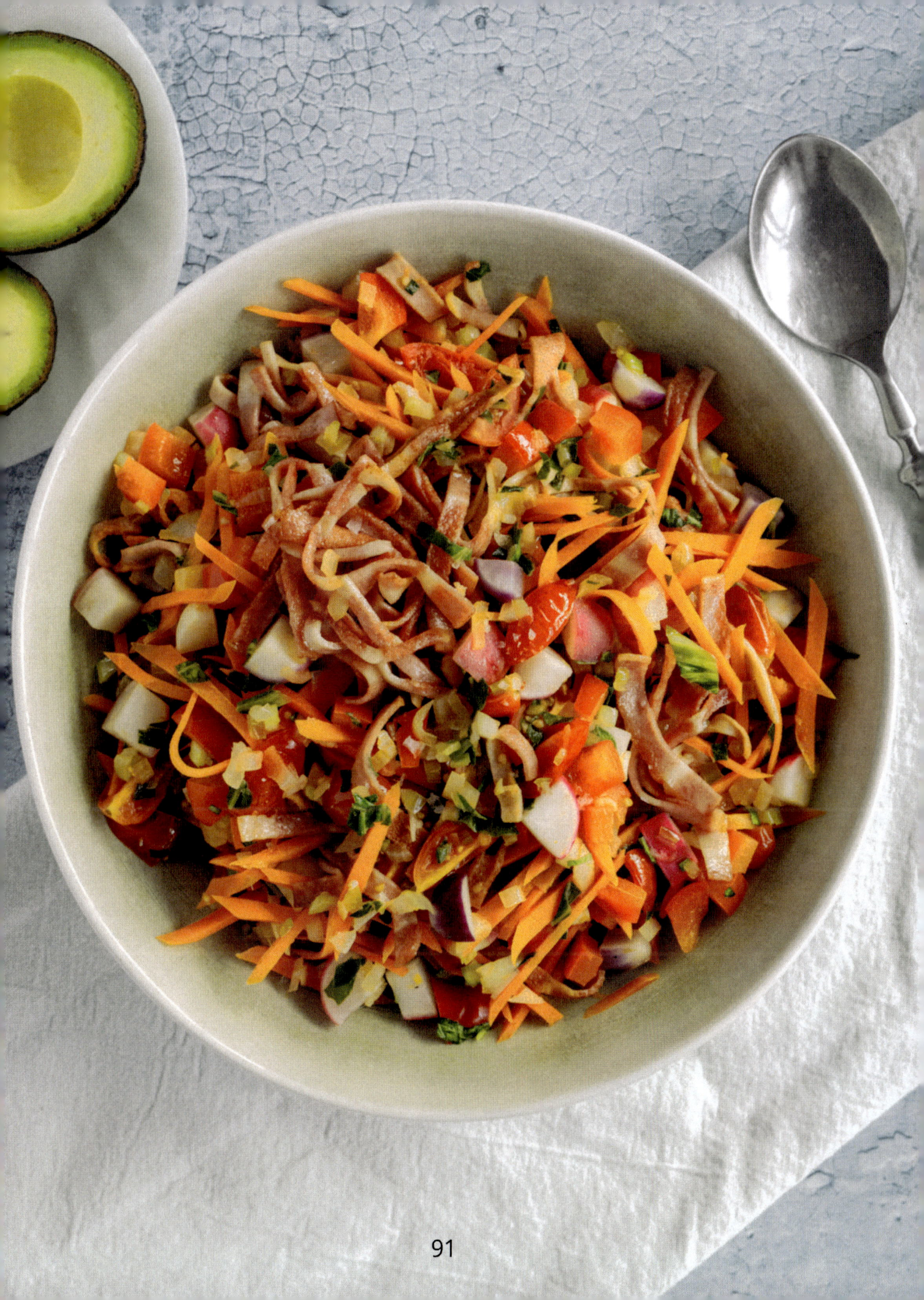

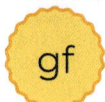

Turkey Bacon Bowl
for a hearty lunch

df gf v

Neville Wright is a bobsledder who represented Canada at the Vancouver 2010, Sochi 2014, and Pyeongchang 2018 Olympics where he raced in the four-man event. Starting out as a successful sprinter, Neville competed in the 2007 IAAF World Championships, but after narrowly missing the qualification for the Beijing 2008 Olympics, he sought out a new sport. Neville's talent was spotted by the Canadian bobsleigh officials, and the rest is history. He is also a speed coach and mentor to Dawn Richards Wilson (check out her recipe on page 145).

Here, Neville shares his crispy turkey bacon bowl. This indulgent and hearty meal is packed with protein, colorful veggies, and served with a side of avocado as a healthy fat.

Makes 1 serving

5 strips of turkey bacon, sliced
1 teaspoon sesame seed oil
1/2 cup of onion, diced
2 cloves of garlic, diced
4-5 stalks of bok choy, minced
1/2 cup of shredded carrots
3 baby red peppers, diced
3 radishes, diced
5-8 cherry tomatoes, sliced
A dash of black pepper
1/2 teaspoon of scotch bonnet hot pepper sauce (optional)
1/2 avocado, sliced

1. In a saucepan, sauté the sliced turkey bacon with the sesame oil until cooked.
2. Mix in and sauté the onion, garlic, bok choy, carrots, red peppers, radishes, and tomatoes.
3. Add a dash of black pepper and stir in the scotch bonnet hot sauce for an extra kick (optional).
4. Cook for 3-5 minutes on medium heat.
5. Serve with half an avocado on the side.

SHAOANG LIU SHAOLIN LIU

Speed Skating

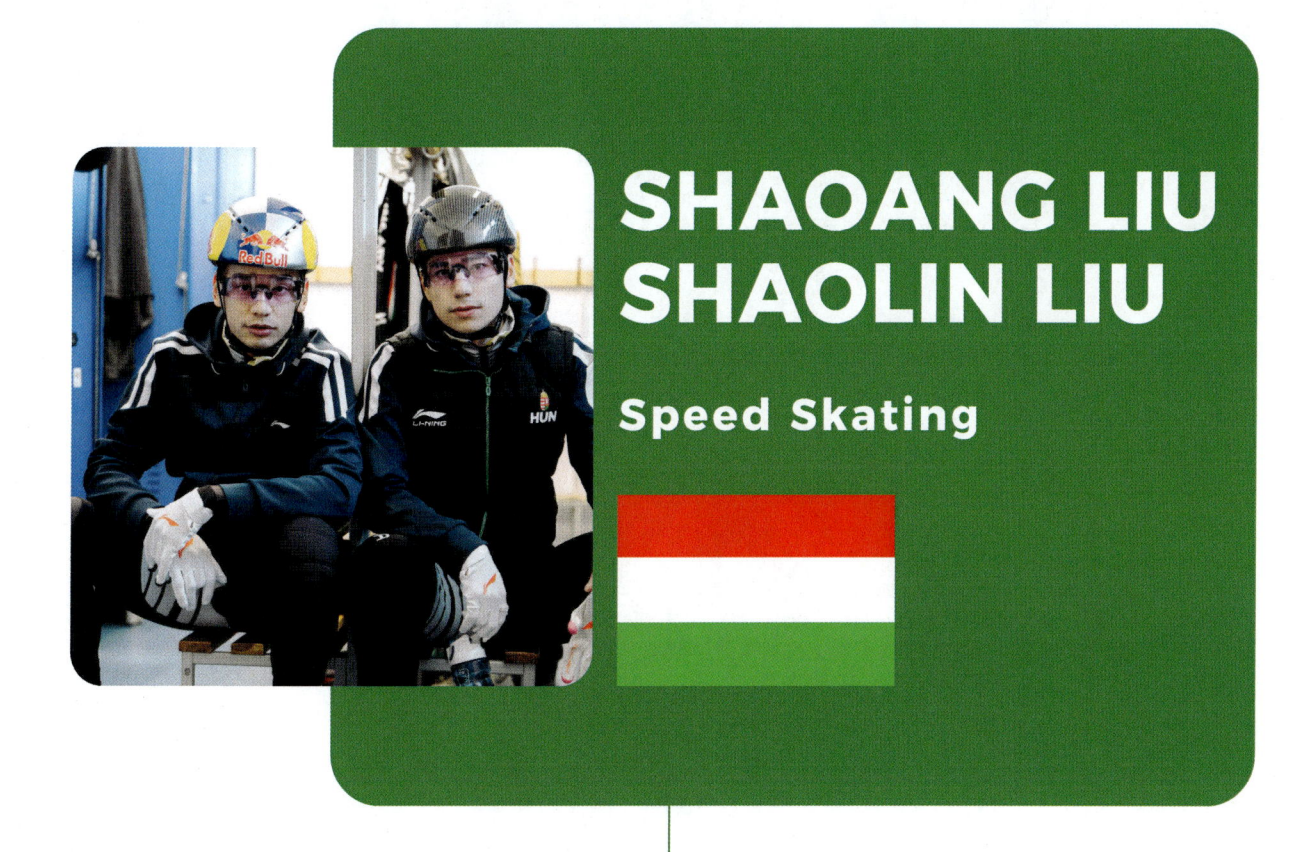

Sleep Habits:

Shaolin: "I try to sleep 9 hours. I love to sleep, typically going to bed around 9-9:30 pm"

Shaoang: "I get 7-8 hours per night."

Olympic Memory:

Shaolin: "The whole Olympics!!"

Shaoang: "Winning my Olympic Gold Medals!"

Recovery Tip:

Shaolin: "I have naps, use Game Ready compression sleeves, or take supplements."

Shaoang: "Massage and stretching."

Morning Routine:

Shaolin: "I wake up one hour before training and I eat right away, about 45 minutes before training"

Shaoang: "7:30 wake up, breakfast, training at 8 am, 9 am ice time, finishing around 11 or 12 pm"

Image by Shaoang and Shaolin Liu

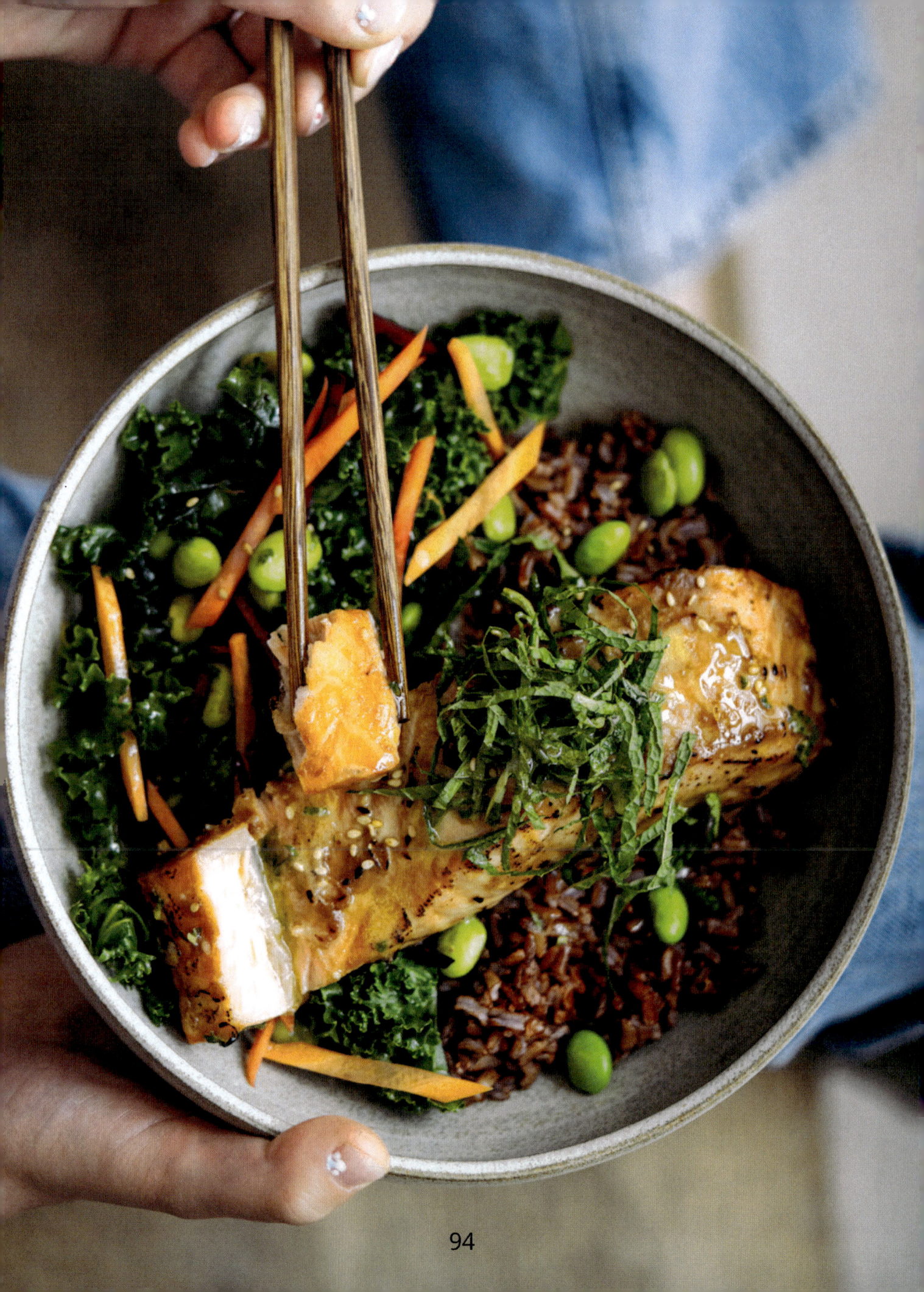

Miso Salmon Nourish Bowl
for strength

gf

Shaolin and Shaoang are brothers and short-track speed skaters who represented Hungary at two Olympic Games. Shaolin is an Olympic Gold Medalist and Bronze Medalist, 10x World Championship medalist, and a 16x European Championship Medalist. Shaoang is a 2x Olympic Gold Medalist, 2x Olympic Bronze Medalist, 13x World Championship Medalist, and 13x European Championship Medalist. That is quite the track record! Beijing was a special Olympics for the brothers: they are half Hungarian and half Chinese, so every medal they won was dedicated to both countries. Their mother stitched the two flags together to support both of their heritages during the competition!

Shaolin and Shaoang eat this Salmon Nourish Bowl for most meals because it is simple, delicious, and includes all of the macronutrients they need for training. NOTE: the salmon can be substituted for any other protein.

Makes 2 servings

Salmon:
- 2 salmon filets
- 2 tablespoons miso paste
- 1 tablespoon soy sauce
- 1 tablespoon mirin
- 1 tablespoon sake
- 1/4 teaspoon sesame oil
- Sesame seeds (optional)

Salad:
- 1 bunch kale (de-stemmed and massaged for 3-4 minutes by hand with 1 tablespoon olive oil and a pinch of salt to soften)
- 1 medium raw beet, grated
- 1 medium carrot, peeled
- 1 cup cooked edamame
- 1 tablespoon white sesame seeds

1. In a bowl, make the marinade by mixing the miso paste, soy sauce, mirin, sake, sesame oil, and sesame seeds.
2. Place the salmon filets in the bowl and use a spoon to coat with marinade. Cover the bowl and let salmon marinate for 30-40 minutes in the fridge.
3. Preheat the oven to 410°F. Line a baking sheet with parchment paper. Lightly scrape off any excess marinade from the salmon and bake it for 10-12 minutes or until slightly browned.

See the next page for further instruction.

4. Make the salad by mixing the massaged kale, beets, carrots, edamame, and sesame seeds in a large bowl, and dress with the Lemon Vinaigrette.
5. Serve with 1/2 cup red rice.

Lemon Vinaigrette
for a zingy flavour

df nf gf

This vinaigrette pairs perfectly with Shaolin and Shaoang Liu's **Miso Salmon Nourish Bowl (page 95)** because the sweet honey and sour lemon in the dressing balance the salty miso. However, this vinaigrette can be used in any salad **(especially the Mediterranean Roast Salad page 89)** or on a protein to add extra flavor.

Makes about 1 cup

1/2 cup freshly squeezed lemon juice
1/2 cup olive oil
2 teaspoons Dijon mustard
2 teaspoons honey (or maple syrup or agave nectar)
8-10 large mint leaves, finely chopped
Ground salt and pepper, to taste

1. Add the lemon juice, olive oil, dijon mustard, honey, mint leaves, salt, and pepper to a glass jar with a lid. Shake until fully combined and emulsified.
2. Pour generously over your favorite salad and toss so that the dressing coats the ingredients evenly.
3. Store in the fridge for up to a week. Shake again before serving. The oil may solidify, so microwave on low until melted.

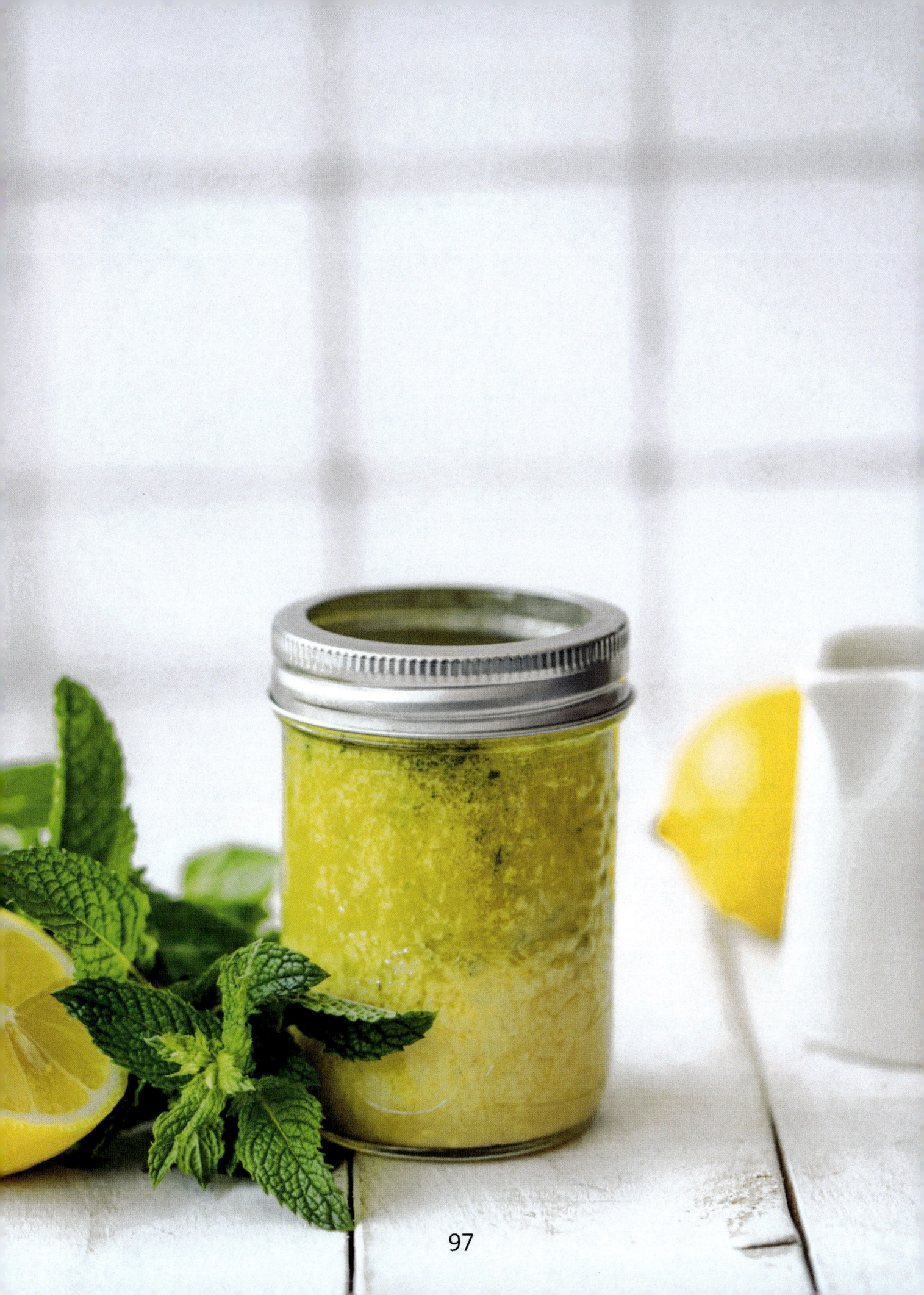

BRITTENY COX

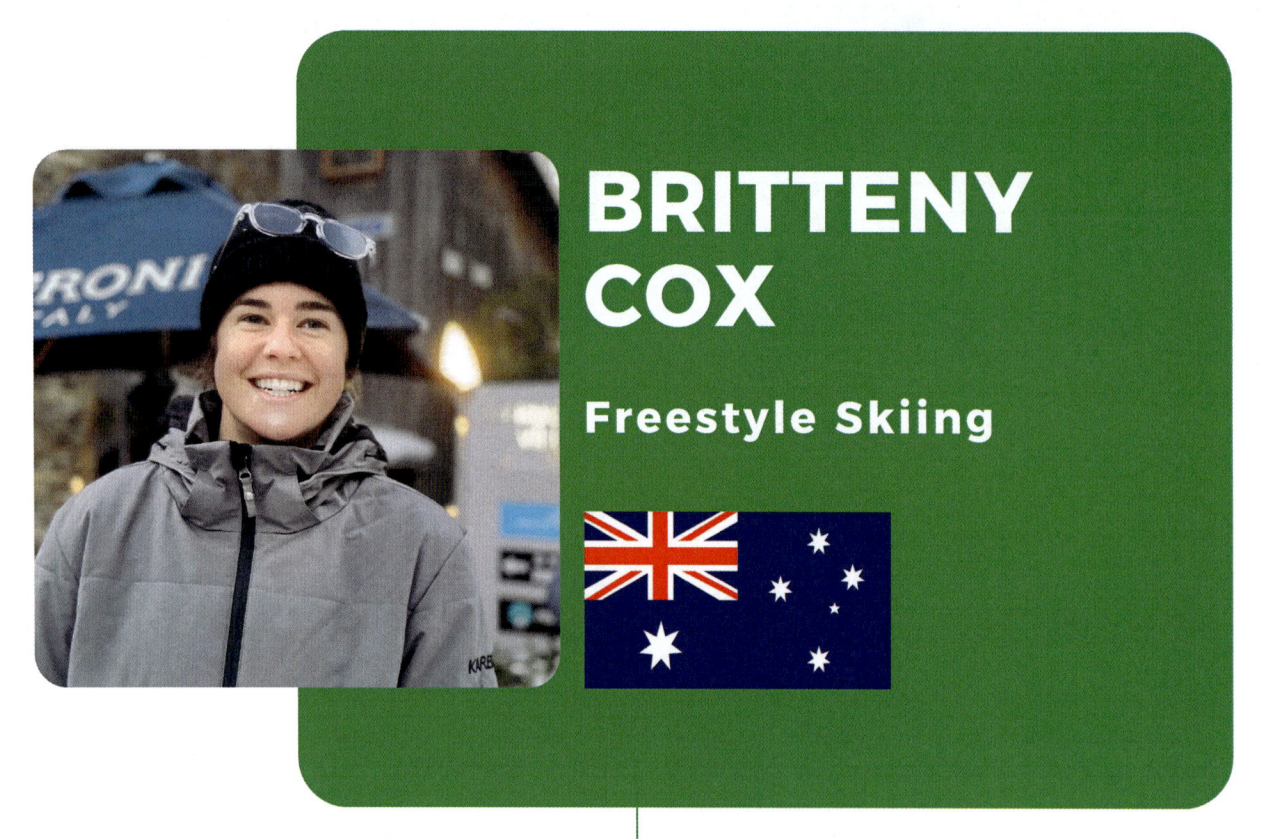

Freestyle Skiing

Sleep Habits:
"I need a minimum 8 hours but preferably more when I'm in the middle of a training camp. If I can't get this at night, I try to squeeze a nap in during the day."

Olympic Memory:
"Being in the start gate with my coach, Kate Blamey, at the 2022 Olympic games and feeling determined, confident, grateful, and proud."

Mental Prep Tip:
"I use the breath-work and meditation techniques from my yoga practice to help bring myself into the present moment. I also use visualization techniques to rehearse my performance and enhance my confidence in the skills I am about to execute."

Recovery Tip:
"I am completely obsessed with yoga, particularly the elements of mindfulness, breath-work, and meditation. I use these practices to ground myself on a big day of training."

Morning Routine:
"I always eat breakfast as soon as I wake in the morning. I don't do any physical activity until I have some fuel in the tank. I use this time to think about my goals and plan for the day, as well as to take a few mindful moments to enjoy my coffee. I then do 25 minutes of yoga to get my body moving before undertaking any specific training. This is followed by a 30-minute warm-up in preparation for on-snow training. I then gear up and head out to ski."

Image by Britteny Cox

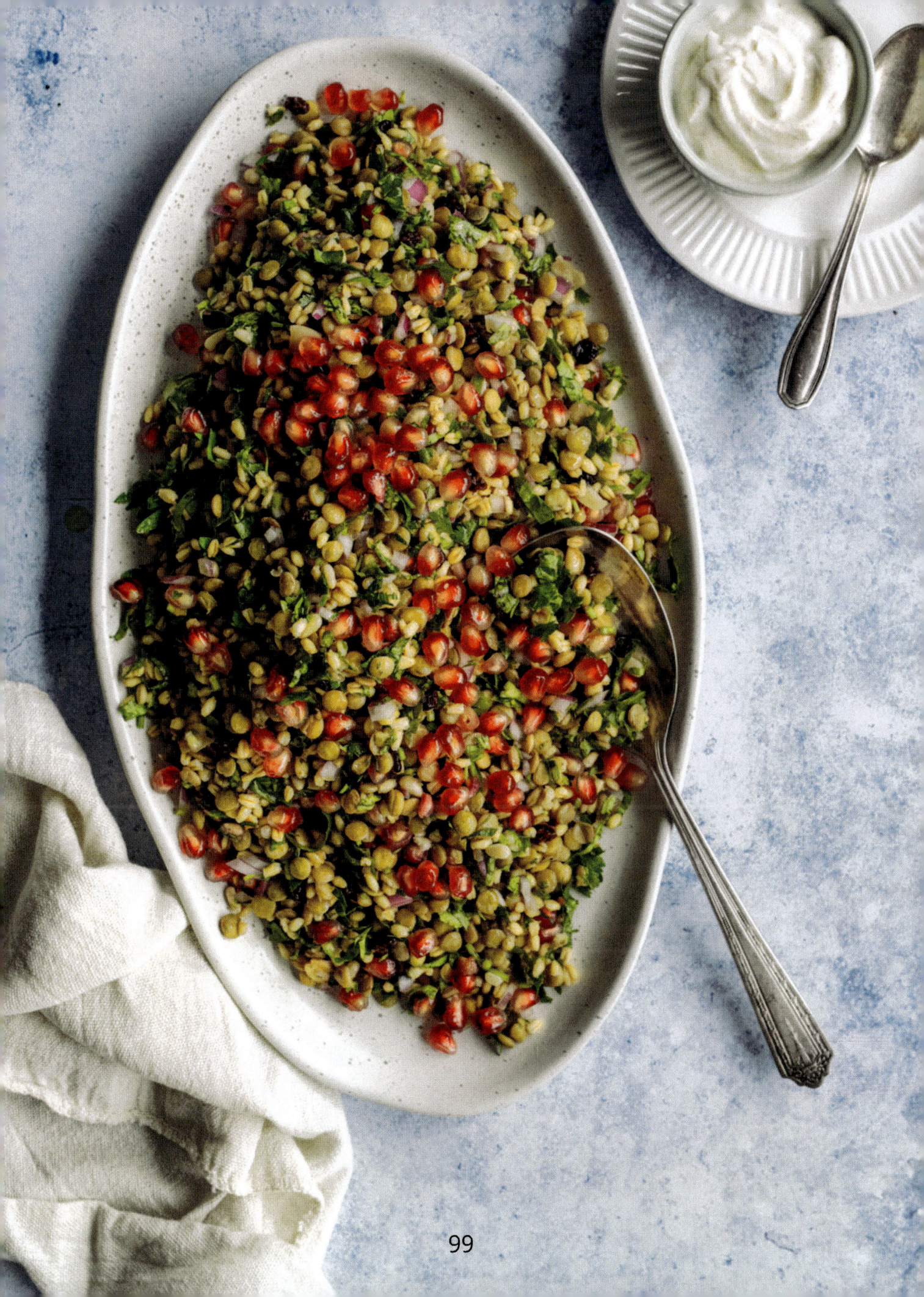

Cypriot Grain Salad
for a sweet and sour treat

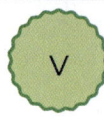

nf gf v df

Britteny Cox is a mogul skier who represented Australia at the Vancouver 2010, Sochi 2014, Pyeongchang 2018, and Beijing 2022 Olympic Games! She called herself the "mother hen" of the Australian mogul team at the Beijing 2022 Olympics. She grew up in a skiing family, and was only 15 years old at the Vancouver 2010 Olympics, making her Australia's youngest Winter Olympian in 58 years. Britt is Australia's first-ever female mogul skier to win a World Cup Medal (Gold and Bronze), and a Crystal Globe. She is more fired up than ever, and her love for the sport still burns bright!

Here, Britt shares this Cypriot Salad recipe. She loves making this for her teammates! Freekeh is an underrated grain that has 6.5g more fiber and 3.5g more protein than brown rice. This salad has an abundance of greens, plant-based protein, and has a nutty flavor with bursts of sweetness from the pomegranate and currants.

Makes 8 servings

1 bunch coriander, chopped
1/2 bunch parsley, chopped
1/2 red onion, finely diced
1 cup freekeh (or quinoa)
1/2 cup green lentils
2 tablespoons pumpkin seeds
2 tablespoons slivered almonds
2 tablespoons toasted pine nuts
2 tablespoons baby capers
1/2 cup red currants
1 cup pomegranate seeds
Juice of 1 lemon
3 tablespoons extra virgin olive

Dressing
1 cup thick Greek yogurt
1 teaspoon ground cumin
1 tablespoon honey

1. In separate pots, blanch the freekeh and lentils in boiling water until cooked. Drain well and let them cool.
2. In a large mixing bowl, add the coriander, parsley, onion, freekeh, lentils, pumpkin seeds, almonds, pine nuts, capers, currants, pomegranate, salt, lemon juice, and olive oil. Mix well.
3. In a small bowl, combine the greek yogurt, cumin, and honey.
4. Place the salad in a serving dish, and top with the yogurt dressing, pomegranates, and a pinch of salt.

101

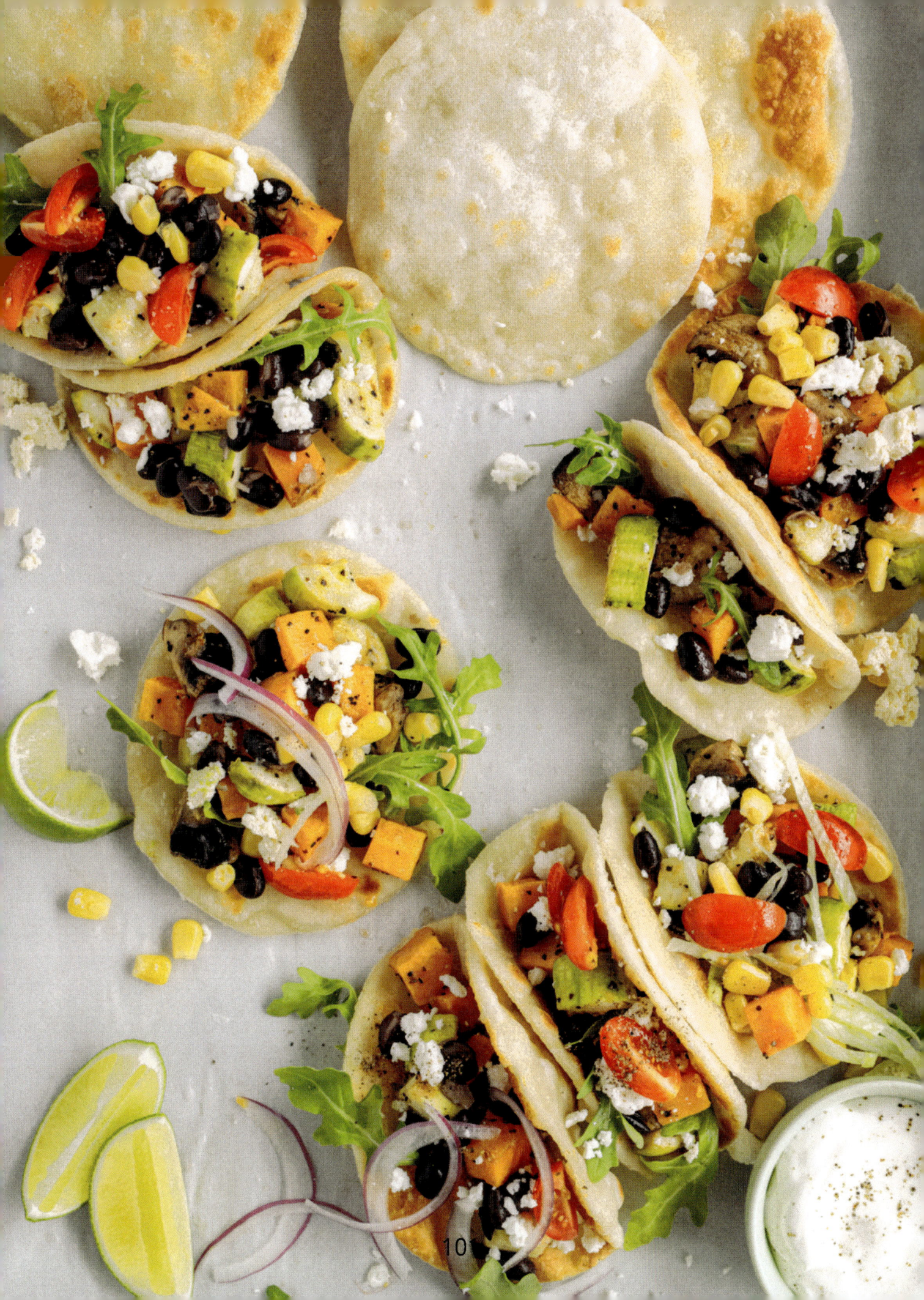

Zucchini Tacos
BONUS RECIPE

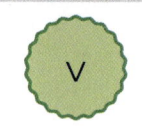

v   gf   nf

Jaelin Kauf is a freestyle skier who represented the USA at the Pyeongchang 2018 and Beijing 2022 Winter Olympic Games. She won silver in Beijing in the freestyle moguls and is also a 2 x World Championship medalist. You go girl!!

Here Jaelin shares her zucchini taco recipe including how to make your own tortillas. "Homemade tortillas might be the secret here, and are super easy to make!" The combination of warm tortillas, tender vegetables, and the tangy queso fresco is out of this world. I mean, she had me at "taco."

Makes 5-7 servings

Taco filling:
3 large zucchinis, chopped
2 sweet potatoes, chopped
4 white mushrooms, sliced
2 tablespoons olive oil
Salt and pepper to season
1 cup arugula
1 can (15 oz) black beans
1/2 cup queso fresco (not if vegan)

Tortillas: makes 16 (4.5" street-sized)
4 cups all-purpose flour (or GF)
2 teaspoons salt
1 1/3 cup warm water
1/4 vegetable oil

Extra topping ideas:
- Peas, corn, lettuce, or avocado
- Diced cherry tomatoes or salsa
- Green onions or cilantro
- Sour cream or guacamole
- Grilled protein: chicken, beef, or tofu

1. Preheat the oven to 400°F. On a baking tray lined with parchment paper, coat the zucchini, sweet potato, and mushrooms with olive oil and bake for 30 minutes. Flip the vegetables after 15 minutes.
2. In a mixing bowl, make the dough by combining the flour and salt. Add the vegetable oil and work it into the flour with your fingertips until it resembles coarse crumbs.
3. Add the warm water and mix until a loose dough forms. Transfer the dough onto a lightly flour-dusted surface (to prevent the dough from sticking), and knead it for about 2 minutes until smooth.
4. Break the dough into 16 equal balls, cover them with cling film, and allow them to rest for 20 minutes.

5. Roll out each dough ball until it is flat and approximately 4.5" wide.
6. Transfer 1-2 tortillas at a time to a large cast-iron skillet and cook on medium heat until the tortillas develop golden brown spots.
7. Fill each taco with vegetables, arugula, black beans, queso fresco, and any other desired toppings.

Guacamole recipe page 132

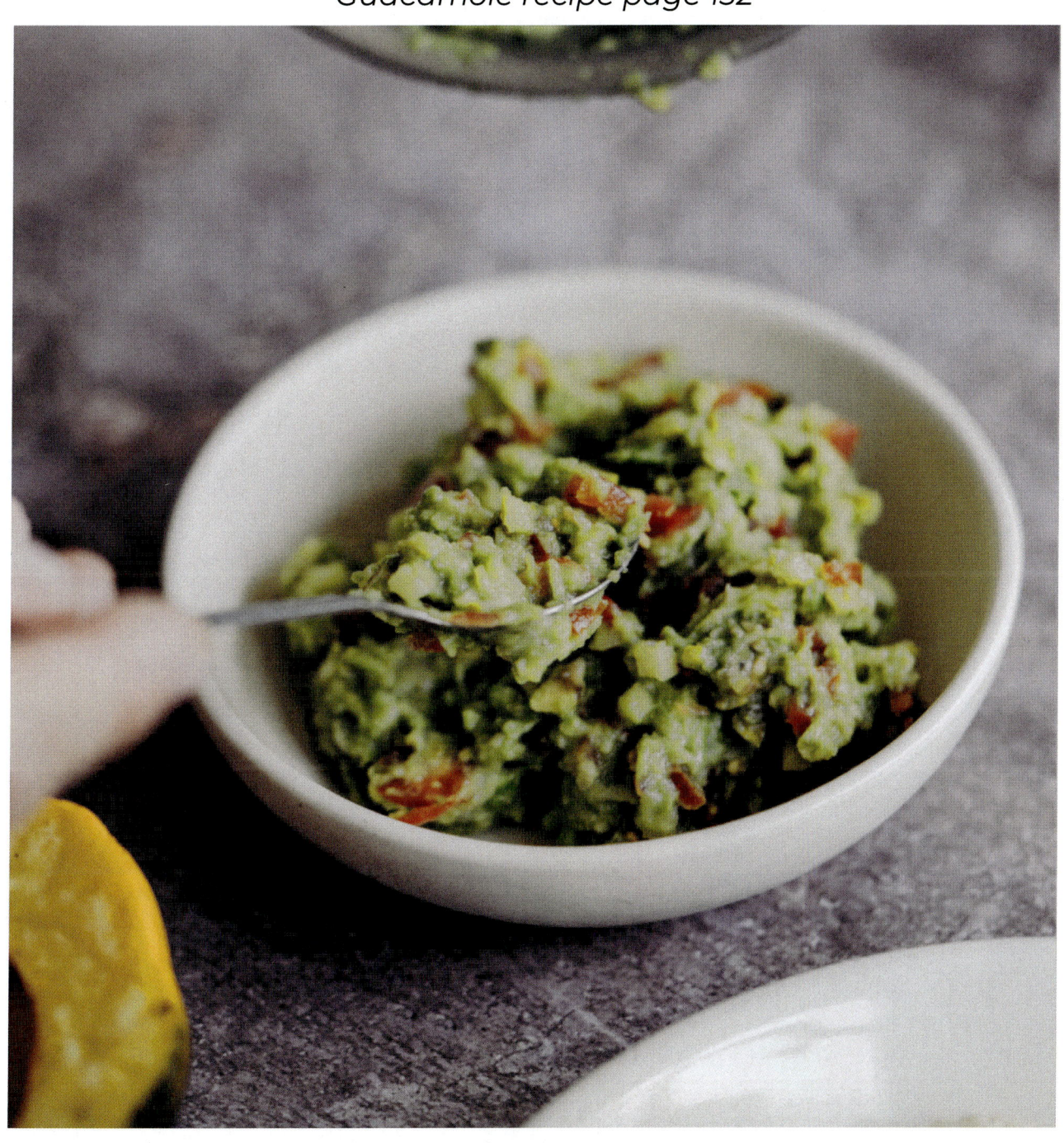

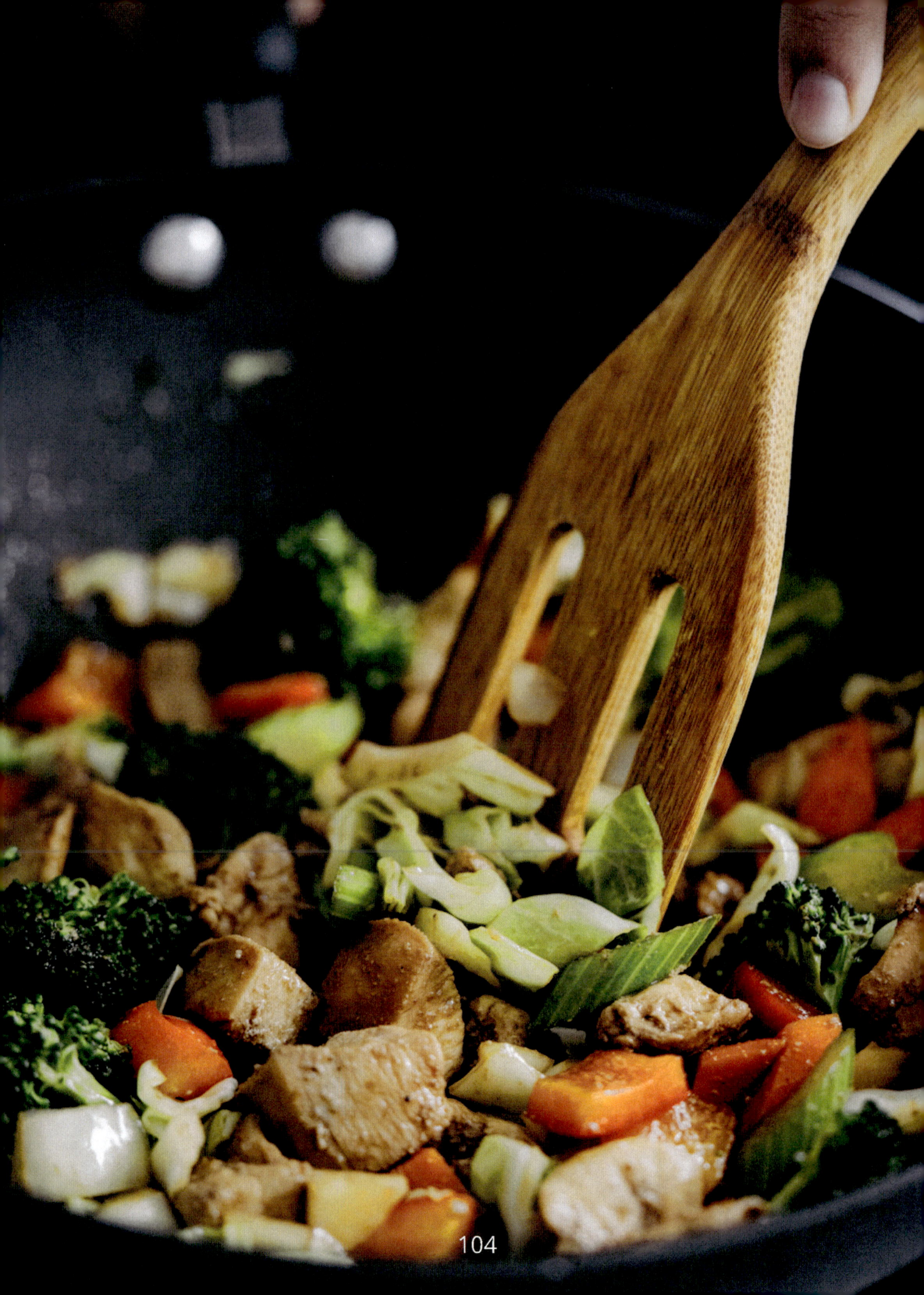

DINNER LIKE A WINNER

The "Instagram" Chicken Fried Rice   106

BBQ Pork Baby Back Ribs   110

Uncle Johnny's Meatballs   113

Shrimp Stir Fry   116

Tempeh Tabbouleh Bowl   119

Chill Out Chili   123

Wholesome Stir Fry   126

BONUS RECIPE: Winner Winner Chicken Dinner   130

BONUS RECIPE: Veggie and Dip Platter   131

BONUS RECIPE: Hollandaise Sauce   134

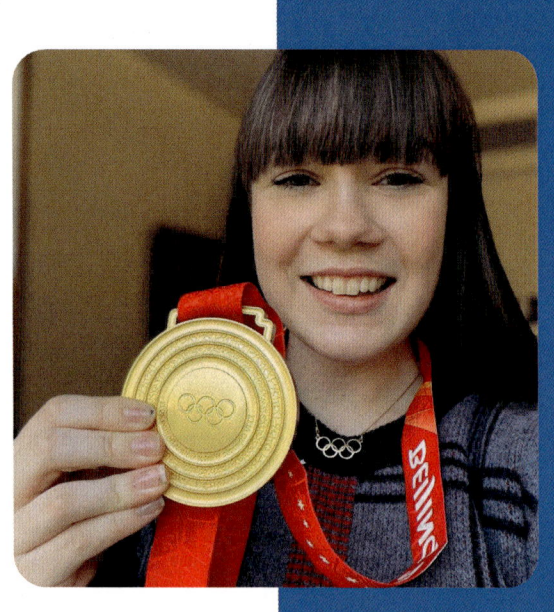

HAILEY DUFF

Curling

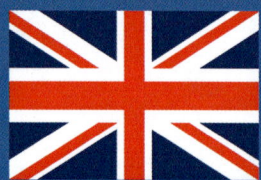

Sleep Habits:
"Roughly 8.5 hours per night. I use a lumie lamp which recreates the natural light of sunset and sunrise. I find it amazing to help me fall asleep and wake up refreshed in the morning!"

Olympic Memory:
"Stepping on the podium was amazing! But also seeing the ice rink for the first time where we would be competing was really cool."

Recovery Tip:
"Eating a lot of food—some protein and carbs. Also stretching and going for a light walk if the weather is good."

Morning Routine:
"Wake up, get ready, and have breakfast. It depends on how much time I have, but it would be either bagel with scrambled eggs or cereal with yogurt and fruit."

Image by Hailey Duff

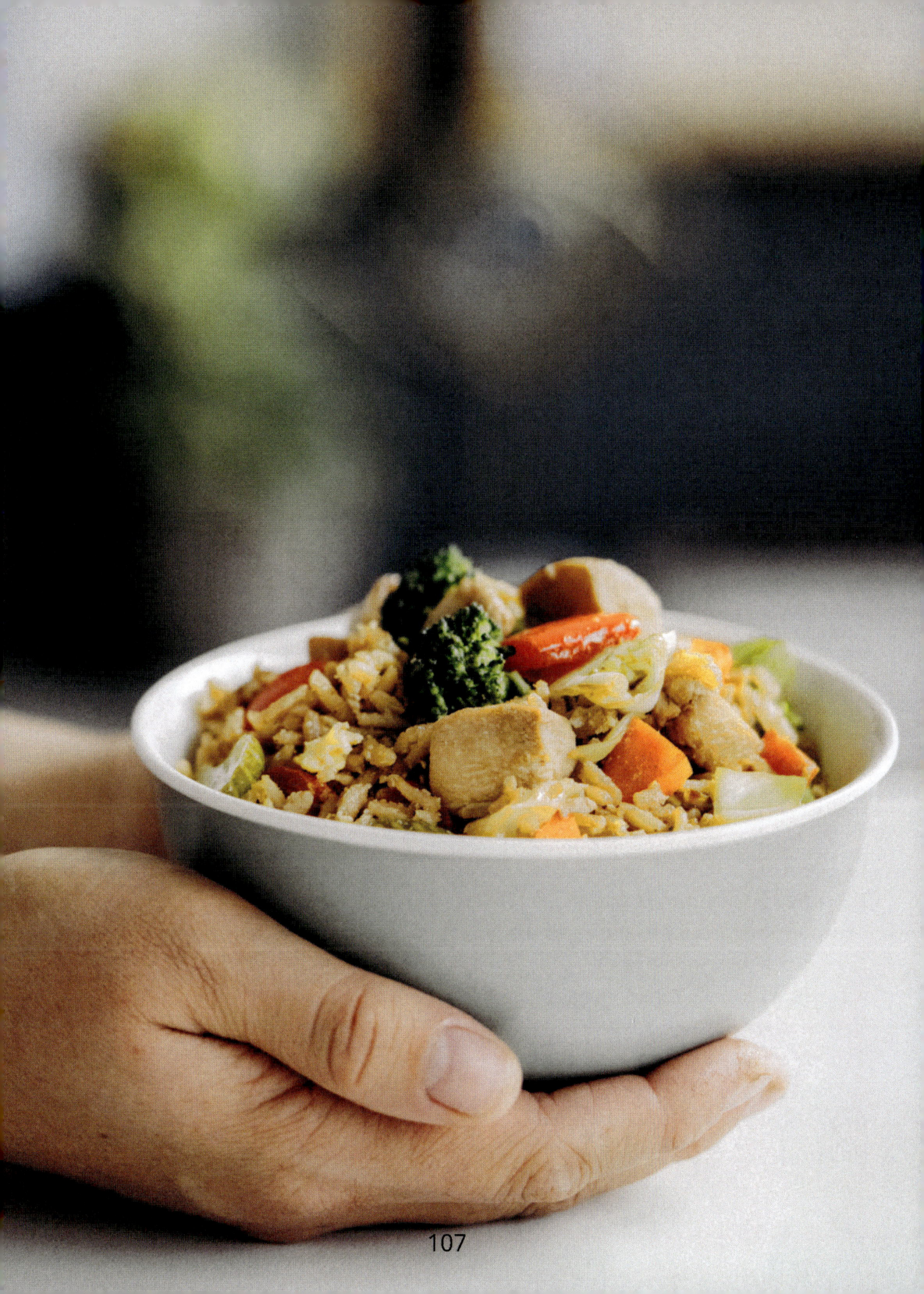

The "Instagram" Chicken Fried Rice
for a quick dinner

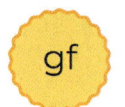

gf df

Hailey Duff is a Scottish curler who represented Great Britain at the Beijing 2022 Olympic Games. She plays lead for skip Eve Muirhead, and her team won GOLD! (I watched it on live TV and was bawling my eyes out).

Here Hailey will share the dinner recipe she makes on repeat. She calls it "The Instagram" stir fry because she saw the recipe on an Instagram reel and loved it! This easy frying pan recipe is perfect for an on-the-go or lazy dinner, as it takes 20 minutes to make and covers all of the nutritional bases. The chicken and egg are full of protein, the rice is a great wholegrain carbohydrate, you get some healthy fats from the safflower oil, and the colorful veggies are packed with vitamins and minerals.

Makes 4 servings

1 cup raw short-grain brown rice
2 tablespoons safflower oil or other high-heat oil
3 tablespoons low-sodium soy sauce
1/2 teaspoon garlic powder
1 tablespoon toasted sesame oil
12 ounces chicken breasts (chopped into 1/2 inch pieces)
Salt and pepper to taste
2 cups cooked mixed chopped vegetables (carrots, onion, celery, peas, broccoli, cabbage, bell pepper)
2 eggs

1. In a pot, cook the brown rice according to the package instructions. Let it cool.
2. Mix the soy sauce, sesame oil, and garlic powder in a small bowl to make the marinade. In a bowl, use 3/4 of the mixture and marinate the chicken.
3. Let the chicken marinate anywhere from 20 minutes to overnight.
4. Heat 1 tablespoon of safflower oil in a large pan over medium heat.
5. Add the chopped chicken pieces into the pan, season with salt and pepper, and cook for 4-5 minutes or until the chicken is cooked through.

6. Add the vegetables to the chicken. Stir fry them with the rest of the marinade,
7. Add the cooked brown rice into the pan with the chicken. Break the rice apart while stir-frying. Push the rice and the chicken to one side of the pan to make room for the eggs.
8. Crack the eggs into the free side of the pan and cook, stirring continuously until scrambled.
9. Turn off heat. Add more sesame oil or soy sauce to serve.

V **Want to make it vegan?** Sub the chicken and egg for tofu.

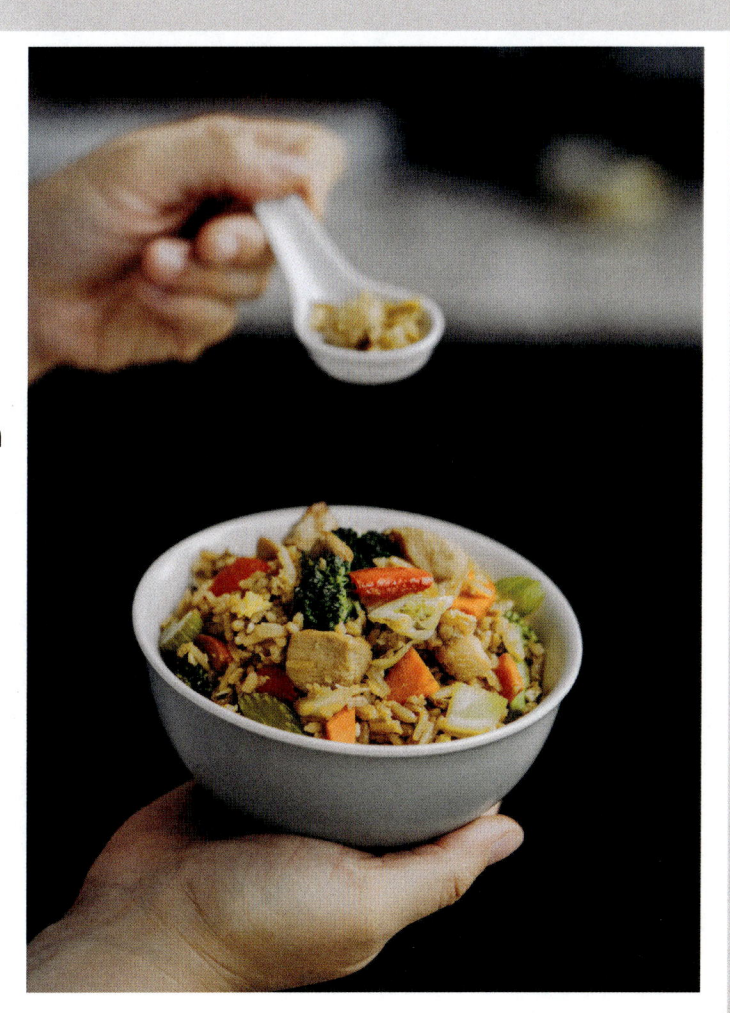

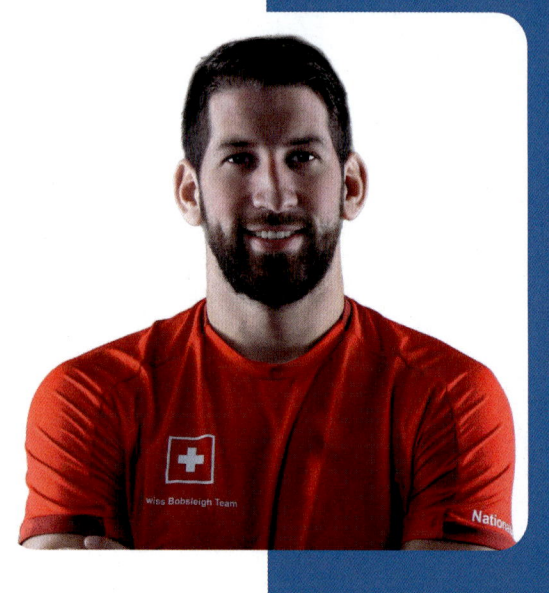

ADRIAN FASSLER

Bobsled 🇨🇭

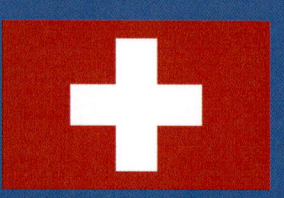

Sleep Habits:
"I usually sleep about 6-7 hours. but should sleep more! I just have this rhythm in my blood."

Olympic Memory:
"The Opening Ceremony when you walk into the stadium and the speaker calls out your country and you walk under the Olympic rings. Goosebumps."

Mental Prep Tip:
"I don't really do anything special: relax, listen to music, and have fun with the other athletes. Let's GO!!"

Morning Routine:
"I get up, drink a coffee and chill a bit, then I get ready. I mostly train alone, so I'm very flexible. I usually never eat before training; if I do, it's at least 2-3 hours before."

Recovery Tip:
"Stretching after a workout. If the time is right, I also like to go for a massage. I love to eat outside and enjoy the beautiful weather. Then the next day I get back to work!"

Image by Manu Naef

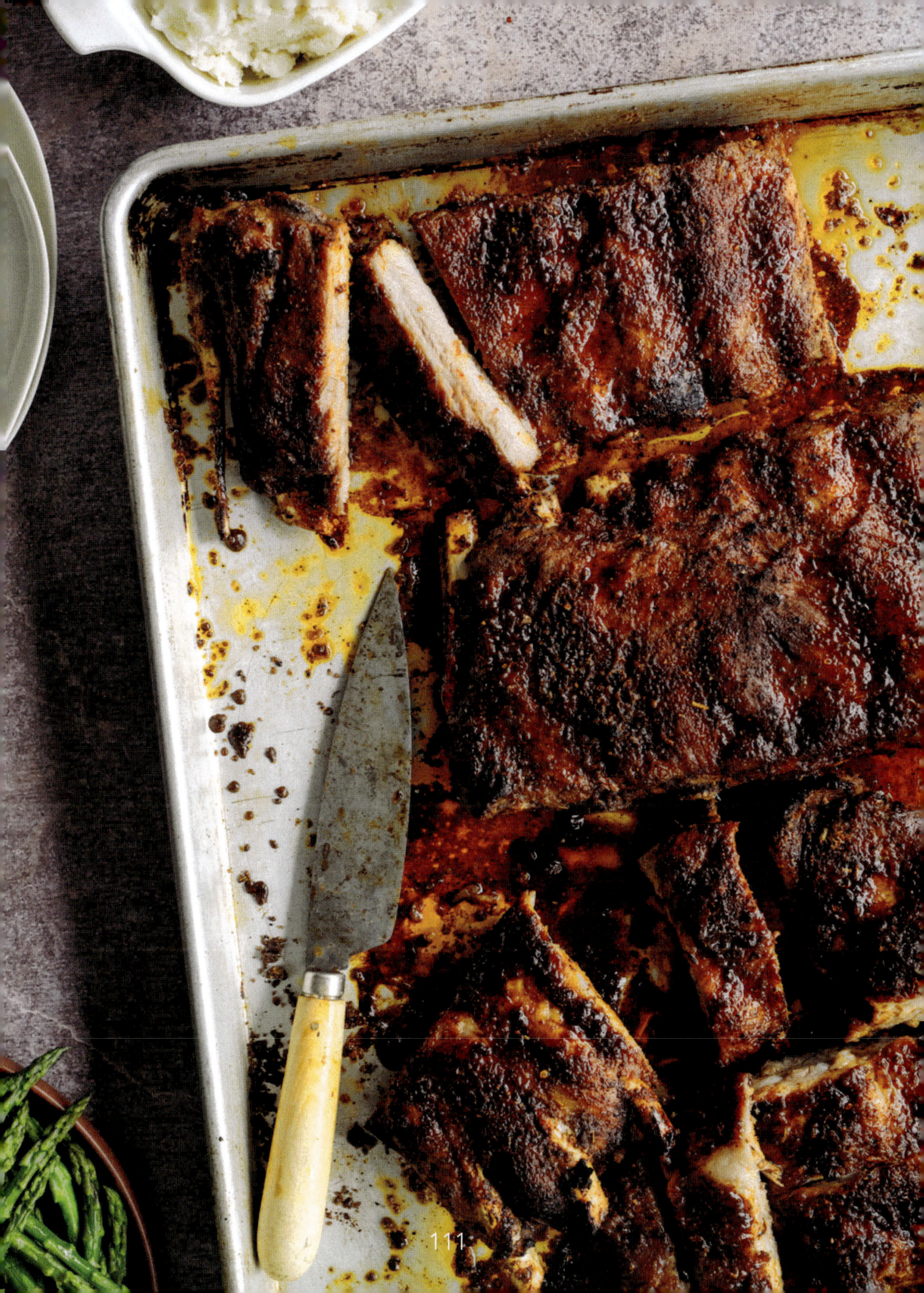

BBQ Pork Baby Back Ribs
for a quick dinner

gf df

Adrian Fässler is a boblsedder who represented Switzerland at the Beijing 2022 Olympics as a brakeman in the four-man event. He also placed 12th at the 2021 European Championships in Winterberg.

Here Adrian shares his BBQ pork spare ribs recipe. Most ribs take hours to prepare, but this recipe provides a shortcut while still giving delicious results! This recipe both boils and grills the ribs because boiling will tenderize the meat and grilling gives them flavor.

Makes 4 Servings

2 rack baby back ribs (about 48 ounces), or spare ribs (cheaper)
Pinch of Kosher salt
1 1/4 cup brown sugar
2 tablespoons chili powder
Dash freshly ground black pepper
1 teaspoon dried oregano
1/2 teaspoon cayenne pepper
1/2 teaspoon garlic powder
1/2 teaspoon onion powder
1 cup barbecue sauce

1. Preheat the grill or grill pan to medium-high heat. Slice the ribs into 3 sections.
2. In a large pot on medium heat, add the ribs, enough water to cover them, and a pinch of salt. Let them boil, then bring to a simmer for 20 minutes. Drain ribs and dry with a paper towel.
3. Make the spice coat by mixing the brown sugar, chili powder, salt, pepper, oregano, cayenne pepper, garlic powder and onion powder. Spoon the mixture onto the ribs and use a brush or your hand to coat them evenly.
4. Place the ribs on the grill pan and cook for 10 minutes, flipping them halfway through. Brush ribs with barbecue sauce and cook for 1-2 more minutes, or until slightly charred.
5. Best served with more barbecue sauce, asparagus, and mashed potatoes.

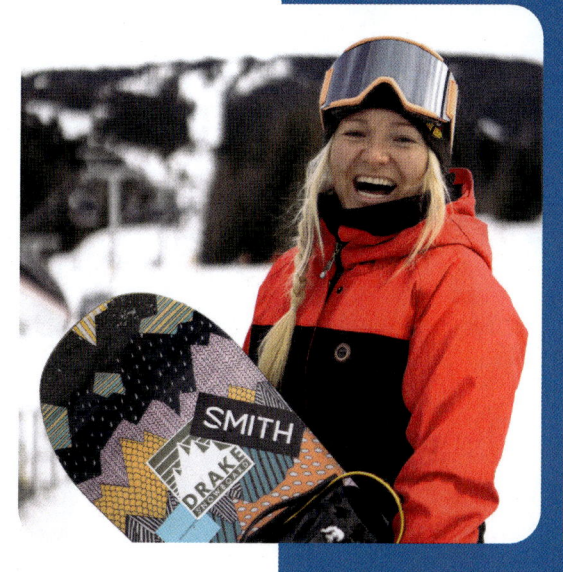

MERCEDES NICOLL

Snowboarding

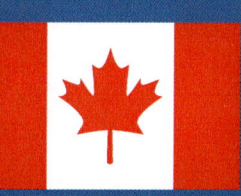

🇨🇦

Sleep Habits:
"I get at least 8 hours. Reading before bed helps me get a good rest."

Olympic Memory:
"When I landed the trick that took me out of sport for 2 years again at the 2018 Winter Games."

Mental Prep Tip:
"I have to believe in myself, remind myself that I can do this!"

Morning Routine:
"Wake up with enough time for breakfast, get all my snowboard gear together, and head out the door. Do a warm-up at the mountain, and go ride!"

Recovery Tip:
"Stretching session, food, and water."

Image by Mercedes Nicoll

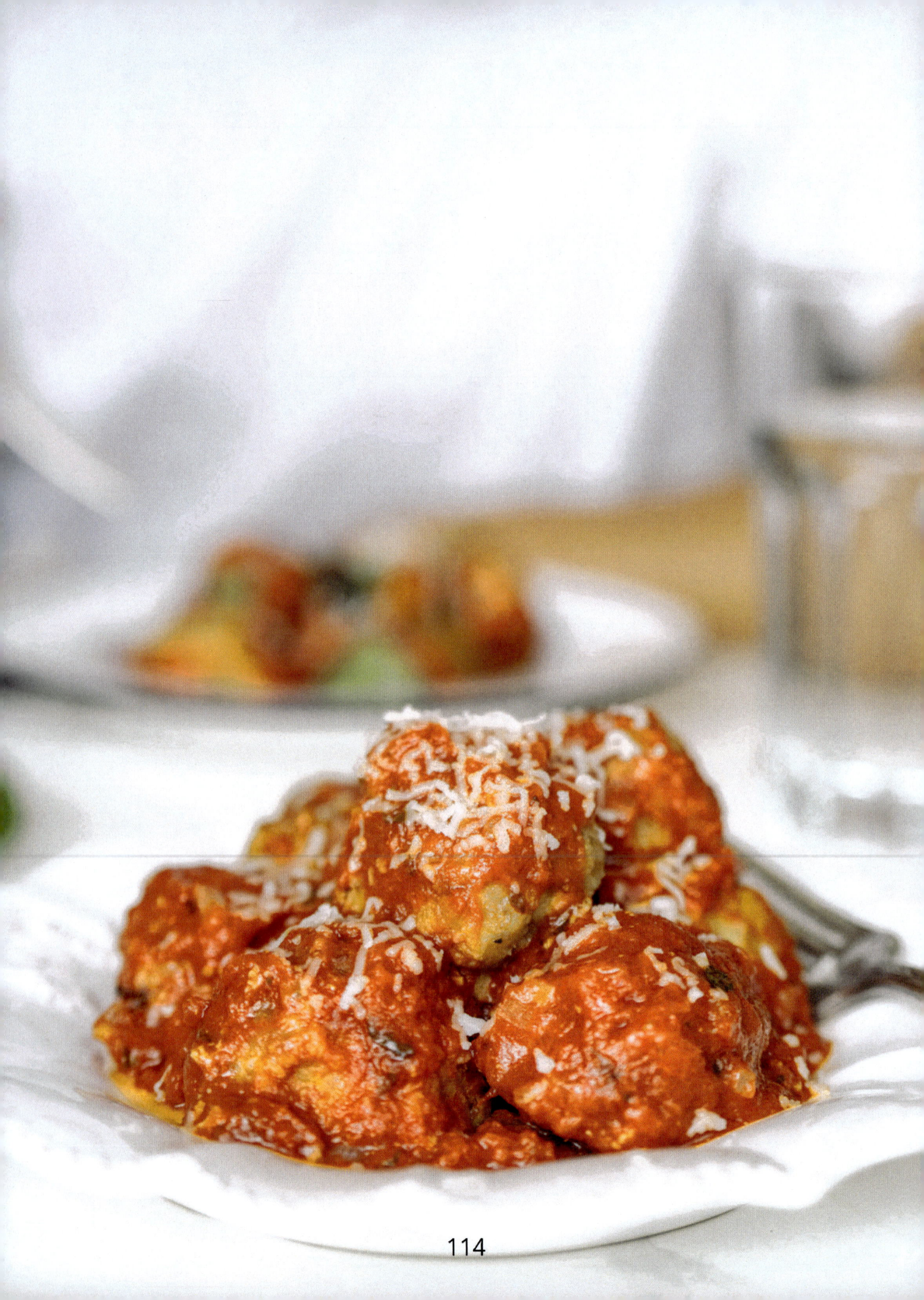

Uncle Johnny's Meatballs
for a hearty Italian dinner

nf gf

Mercedes Nicoll is a snowboarder who represented Canada at the Turin 2006, Vancouver 2010, Sochi 2014, and Pyeongchang 2018 Olympics in the halfpipe event. She had an outstanding performance in Vancouver 2010 where she placed 6th (the second-best Olympic result ever by a male or female Canadian halfpipe snowboarder). She has 8 World Cup medals and is a 5x Canadian National Champion.

Mercedes loves meatballs, so I knew I needed to feature my Uncle Johnny's famous homemade meatball recipe! This crowd-pleasing classic meal feeds a big family or is perfect for big batch meal prep.

Makes 25-30 meatballs

Sauce:
1/4 cup olive oil
1 medium onion, minced
4-5 garlic cloves, minced
2 28-ounce cans Italian crushed tomatoes
6 leaves fresh basil, finely chopped
Pinch of dried oregano
Salt and ground black pepper

Meatballs:
2 eggs
1/3 cup water
1/3 cup olive oil
1 1/2 cup breadcrumbs (GF if sensitive)
1 cup Romano cheese, grated
1 teaspoon oregano
3 garlic cloves, diced
32 ounces ground pork
Serve with more Romano cheese

1. Sauté onion and garlic with olive oil in a pan on medium heat for 3 minutes or until translucent and softened. Add the tomatoes and their juices and bring to a boil.
2. Reduce the heat, let it simmer and thicken for 45 minutes. Add basil, oregano, and black pepper. Cook for 1 more minute.
3. In a bowl, beat the eggs, water, and olive oil until combined. In another bowl, mix the breadcrumbs, cheese, oregano, and garlic.
4. In a large bowl, add the egg mixture and breadcrumb mixture to the ground pork. Use a wooden spoon or your hands to combine.
5. Roll up into balls. Preheat oven to 350°F, and bake the balls for 30 minutes.
6. Add meatballs and excess fat from the pan to the sauce. Let it simmer on low heat for 45 more minutes.

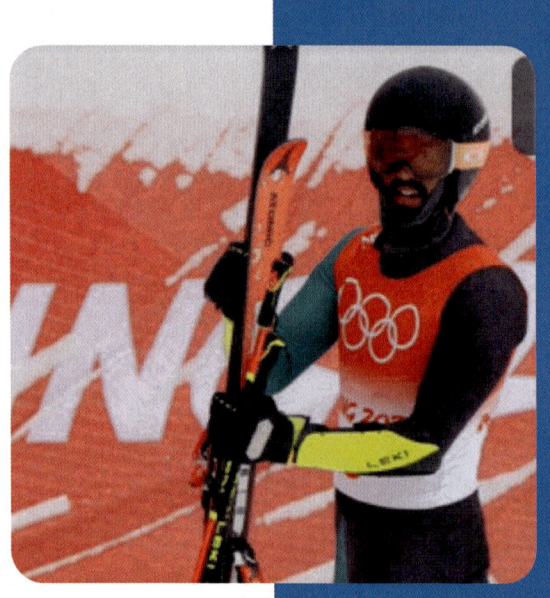

BENJAMIN ALEXANDER

Alpine Skiing

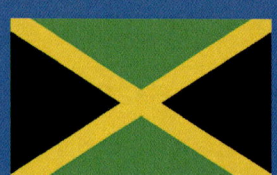

Sleep Habits:

"I try to get as much as possible. If I'm exhausted at 5 pm and I have nothing pressing to get done, I'll happily try to get a full 12 hours of sleep in. #1 tip: get it while you can! Don't check your social media before bed."

Olympic Memory:

"Walking out into the opening ceremony as the 15th person to ever qualify for Jamaica in the Winter Games (and as the flag-bearer) was insane. A moment I'll never forget."

Mental Prep Tip:

"I smash my chest a few times to get the adrenaline flowing; you really need to be mentally prepared to fight for every single turn to succeed." (See more on page 213).

Morning Routine:

"A few push-ups just to get the blood flowing, nothing too intense. A huge glass of water, coffee, and a bowl of cereal. I get my stretching done on the ride up the mountain."

Recovery Tip:

"Hot tub - we have an epic tub that I consider my sanctuary; I get at least an hour in it every day."

Image by Noah Wallace

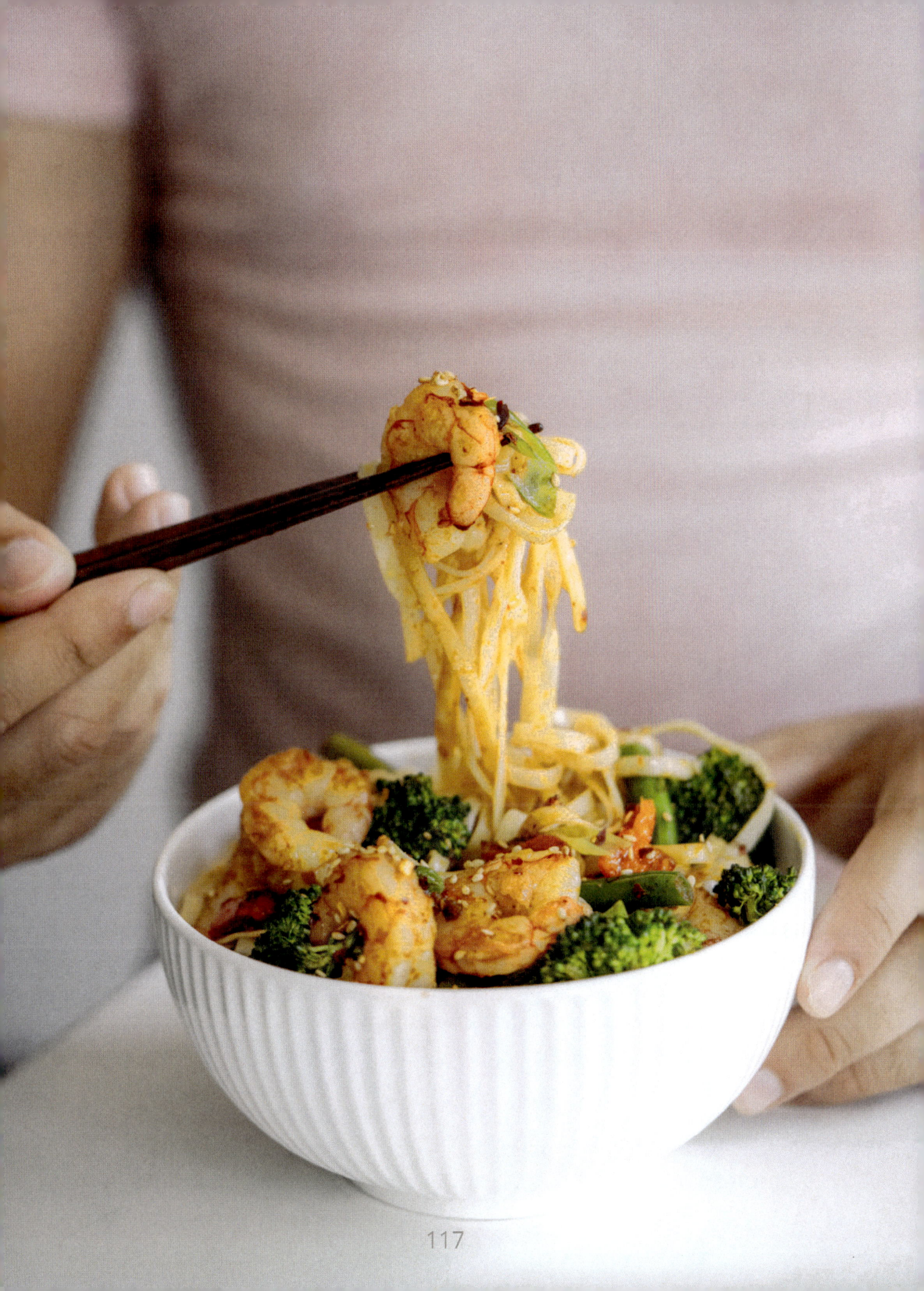

Shrimp Stir Fry
for a spicy supper

df nf gf

Benjamin Alexander is the first-ever Jamaican alpine skier who competed at the Beijing 2022 Olympics. With a mother from Great Britain and a father from Jamaica, Benjamin saw an opportunity to compete for his father's homeland. He got a Jamaican passport and only started skiing pro in 2019. Formerly, Benjamin was a DJ, touring 30 countries and performing at the famous Burning Man Festival, and he co-founded the award-winning music festival Further Future. Benjamin is truly inspiring and demonstrates that hard work pays off.

Makes 2 servings

1 tablespoon sesame oil
9 ounces shrimp, peeled and deveined
1 1/2 cup broccoli florets, chopped
1/2 red bell pepper, chopped
1 cup green beans
2 scallions, chopped
Salt and pepper to taste
Rice or noodles to serve (or GF)
1 teaspoon crushed red pepper flakes or sesame seeds to taste

Spicy sauce:
2 tablespoons sesame oil
1 tablespoon soy sauce
1/2 tablespoon garlic powder
1/2 tablespoon honey
1/2 teaspoon ginger
1 tablespoon rice wine vinegar
1 tablespoon chili powder
1/4 cup chicken broth
1/2 tablespoon cornstarch (mixed with 1/2 tablespoon water)

1. On medium heat, pour the sesame oil into a pan. Add the shrimp and cook for 1-2 minutes per side (or until pink). Remove from pan and set aside.
2. Use more oil if needed. Add broccoli, pepper, green beans, and scallions. Cook until softened.
3. Make the sauce: whisk together the sesame oil, soy sauce, garlic powder, honey, ginger, rice wine vinegar, chili powder, and chicken broth in a bowl.
4. Add sauce into the pan with the vegetables, stir, and bring it to a boil. Let it simmer for 2-3 minutes.
5. Add the corn starch and water mixture and stir. It should quickly thicken.
6. Add the shrimp back into the pan, and let them cook through with the vegetables and sauce for another 2 minutes.
7. Serve with cooked noodles or rice, and garnish with sesame seeds and red pepper flakes.

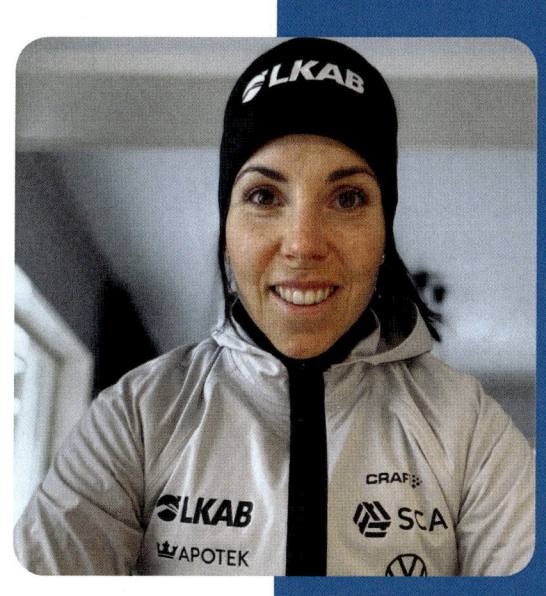

CHARLOTTE KALLA

Cross Country Skiing

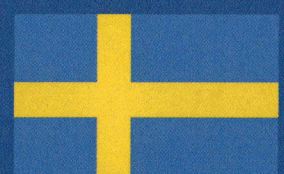

🇸🇪

Sleep Habits:

"I get 8-9 hours sleep. It's dark and cool in my room; sometimes I wear earplugs. No screens the last hour before I go to bed, and I get up at the same time every day."

Olympic Memory:

"Taking the gold medal in Pyeongchang 2018 in the first competition of the Olympics. I felt really strong that day and it was wonderful to be in the zone and feel that my body responded!"

Recovery Tip:

"Spending time with family and friends. Also, I think it's important to have routines. I eat directly after my training, go to bed early to get at least 8 hours of sleep, and I often take a nap in the afternoon."

Mental Prep Tip:

"I have a talk with my coach the evening before to make a race plan. I have a phone call with my psychologist in the morning just to remind me of my race plan and to focus on what I can control."

Morning Routine:

"I get up at 6:40 am and eat breakfast with my partner before he goes to his office. Usually, I eat porridge and a sandwich with a boiled egg, and I drink a cup of coffee. I do some stretching and activating exercises. If I go roller skiing, I look at some technique videos to remind me about where I want to put my focus."

Image by Charlotte Kalla

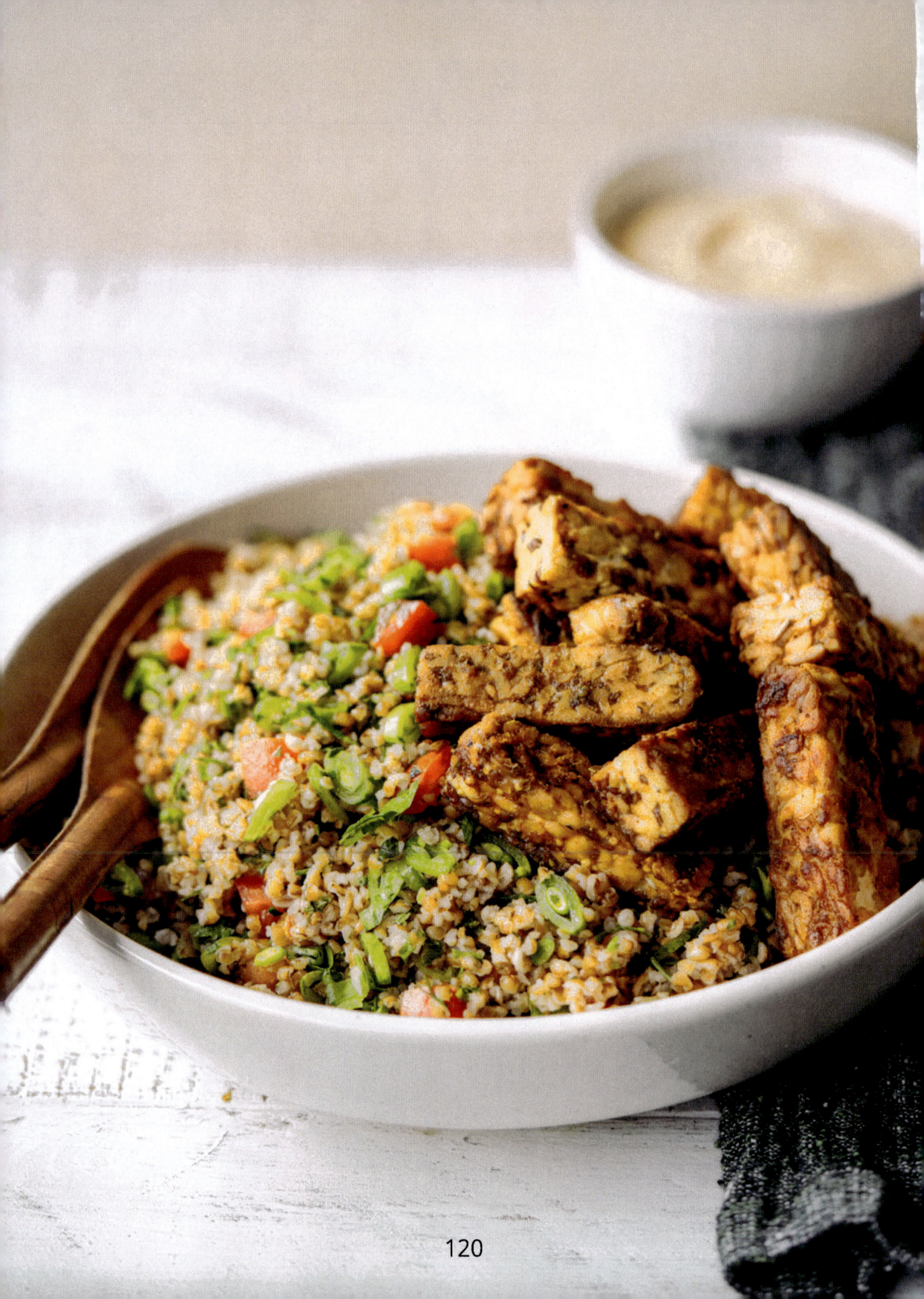

Tempeh Tabbouleh Bowl

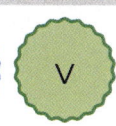

for a fresh and filling meal

Charlotte Kalla is a 4x Olympian and is Sweden's most successful female cross country skier of all time. She has won 9 Olympic medals (3 Gold, 6 Silver) and 13 World Championship medals (3 Gold, 6 Silver, 4 Bronze). She is a legend in Sweden and continues to push the boundaries in her sport.

Charlotte's favorite recipe is this fresh tempeh bowl, served with a tabbouleh salad and bean cream which is a great option for lunch or dinner. The protein from the tempeh and bean cream is perfect for vegans or vegetarians, and there are plenty of beneficial nutrients and minerals in the vegetable packed tabbouleh salad base.

Makes 2 servings

14 ounces tempeh
2 garlic cloves, grated
1 tablespoon ground cumin
1 tablespoon smoked paprika powder
1 tablespoon dried oregano
1 tablespoon Japanese soy
1 tablespoon organic grapeseed oil
Dash of black pepper

Parsley Tabbouleh
1 1/2 cups organic bulgur wheat
1 tablespoon vegetable stock
3 tomatoes, diced into small cubes
5 ounces sugar snap peas
1 handful of mint, finely chopped
7 ounces fresh parsley, finely chopped
3 garlic cloves, finely chopped
1 tablespoon olive oil
1 1/2 lemon, juiced
Salt and black pepper

Bean Cream
1 can (13.5 ounces) cannellini beans
2 garlic cloves, coarsely chopped
1 teaspoon olive oil
1 teaspoon cumin
1 teaspoon smoked paprika powder
1/2 lemon juice or 1 tablespoon white wine vinegar
Salt and black pepper

1. Cut the tempeh into 1/2 inch thick slices. Put tempeh, garlic, cumin, paprika powder, oregano, soy, grapeseed oil, and pepper in a tight plastic bag and let marinate for at least 1 hour.
2. To make the tabbouleh, boil the bulgur wheat according to the package instructions, but use the vegetable stock instead of salt in the boiling water.

3. Rinse, finely chop, and mix the tomatoes, sugar snap peas, mint, parsley, and garlic in a large bowl.
4. Add the boiled bulgur wheat into the bowl with the vegetables. Pour in the olive oil and lemon juice and stir. Add a few pinches of salt and pepper to taste.
5. To make the bean cream, rinse the beans in cold water and strain them. Peel and coarsley chop the garlic. Mix the beans, garlic, olive oil, cumin and paprika powder in a blender, food processor, or with a hand mixer until it turns into a smooth sauce. Add lemon juice, salt, and pepper to taste.
6. Pour the marinated tempeh and the entire contents of the bag into a hot frying pan. Fry the tempeh in the marinade until it has a crispy brown color on both sides. Serve tempeh with tabbouleh and bean cream.

JON ELEY

Speed Skating

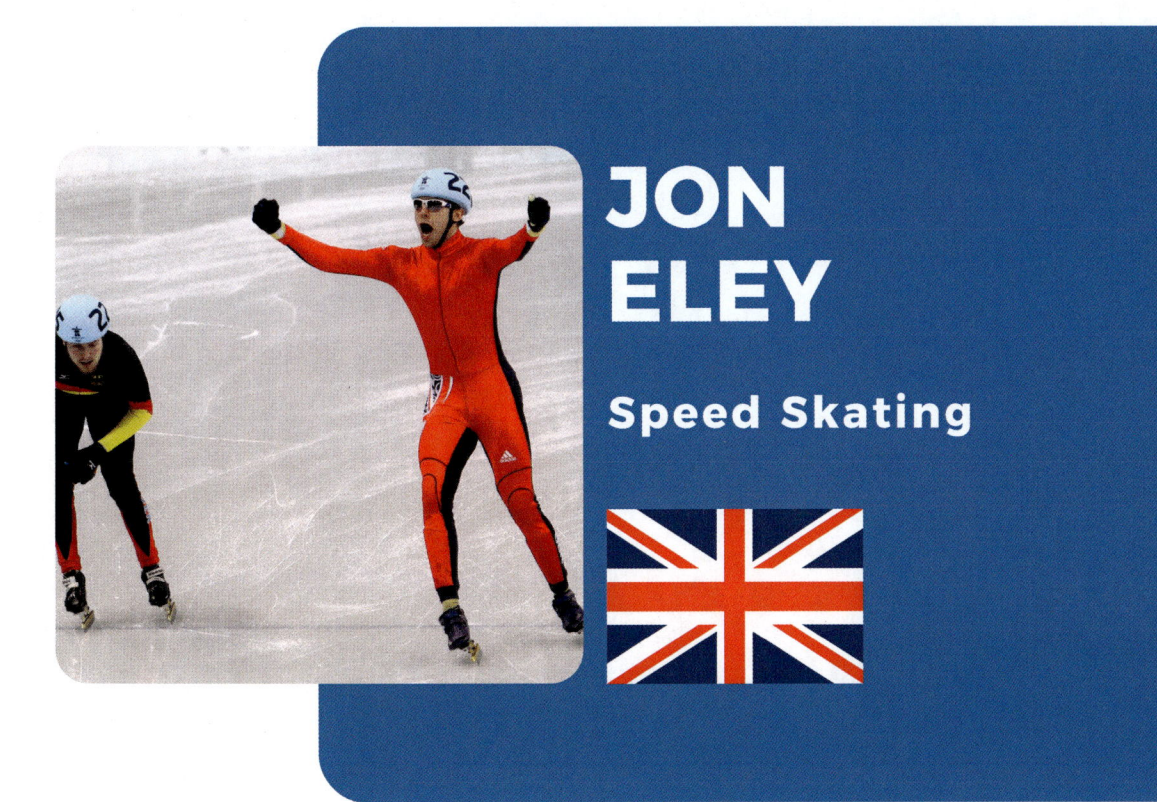

Sleep Habits:

"I always tried to have 8 hours sleep a night, I would also have an afternoon nap between training sessions. My number 1 tip for sleeping is having a good pillow, which I always traveled with."

Olympic Memory:

"Competing in the Olympic 500m final at my first Games, the atmosphere was amazing and it was what I had dreamed of and prepared so hard for—I was living the dream. My other favorite memories have come in the relay, competing as a team, achieving as a team, and being able to celebrate as a team was always the best feeling in my career—sharing in each other's hard work and success."

Image by Paul Shoebridge

Mental Prep Tip:

"I would use visualization to focus on my performance, how I would race my race, and picture my opponents' strengths and weaknesses. In the final moments before I would step onto the ice, I would use self-talk and embrace the atmosphere in the arena to convince myself this was my stage and I was going to own it." (See more on page 215).

Morning Routine:

- Wake up at 6:15 am and shower.
- Breakfast: a bowl of porridge with blueberries and a banana.
- Journaling: complete a daily monitoring app (readiness for training), and write my training goals for the day.
- Go to the rink at 7 am, sharpen my skates for training,
- Start off-ice warm-up at 7:30 am before going onto the ice for training at 8.30 am.

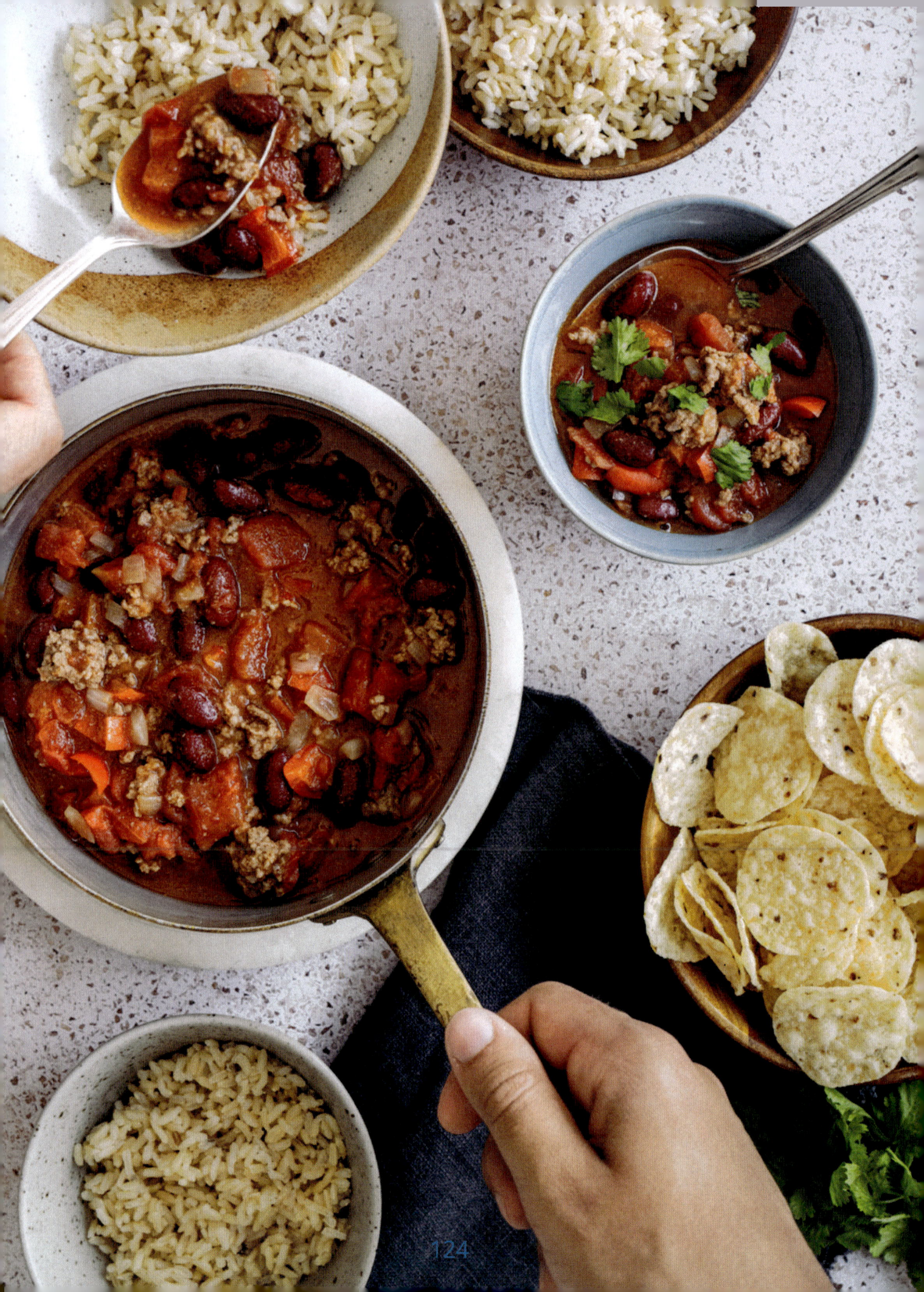

Chill Out Chili
for comforting nourishment

gf

Jon Eley is a short track speed skater who formerly represented Great Britain at the 2006, 2010, and 2014 Winter Olympic Games. He was the flag-bearer for Great Britain at the 2014 Sochi Olympics and was part of the British 5000m team that broke the World Record in 2011. Jon has been an amazing team leader and support system for me at World events, and he is a huge asset to British Ice Skating.

Jon's favorite dinner recipe is this spicy chili, which is the perfect comfort food after a long training day (or week!). Create your own chili bowl, or try adding the chili and rice into a soft burrito or hard taco shell for variety and an extra crunch.

Makes 2 Servings

1 tablespoon olive oil
1 onion, diced
1 teaspoon mild chili powder
2 teaspoons ground cumin
8.8 ounces lean ground beef
2 chopped red peppers
14 ounces canned diced tomatoes
1 can (15 oz) red kidney beans, rinsed
1 cup cooked brown rice, to serve
Salt and pepper to taste
Handful of tortilla chips, to serve
Optional: garnish with cilantro

> How to make your own tortilla chips:
> 1. Slice a few tortillas (corn or regular) into 6 triangle-shaped wedges and spread them out on a baking sheet.
> 2. Bake at 350°F for 6 minutes.
> 3. Use a fork to flip them over, sprinkle them with salt, and bake for another 6-9 minutes until golden brown.

1. Pour the olive oil into a pan, and gently fry the onions with the chili powder and ground cumin for 2 mins.
2. Add in the ground beef and cook on medium heat until browned.
3. Add the peppers into the pan and cook for 2-3 mins.
4. Pour in the tomatoes and the red kidney beans (including the sauce).
5. Turn the heat to low and let the chili simmer for 10-20 mins.
6. Serve with cooked rice and season with salt and pepper. If it's been a heavy training day or week, top with Doritos Dippers Lightly Salted Tortilla Chips or make your own!

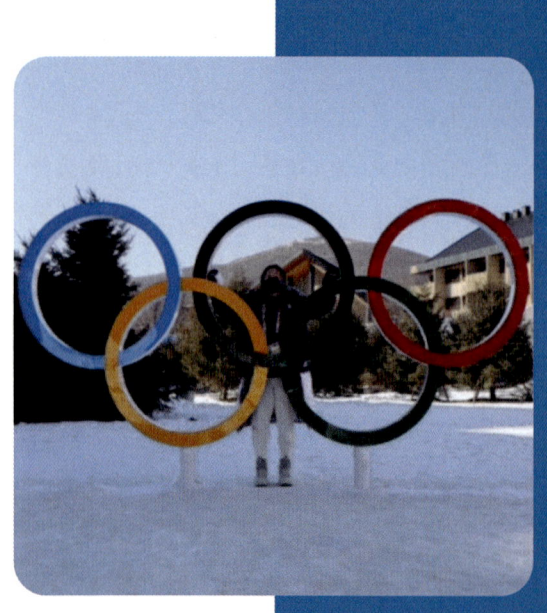

KAI OWENS

Freestyle Skiing

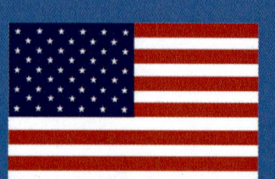

Sleep Habits:

"I sleep 10 hours minimum when I'm training. Plus afternoon naps. #1 way to help me sleep is to have a good night routine. I like to foam roll, then stretch, then shower. I use the Normatec compression pants and watch a light show or read. Doing all of this with calming music on and dimmed lights helps prepare my mind for sleep."

Olympic Memory:

"Favorite memory of the Olympics was skiing the course at night for the first time."

Mental Prep Tip:

"I like to journal and talk to my sports psych. I journal about what I'm confident in, and remember to trust myself and my abilities. If I am not confident and nervous I like to acknowledge those feelings and say to myself that everything I feel is okay."

Morning Routine:

"Wake up, get dressed, eat breakfast, warm up for skiing, drive to hill, get ski clothes on and go skiing."

Recovery Tip:

"I typically like to foam roll, stretch and use Normatec. In the summers and on a heavy lifting days I take ice baths."

Image by Kai Owens

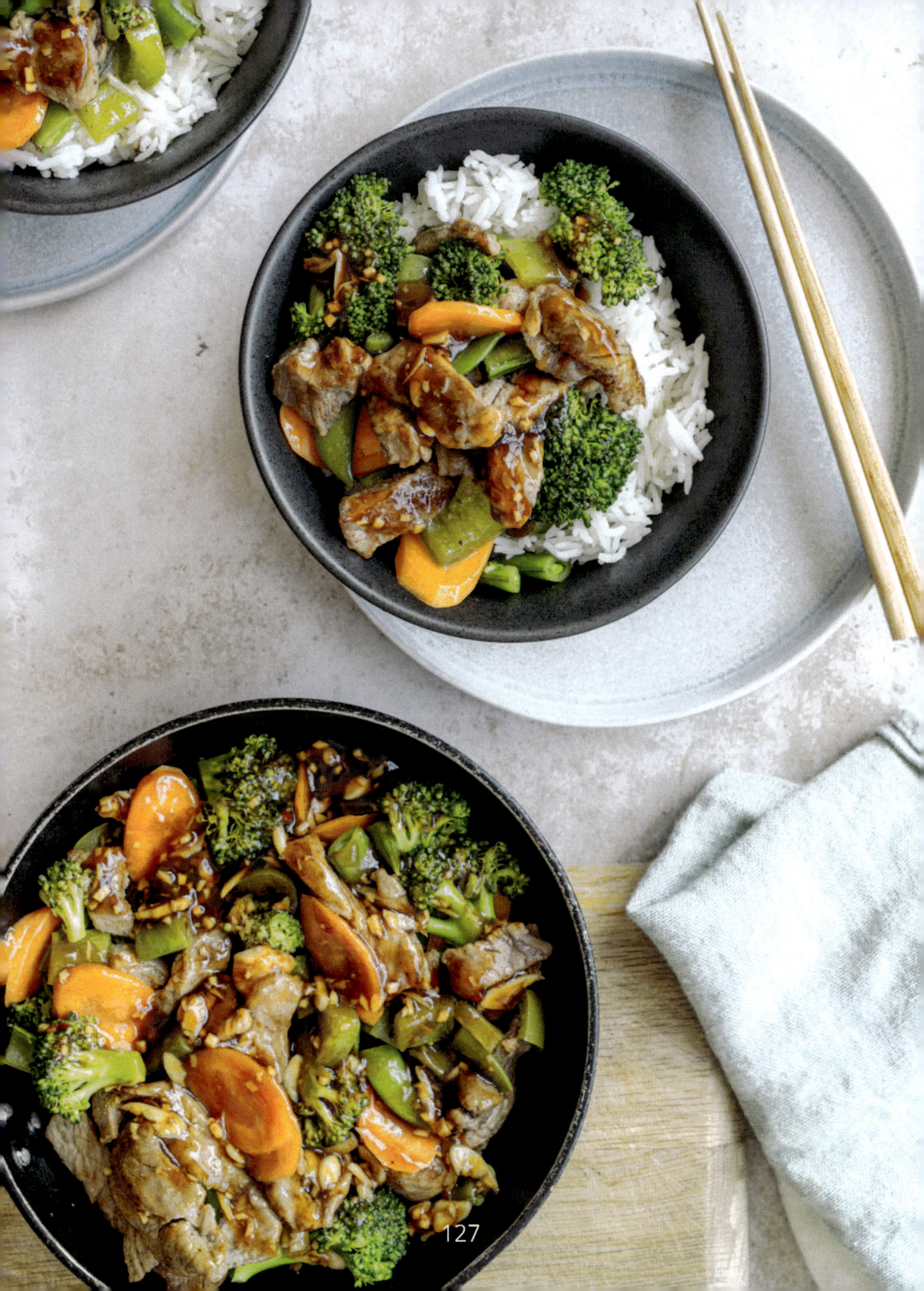

Wholesome Stir Fry
for a comforting dinner

gf

Kai Owens is a force to be reckoned with. Kai lives up to her name, which means "victorious." She is a 17-year-old freestyle skier who represented the USA at the Beijing 2022 Olympics. She is also a 2x NorAm Cup Winner, a World Cup medalist, and at 14 she was named the youngest American to win a Continental Cup. Born in China but adopted and raised in the USA, Kai got to return to her homeland to compete at the Olympics and showed true grit, determination, and love for her sport.

Here Kai shares her stir fry recipe, which is super versatile and great for meal prep because you can switch up the protein and vegetables to make it feel like a completely different meal!

Makes 7-8 servings

4 large carrots, chopped
1 cup snap peas
2 bell peppers, chopped
3 small heads of broccoli, chopped
48 ounces of ground protein: chicken, beef, tofu, for example
Olive oil for cooking
1.5 cups uncooked rice
6 cups water

Sauce:
1.5 cups teriyaki sauce
1 tablespoon soy sauce
1-2 tablespoons corn starch
1 teaspoon garlic, minced
1 teaspoon ginger root, minced
More teriyaki sauce to taste

Extra flavour:
Sirracha
Sesame Oil

1. Cut the vegetables into small pieces. Slice the meat into a similar size as the vegetables.
2. On medium heat, add a drizzle of olive oil to a large saucepan and add meat. Cook the meat fully. If you only have one pan, put meat in a bowl off to the side. Rinse out the pan and add olive oil, then cook vegetables.
3. Once the water begins to boil, add the rice and follow instructions on rice packet.
4. Once vegetables are cooked, combine the meat and vegetables in one pan, and cook on the lowest heat.
5. Combine the ingredients under "sauce" in a small bowl. Add sauce to the meat and vegetables and stir to combine. Serve with rice.

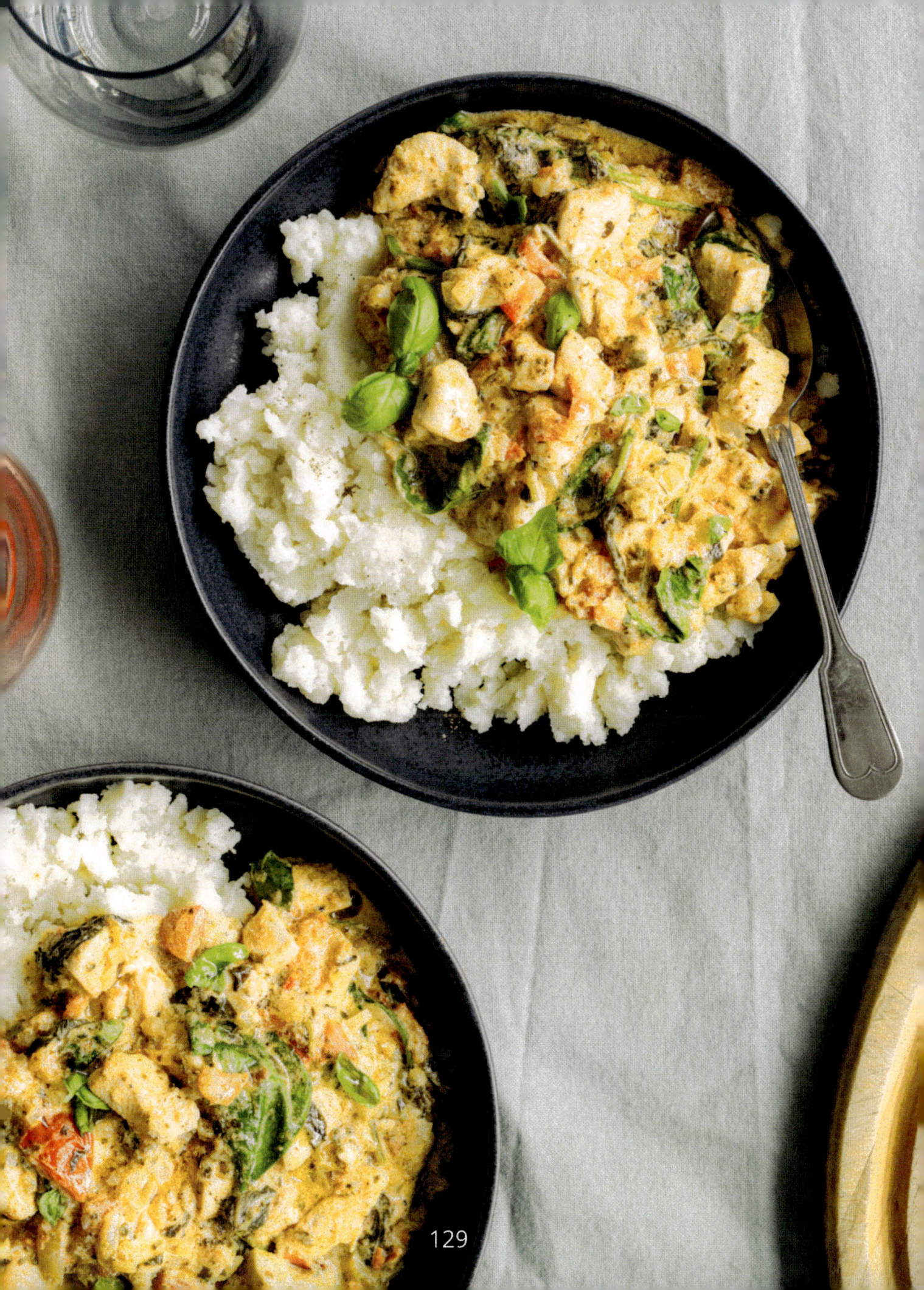

Winner Winner Chicken Dinner gf
BONUS RECIPE

Marcus Wyatt is a skeleton racer who represented Great Britain at the Beijing 2022 Olympics, and he is also the first British Men's World Cup Medalist since 2013.

This chicken recipe is easy to make, and one Marcus "keeps coming back to over and over again." Sometimes simple is best. All of the nutritional bases are covered because you get protein from the chicken, healthy fats from the pesto, a variety of vitamin-rich vegetables, and complex carbohydrates from the potatoes or pasta. *insert chef's kiss*

Makes 2 servings

1 cup mashed potato or brown-rice pasta (or GF if sensitive)
2 medium chicken breasts, diced
Salt and pepper to taste
1 onion, finely chopped
10 cherry tomatoes, diced
3 tablespoons pesto
5 tablespoons crème fraîche
2 handfuls spinach
Fresh basil to taste

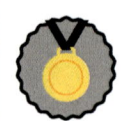

Want to take this recipe to the next level? Add a sprinkle of mozzarella or parmesan cheese to achieve a pizza-like taste!

1. Add the potatoes or brown-rice pasta to a pot and pour over enough water to cover the potatoes or pasta by 1". Cook the potatoes for 12-15 minutes and the pasta for 8-12 minutes. Rinse and set aside.
2. Season the chicken breasts with salt and pepper. Place the chicken into a medium saucepan. Cook on high heat for 5 minutes.
3. While the chicken is cooking, add the finely chopped onion to the pan with the chicken. Let it all cook for 4 more minutes.
4. Add the tomatoes, pesto, and crème fraîche into the pan and mix everything together.
5. Lower the heat, add the spinach, and cook it until it is wilted. Once the chicken is cooked through, remove the pan from the heat and serve with potato or pasta, extra salt, pepper, and basil.

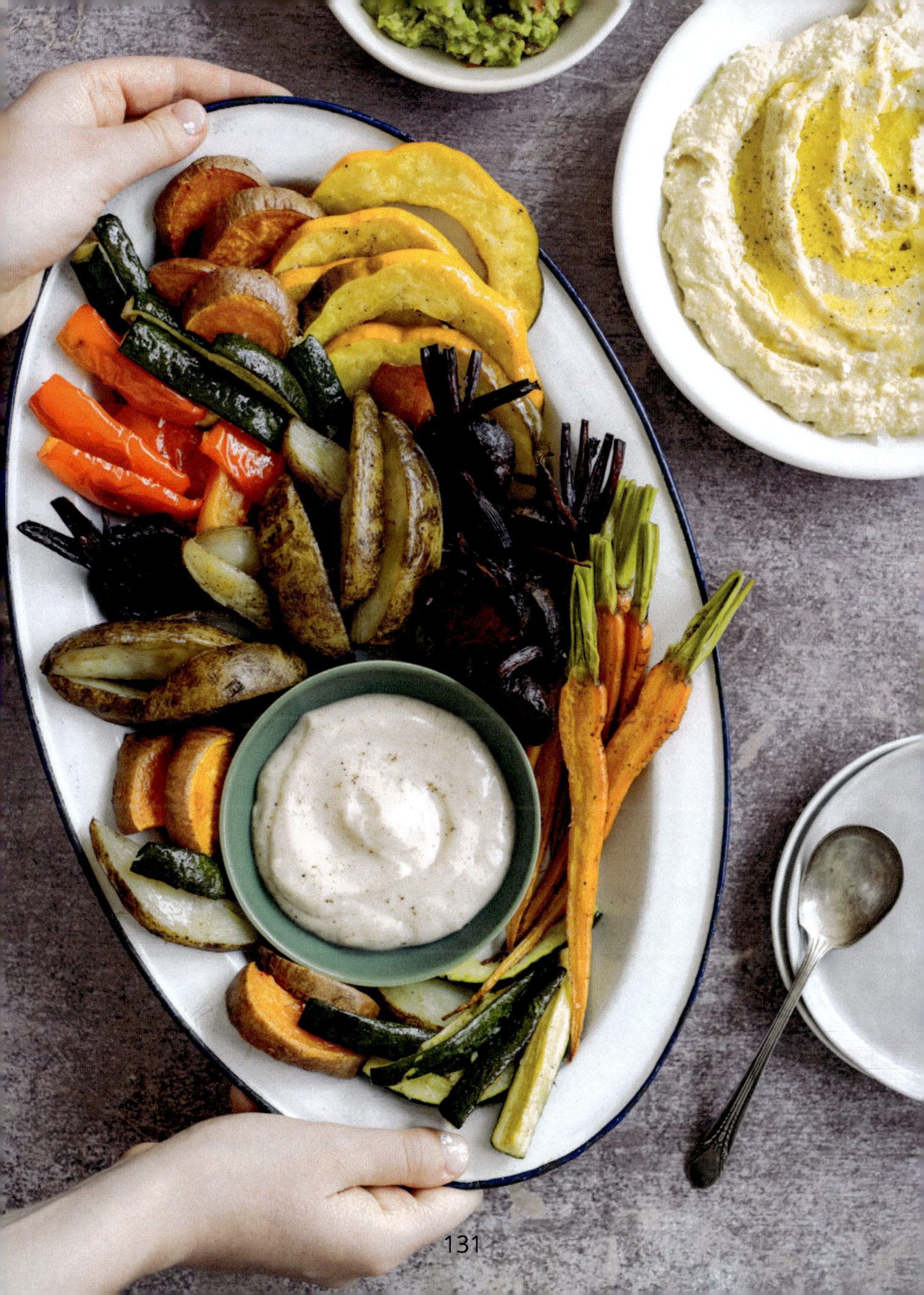

Veggies and Dip Platter
BONUS RECIPE

df gf v

Anna Fernstädt is a Czech-German Skeleton racer who competed at the Pyeongchang 2018 Olympics representing Germany, and at the Beijing 2022 Olympics representing the Czech Republic. After switching to Team Czech Republic, she needed to compete at lower levels to earn her World Cup quota spot, so she dominated the field by becoming the 2018, 2019, and 2020 Junior World Champion, as well as the World Mixed Team Bronze Medalist in 2017.

Czech out this recipe!! (Sorry Anna, I had to). Here Anna shares her recipe for roasted vegetables with a variety of dips. This platter is great for larger groups or parties and makes having vegetables a whole lot more exciting and delicious.

Makes 3 Servings

Vegetables: whatever is in season
Hokkaido pumpkin (her absolute favorite!)
Sweet potato
Potato
Bell pepper
Beetroot
Zucchini
Carrots, washed and peeled
Any other vegetables you like
Season with olive oil, salt, and pepper

Dip 1: Yogurt Dip
1 cup unsweetened almond yogurt
1 squeeze lemon juice
1/8 teaspoon salt
1/8 teaspoon pepper
Optional: garlic powder, onion powder, thyme

Dip 2: Guacamole
1 avocado, mashed with a fork
5 cherry tomatoes, finely diced
1/4 cup cucumber, finely diced
2-3 small pickles (optional), finely diced
1 squeeze lemon or lime juice
1/8 teaspoon salt
1/8 teaspoon pepper
2-3 tablespoons unsweetened almond yogurt (optional)

Dip 3: Hummus
5.3 ounces chickpeas
1 squeeze lemon juice
1/8 teaspoon salt
1/8 teaspoon pepper
1-2 cloves cooked garlic, or 1/4 teaspoon garlic powder
1.5 teaspoons tahini

1. Preheat the oven 390°F. Wash and cut the pumpkin, sweet potatoes, potatoes, bell peppers, beetroot, zucchini, carrots, and any other vegetables into strips.
2. In a large mixing bowl, season the vegetables with olive oil, salt, and pepper.
3. Spread the vegetables on a baking tray lined with parchment paper, bake for 20-40 minutes as some vegetables cook faster than others.
4. Make the hummus by blending the chickpeas, lemon juice, salt, pepper, garlic, and tahini until smooth. Drizzle with olive oil to serve, or store in an airtight container in the fridge for up to a week.
5. Make the guacamole in a bowl by mixing the mashed avocado, finely diced tomatoes, cucumber, pickles, lemon juice, salt, and pepper. Optional: add the unsweetened almond yogurt to make it lighter.
6. Make the yogurt dip in a bowl by mixing the unsweetened almond yogurt, lemon juice, salt, and pepper.

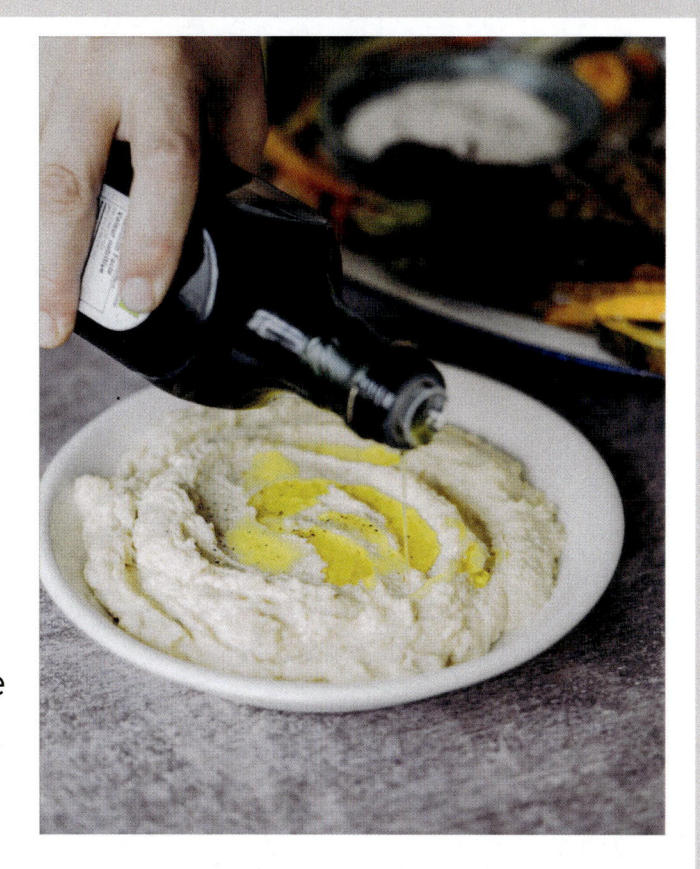

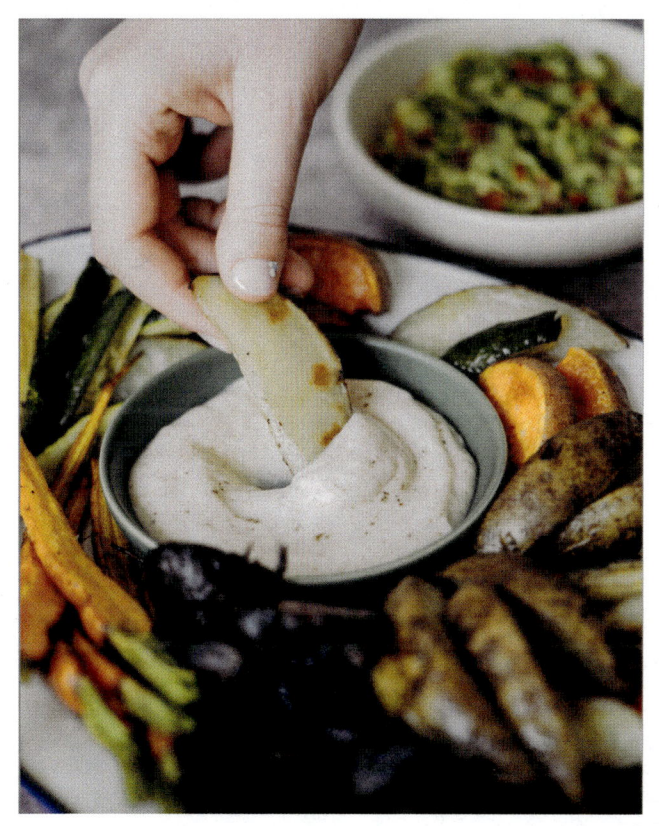

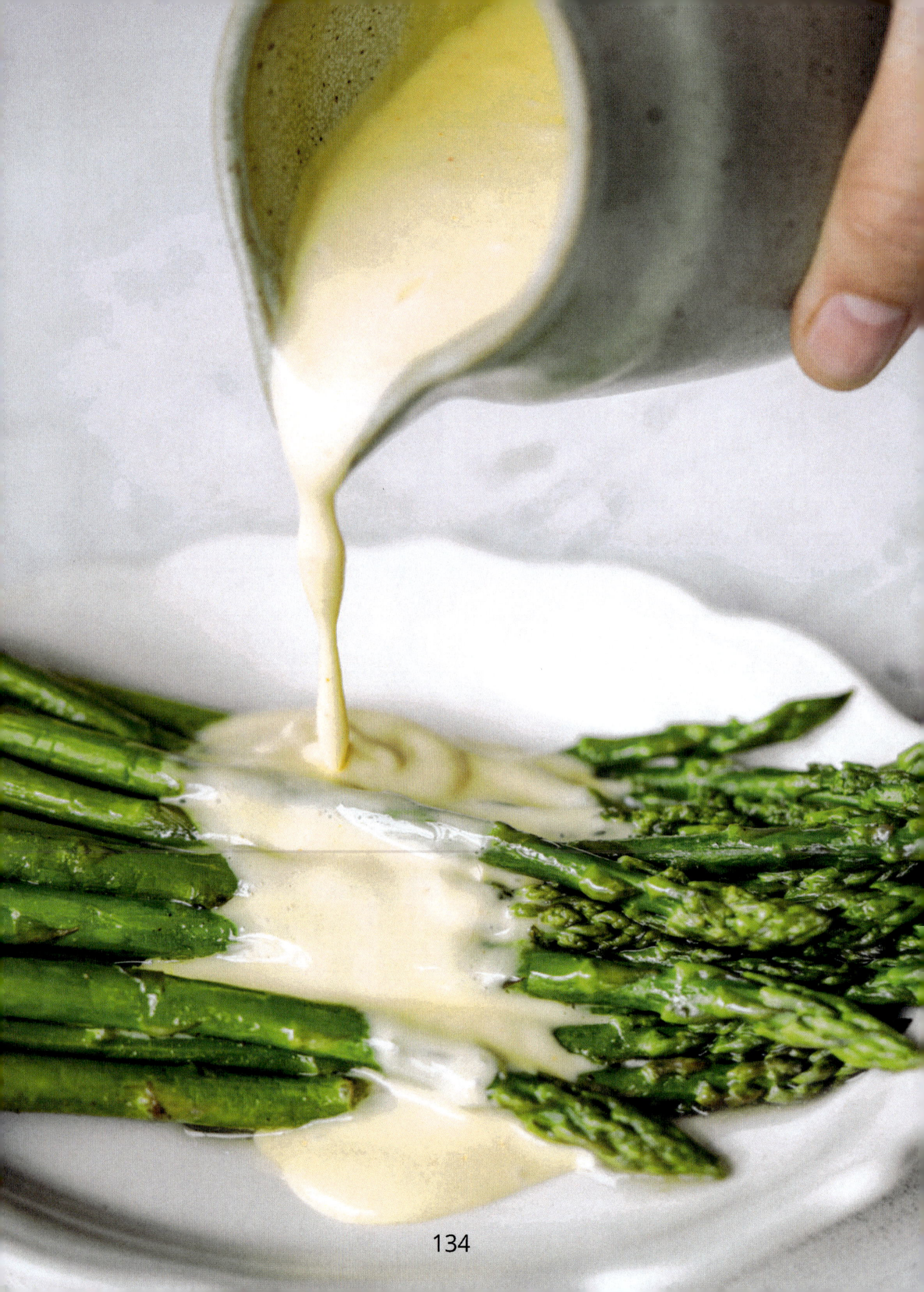

Hollandaise Sauce
BONUS RECIPE

nf gf

Dawn Richardson Wilson is a bobsledder who represented Canada at the Beijing 2022 Olympics, where she placed 8th in the two-woman event alongside Cynthia Appiah. Dawn was born in Accra, Ghana, and emigrated to Canada when she was two years old. She first started the sport in 2018 and is now a full-time World Cup brakewoman for Team Canada.

Here Dawn shares her Hollandaise sauce recipe. This sauce would go great on the **Turkey Bacon Bowl** (page 92), the **Avocado Toast with Poached Eggs** (page 58), and the **Veggie and Dip Platter** (page 132) to name a few.

Makes 2-3 servings

3 egg yolks
1 tablespoon lemon juice
1 teaspoon Dijon mustard
1/4 teaspoon salt
Cayenne pepper (to your liking)
1/2 cup melted butter

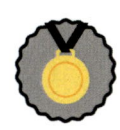

> Your butter needs to be hot, not just melted. The recipe will not emulsify with lukewarm butter.

1. In a bowl, combine the egg yolk, lemon juice, dijon mustard, salt, and pepper in a blender for 5 seconds.
2. Melt the butter in the microwave until it is hot.
3. Turn the blender to medium speed and slowly pour in the hot butter to the mixture as it blends.
4. Store in the fridge in an airtight container for up to a week.

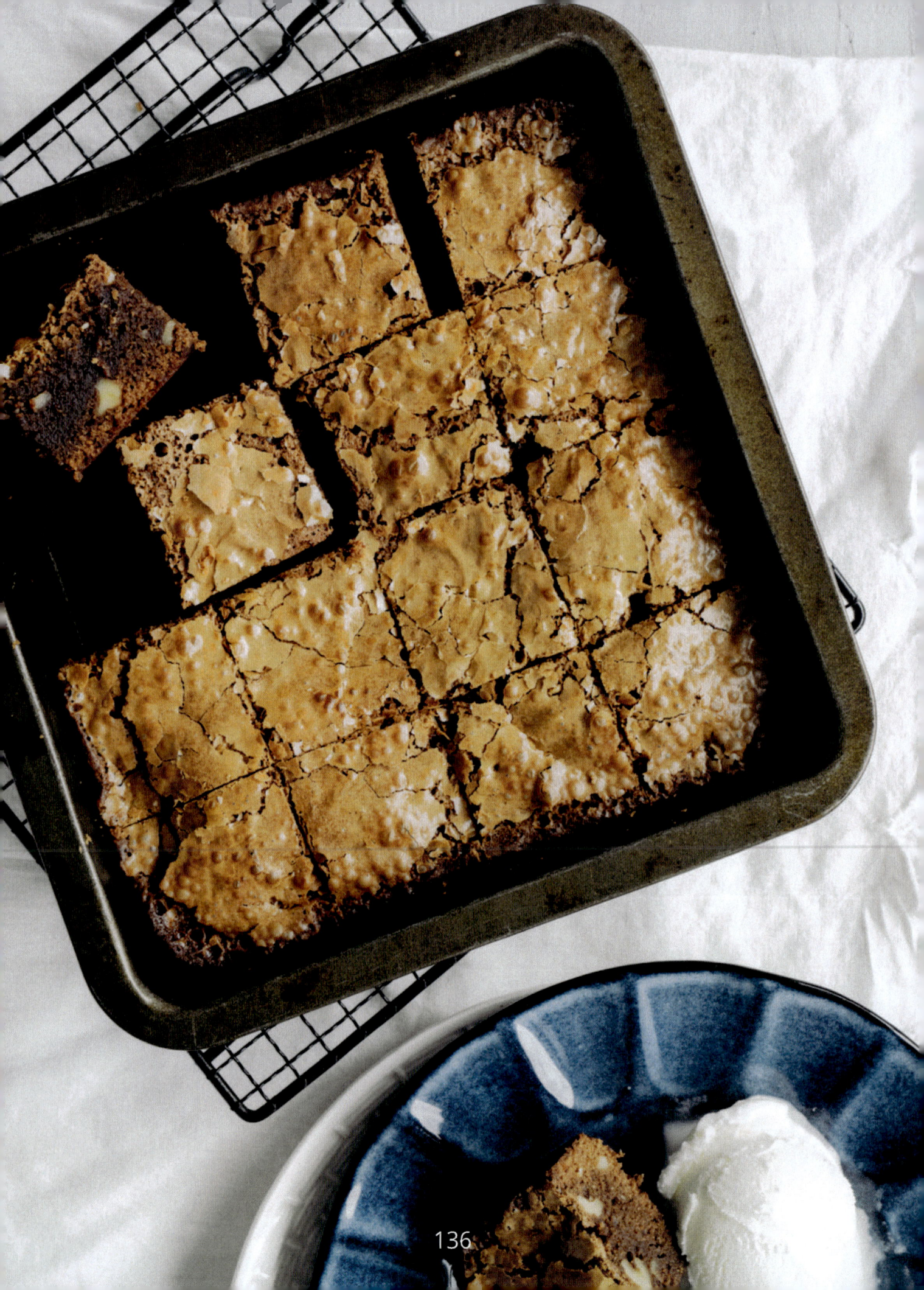

ELITE SNACKS AND SWEETS

Almond Butter Banana Bites   138

Nice Cream   141

Walnut Brownies   145

BYOYP (Build Your Own Yogurt Parfait)   148

Sugar Mint Pineapple   154

Caramelized Pears   157

Ultimate Power Cookies   160

BONUS RECIPE: Lemon Chia Energy Balls   162

BONUS RECIPE: Cookie-Dough Power Balls   164

BONUS RECIPE: Apple and Blackberry Crumble   166

BONUS RECIPE: Race Ready Rice Pudding   168

BONUS RECIPE: Millionaire Shortbread   170

BONUS RECIPE: Zucchini Banana Bread   172

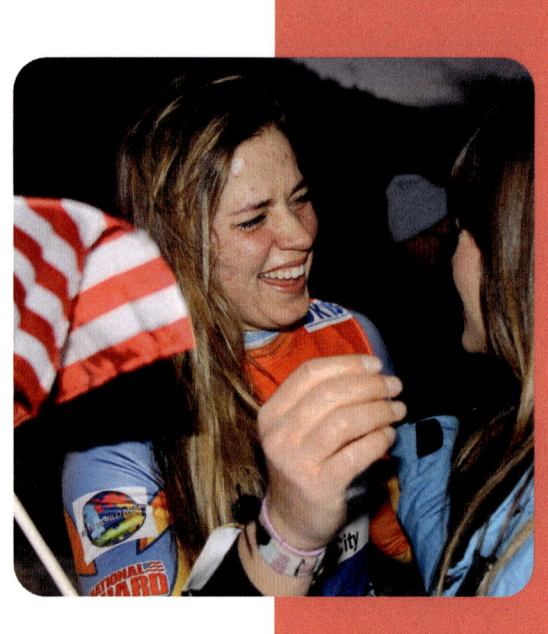

KATE HANSEN

Luge

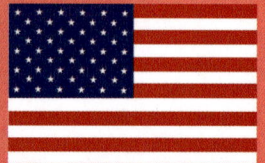

Sleep Habits:
"I get at least 8 hours, preferably 9. My tip is to put valerian oil on my forehead at night." (It is supposed to help with calmness and interact with the receptors engaged in mood and sleep).

Olympic Memory:
"Walking into opening ceremonies and bursting into sobs, it was incredible, and what a release that I finally made it."

Mental Prep Tip:
"I use tapping techniques and say affirmations while I do them. I prime my body for what I need it to do. Right before I slide, I think of the best wave I ever caught surfing which puts a big smile on my face. Then I'm ready." (see more on page 215).

Morning Routine:
"I eat breakfast an hour before training, write in my journal, read, stretch, then head to training."

Recovery Tip:
"I put on the recovery compression pants, go to my sports medicine clinic, and ice. It is also good to be in nature."

Image by Fredrik Von Erichsen (Getty)

139

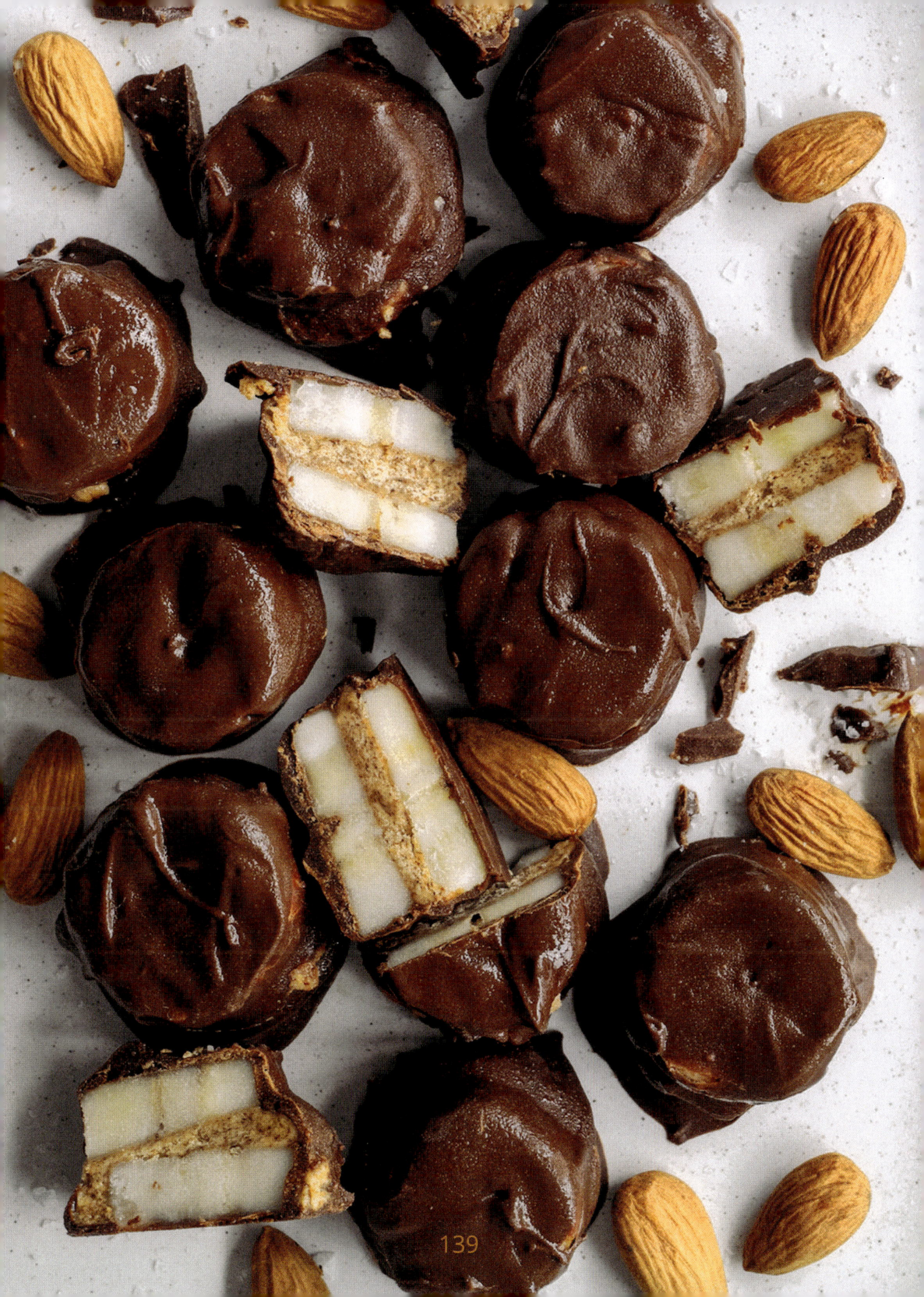

Almond Butter Banana Bites
for a sweet and salty bite

df gf v

Kate Hansen is a luger who represented the USA at the Sochi 2014 Olympics, where she came in 10th place. In 2008, when she was only fifteen years old, Kate became the youngest Junior World Champion. She loves to listen to Beyoncé pre-competition, and her dance warmup became her trademark. Her dance was re-posted on Beyoncé's Facebook page as a good luck message to Kate before the Sochi Olympics.

Here Kate shares her go-to pre-workout snack: almond butter and banana. Smack two banana slices together with almond butter and a drizzle of dark chocolate, freeze it, and BOOM you have a mini "ice cream" sandwich bites. These are perfect as a frozen snack, but taste so good they could be dessert!

Makes 12-15 sandwiches

2 large bananas
6 tablespoons almond butter
1/2 cup dark chocolate, melted

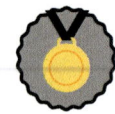

Want it to taste like a snickers bar?
Use peanut butter instead of almond butter.

1. Peel and slice the bananas into rounds, about a half-inch thick.
2. Place half of the banana slices onto a baking sheet lined with parchment paper.
3. Spread 1/2 tablespoon of almond butter onto each banana slice and place another banana slice on top to create a mini banana sandwich. Do this until all banana slices are used and you have about 12-15 sandwiches.
4. Melt 1/2 cup dark chocolate in the microwave and use a tablespoon to coat each banana slice with dark chocolate.
5. Freeze for 1 hour or overnight. Store in the freezer for 1-2 months.

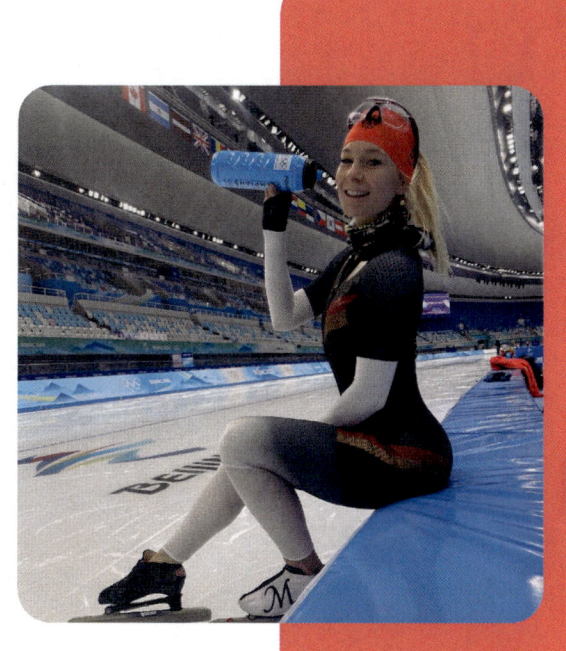

MICHELLE UHRIG

Luge

🇩🇪

Sleep Habits:

"I sleep 8 hours minimum."

Mental Prep Tip:

"Always tell yourself your goals while training. Give yourself positive vibes, like telling yourself 'you got this!' and you will show your best."

Olympic Memory:

"Walking into the Olympic Stadium in the Opening and Closing Ceremonies."

Morning Routine:

"For breakfast, most of the time I have an egg and some bread and pea milk coffee."

Recovery Tip:

"Hot showers and ice baths."

Image by Michelle Uhrig

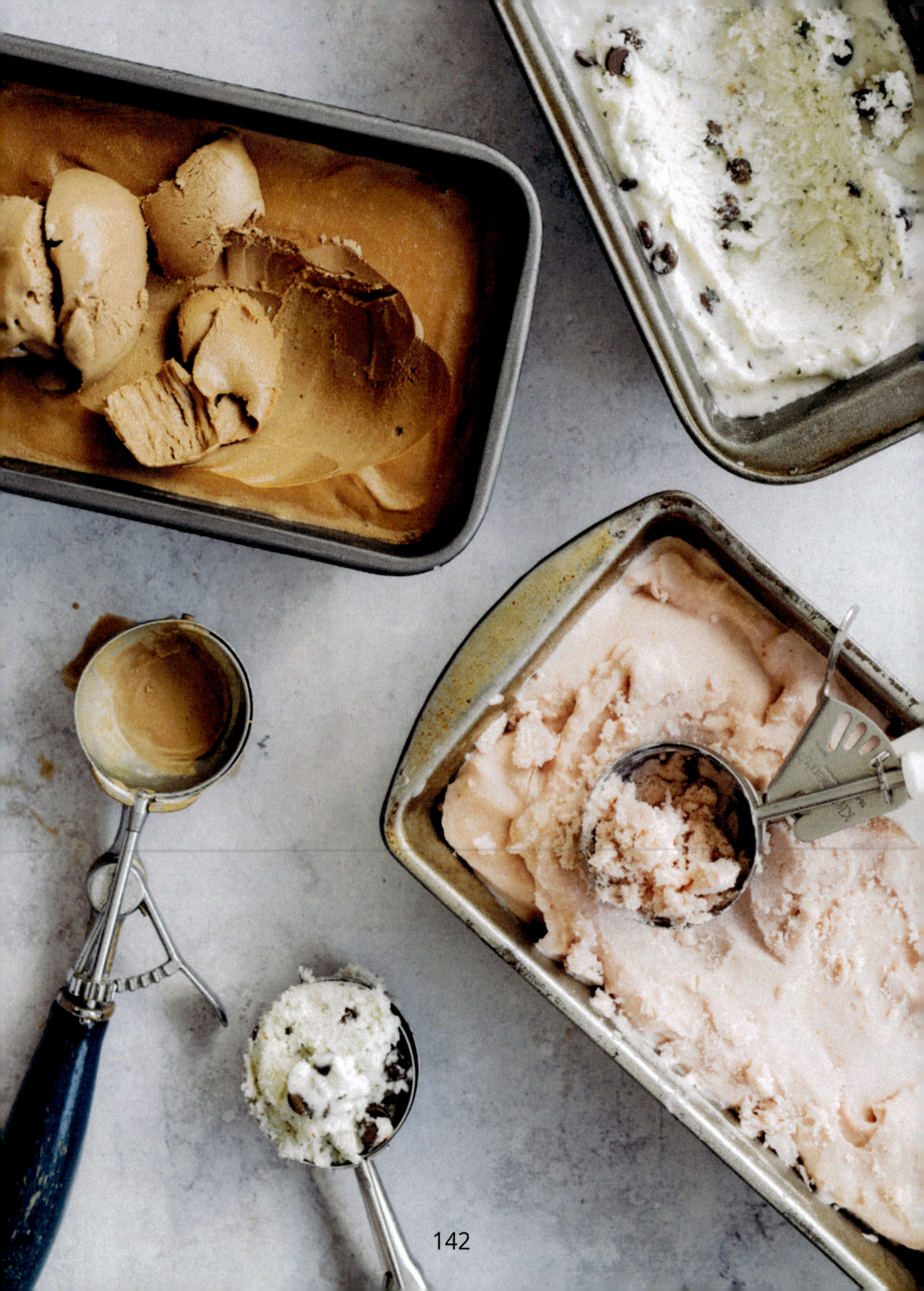

Nice Cream
for a refreshing treat

df gf v

Michelle Uhrig is a speedskater who represented Germany at the Pyeongchang 2018 and Beijing 2022 Olympics in the 1000m event. She is a World Cup silver medalist, European bronze medalist, a 7x German Champion, and she is also part of the Federal Police.

Here, Michelle shares her coconut milk "nice" cream recipe that uses simple, whole-food ingredients and is refreshing after a sweaty training session.

Makes 6 Servings

For strawberry lovers:
3 cups frozen strawberries (or other berries)
1 can (13.5 oz) full-fat coconut milk
1 teaspoon linseed oil
3 tablespoons maple syrup
2 tablespoons cashew butter
2-6 tablespoons unsweetened almond milk

For chocolate lovers:
1 can (13.5 oz) full-fat coconut milk
1/2 cup cocoa powder
3/4 cup maple syrup
1 teaspoon vanilla extract
(optional but worth it: 2 tablespoons peanut butter and 1 frozen banana).
2-6 tablespoons unsweetened almond milk

For mint chip lovers:
1 can (13.5 oz) full-fat coconut milk
1/4 teaspoon peppermint extract
1/4 cup maple syrup
1 1/2 teaspoon vanilla extract
10-15 fresh mint leaves
Pinch of salt
2-6 tablespoons unsweetened almond milk
1/2 cup dark chocolate chips

Topping ideas:
- Drizzle of honey
- Fresh fruit
- Granola (see pages 44, 47)
- Coconut flakes
- Dark chocolate chips
- Nuts and seeds (whole or butters)

1. Transfer the coconut milk mixture into an ice cube tray (should make 14-16 ice cream cubes) and freeze for at least 6 hours.
2. Pick your ice cream flavor and blend the ingredients together on a high speed until smooth. If making mint chip ice cream, do not add chocolate chips at this stage.
3. Add all of the coconut milk ice cubes and 2 tablespoons of unsweetened almond milk to a high-speed blender or food processor, and blend until thick and smooth. Add an extra 1 tablespoon of almond milk at a time until smooth.
4. If making mint chip, add the chocolate chips now and blend until combined and in small pieces.
5. Enjoy right away for the best soft serve consistency, or store in the freezer in an airtight container for a firm, scoopable texture.

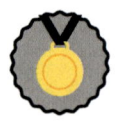

Use a room temperature, smooth and creamy brand of coconut milk for the best results.

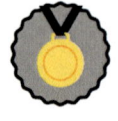

Try putting the coconut milk mixture into popsicle molds for a summer treat.

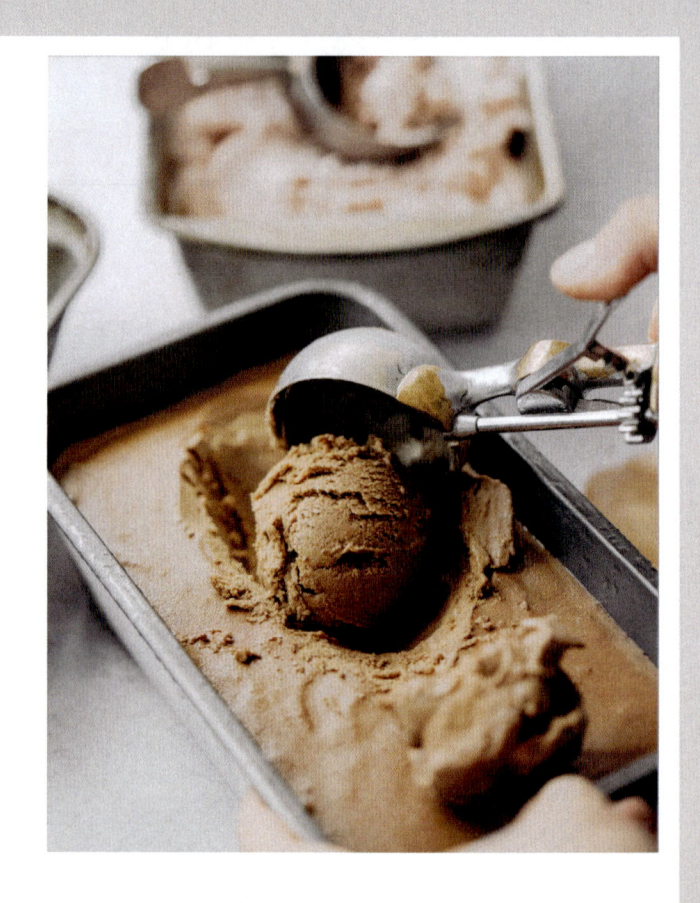

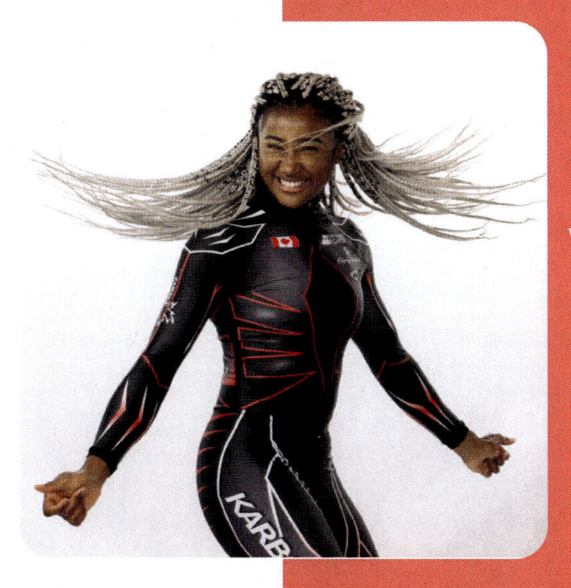

DAWN RICHARDSON WILSON

Bobsled

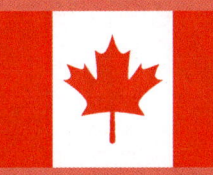

Sleep Habits:
"I aim for 7-8 hours. Quality over quantity is a big game-changer. Optimize your bedroom environment, by reducing the use and exposure of external lights and bringing the temperature down."

Olympic Memory:
"There are two moments that tie as my favorite, one being when the Olympic team was announced, and the other was walking into The Birds Nest in Beijing. The closer I got, the more my heart quickened and the tears I swore I wouldn't cry began to fall, it was as if all the years of hard work were replaying with every step I took."

Recovery Tip:
- Solidify training notes in a journal.
- Showers should be followed by a stretching and rolling session.
- End the night with a good movie or a board game with friends.

Mental Prep Tip:
"I try to keep competition day similar to the day I had a great performance in practice. For example, I start my morning with gospel music, get ready for the day, and switch it over to more motivational speeches as I get closer to game time. I review videos and notes regarding the track. Above all things, I personally believe in a positive self-speech, and I have a mantra that I say during tough times, competition days, or days where I just need a boost. My mantra is "I am strong, powerful, and aggressive. I can and will do anything I put my mind to."

Morning Routine:
- Wake at 6:30 am. Lie there, breathe, and get the mind ready with a motivational speech.
- Breakfast #1 and get dressed.
- Breakfast #2 and answer emails.
- Drive little siblings to school.
- 9:30 am sprint session (1/2 sessions of the day).

Image by Dawn Richardson Wilson

146

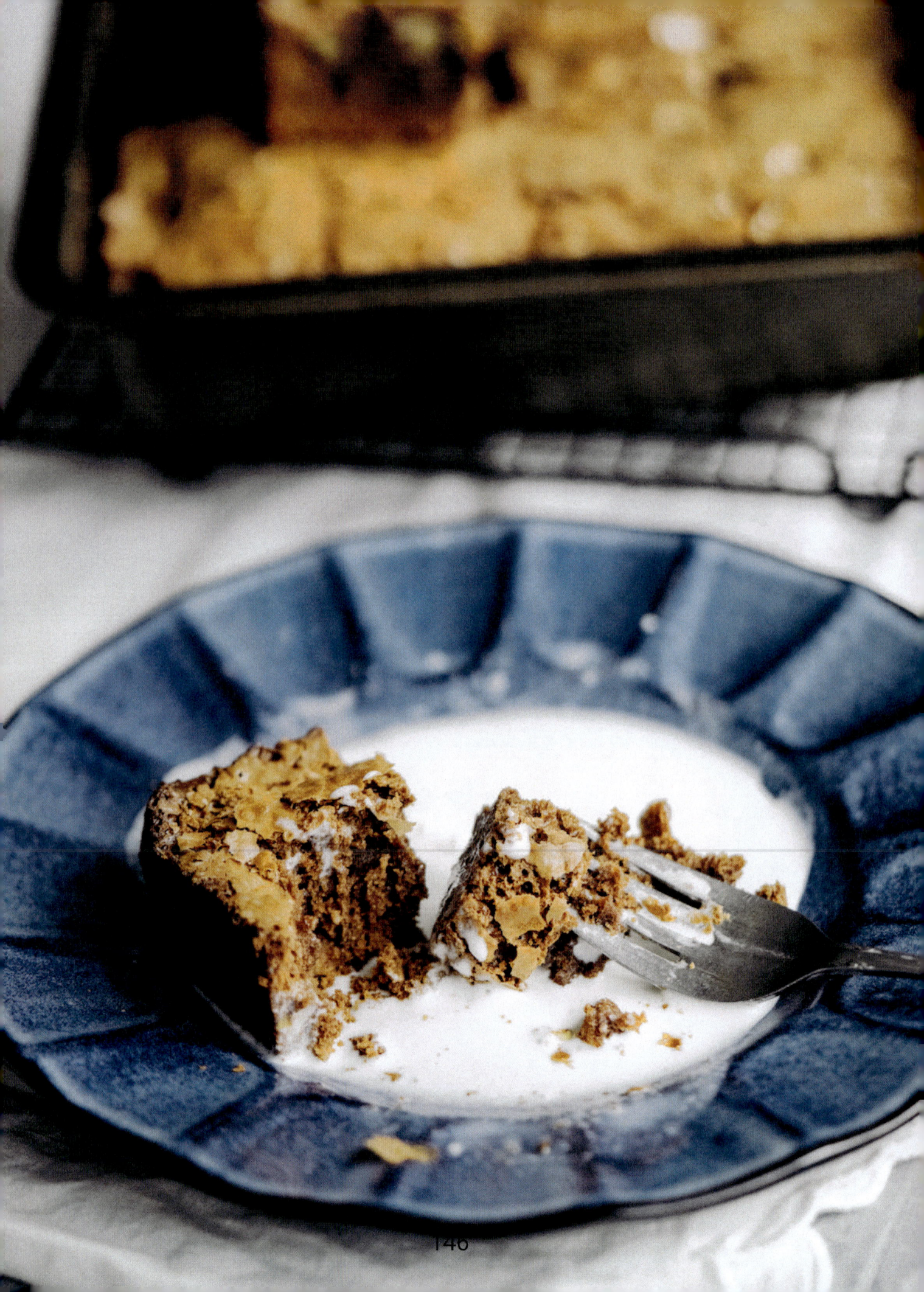

Walnut Brownies
for a decadent dessert

df

Dawn Richardson Wilson is a bobsledder who represented Canada at the Beijing 2022 Olympics, where she placed 8th in the two-woman event alongside Cynthia Appiah. Dawn was born in Accra, Ghana, and emigrated to Canada when she was two years old. She first started the sport in 2018 and is now a full-time World Cup brake woman for Team Canada.

Dawn's go-to dessert is homemade brownies served with vanilla ice cream and fresh berries. These gooey chocolatey brownies melt in your mouth and the walnuts add a crunch at every bite. Your house will smell so good, so don't be surprised if your neighbors come over for a slice!

Makes 16 Servings

2/3 cup butter
1 cup unsweetened baking chocolate, cut into pieces
3/4 cups sugar
2 teaspoons vanilla
3 eggs
1/2 cup all-purpose flour
1 cup chopped walnuts

1. Preheat the oven to 350°F and grease the bottom and sides of a 9x9 inch square pan.
2. On the stove, heat the butter and chocolate and stir continuously until melted. Let it cool slightly.
3. In a large mixing bowl, beat the sugar, vanilla, and eggs with an electric mixer on high speed for about 5 minutes or until light and fluffy.
4. Beat in the chocolate mixture on low speed. Beat in the flour until just blended (don't over-mix). Stir in the walnuts.
5. Spread the mixture in a pan and bake for 40-45 minutes or until the edges of the brownies pull away from the pan.
6. Best served warm with vanilla ice cream and fresh berries!

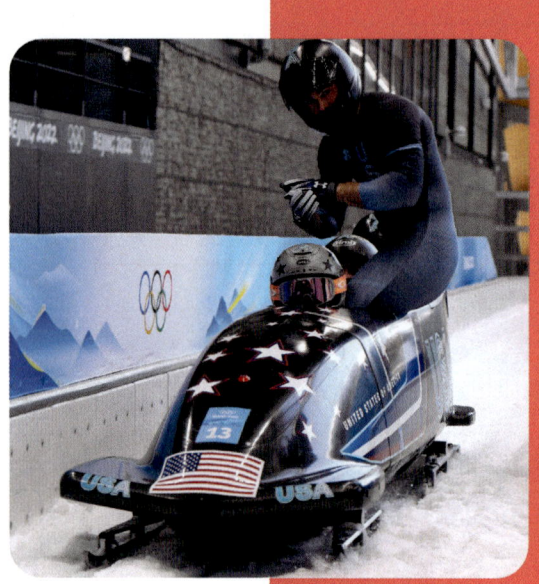

JOSH WILLIAMSON

Bobsled

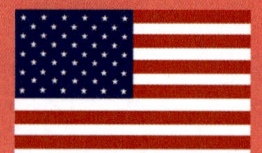

Sleep Habits:

"I get 7-9 hours most nights. The earlier I wind down and get away from screens, the more tired I get, so the better I sleep! I also keep my room really cold, like 66-68°F"

Olympic Memory:

"Walking into the Olympic Stadium in the Opening and Closing Ceremonies."

Recovery Tip:

"I like to shower, get in something comfy, light a candle, get a large glass of water, and read."

Mental Prep Tip:

"I try to do things that make me feel confident, play music that makes me confident, wear clothes that make me confident, and drink a lot of caffeine to get excited!" (See more on page 214).

Morning Routine:

"Get up, shower, shave, quick breakfast. I'll usually journal and then get as much work done as I can before training. If I have time after work I read a bit. I try to stick to quick breakfast ideas like hard-boiled eggs, overnight oats, or fruit. My goal is to get all my work done before I workout, so after training, I can relax!"

Image by Josh Williamson

149

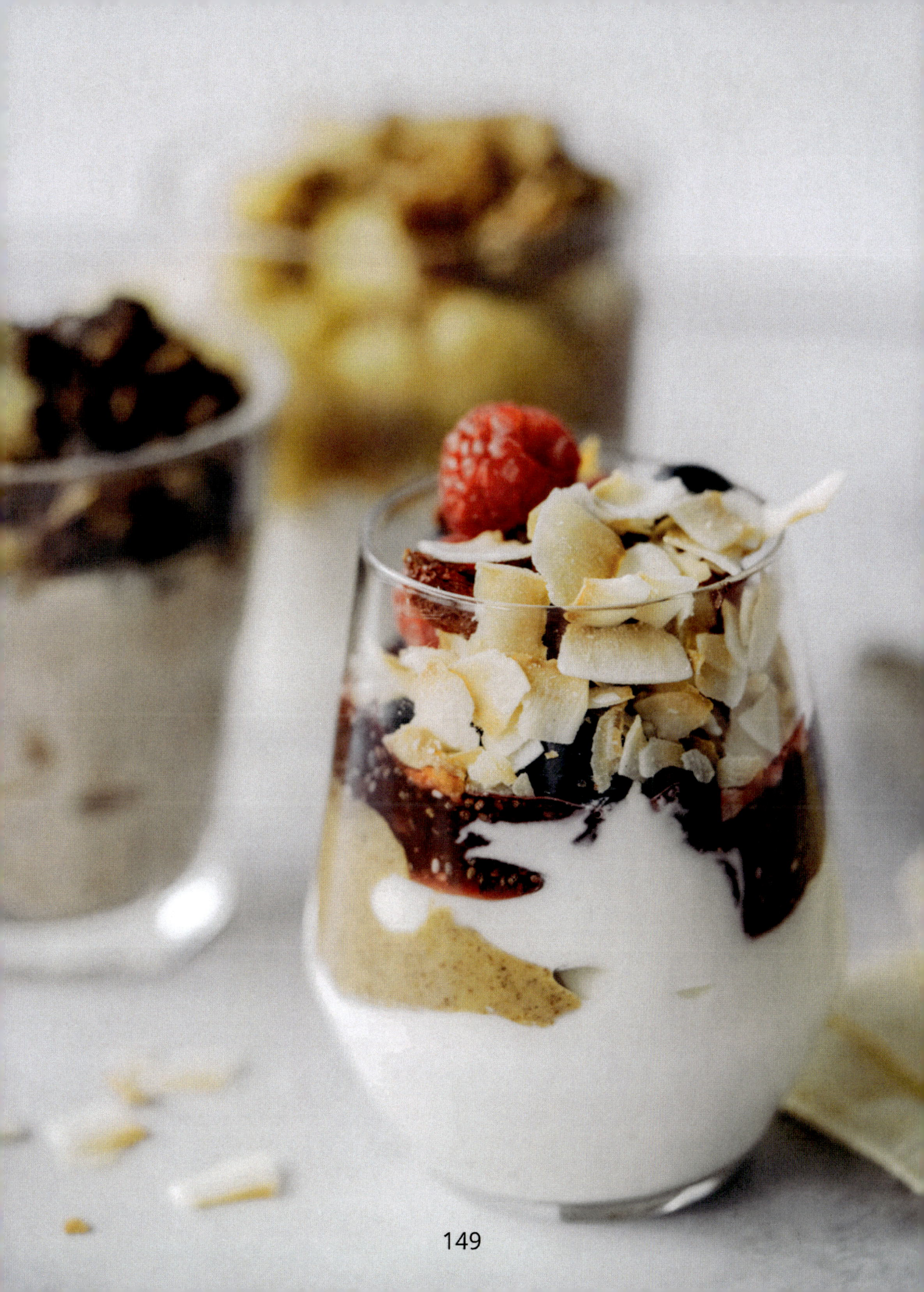

BYOYP (Build Your Own Yogurt Parfait)
for a sustaining snack

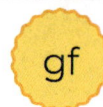

gf

Josh Williamson is a bobsledder who represented the USA at the Beijing 2022 Olympics, where he placed 10th in the four-man event, and he is also a 2x World Cup medalist. Josh didn't know bobsled even existed until he saw an Instagram ad for "The Next Olympic Hopeful" TV show that looks to find talent in niche Olympics Sports. Since he had the perfect build and skills for bobsled, Josh won the competition and was sent to the 2018 Olympic qualifiers. After four years of transitioning to bobsled and training hard, Josh showed up in Bejing as an Olympian.

Unsweetened, plain, Greek yogurt is one of the most delicious and versatile sources of protein. It can be added to smoothies, frozen into popsicles for dessert, or added to breakfast oatmeal and pancakes for a protein boost. Josh's go-to afternoon snack on training days is a yogurt parfait, and it tastes so good it can even be an after-dinner dessert. The combination of yogurt, fresh fruit, nut butter, and extra toppings like seeds, honey, granola, or dark chocolate chips is so delicious it feels deceiving!

Here you can Build Your Own Yogurt Parfait to create a nutritionally balanced and personalized snack. Simply choose a yogurt base; a healthy carbohydrate like seasonal fruit; and a healthy fat like nut butter, whole nuts, or seeds. We recommend using a plain yogurt with no added sugar. Flavored yogurts contain high levels of added sugar, meaning that eating them is like having a few scoops of ice cream! For those of you who need inspiration, there are three pre-made recipes on page 152 that will most definitely satisfy all of your cravings.

Josh's yogurt parfait combination:

- 1/2 cup whole milk Greek yogurt
- 1 tablespoon heavy whipping cream
- 1 tablespoon dark chocolate chips (higher the % the better)
- 1 scoop of protein powder if you're low on your protein for the day!
- 2 tablespoons sliced almonds
- 1 tablespoon honey

Makes 1 serving

Choose your base: 1/2 cup yogurt

- [ ] Plain greek yogurt
- [ ] Plain whole milk yogurt
- [ ] Plain coconut yogurt (dairy-free)

If you are a chocolate lover, mix in 1/2 teaspoon cocoa powder with your yogurt of choice to give it a chocolatey taste.

Choose your fruit: 1 cup fruit

Seasonal fruit:

Winter:	Spring:	Summer:	Fall:
☐ Kiwi	☐ Cherries	☐ Berries	☐ Apples
☐ Orange	☐ Apricots	☐ Grapes	☐ Figs
☐ Kumquat	☐ Peaches	☐ Pineapple	☐ Pear
☐ Grapefruit	☐ Banana	☐ Watermelon	☐ Plums

Choose your healthy fat: 1 tablespoon

Nuts/nut butters and seeds/seed butters (crunchy or smooth):

- [ ] Peanuts / Peanut Butter
- [ ] Almonds / Almond Butter
- [ ] Cashews / Cashew Butter
- [ ] Hazelnuts / Hazelnut Butter
- [ ] Macadamias / Macadamia Nut Butter
- [ ] Tahini (nut-free)
- [ ] Hemp seeds
- [ ] Flax seeds
- [ ] Chia seeds
- [ ] Sunflower seeds or Sunflower Butter (nut free)

Extras:

- [ ] Unsweetened coconut flakes
- [ ] Goji berries
- [ ] Ground cinnamon
- [ ] Cacao nibs

Have a sweet tooth?

- [ ] Dried fruit: raisins, apricots, dates
- [ ] Dark chocolate chips
- [ ] Drizzle of honey or maple syrup
- [ ] Sprinkle of granola (pages 44, 47)

Yogurt parfait inspiration:

makes 1 serving

The Chunky Monkey: for peanut butter cup lovers.

1/2 cup Chocolate yogurt (1/2 cup yogurt of choice mixed with 1/2 tablespoon cocoa powder).
1/2 banana sliced (tip: freeze the banana slices for 1 hour to create an ice cream-like taste and texture)
1 tablespoon peanut butter
1 tablespoon chocolate granola (pages 44, 47)
1 tablespoon chia seeds
Optional (but, not really): sprinkle of dark chocolate chips.

Mix 1/2 cup yogurt and 1/2 tablespoon cocoa powder into a cereal bowl. Top the yogurt with the banana, peanut butter, chocolate granola, chia seeds, and (optional) chocolate chips.

Summer Berry Bowl: for mixed berry tart lovers.

1/2 cup yogurt of choice.
1 cup fresh berries or frozen berries
1 tablespoon almond butter
1 tablespoon homemade raspberry chia jam (see page 153)
1 tablespoon goji berries
1 tablespoon unsweetened coconut flakes
Drizzle of honey

Add 1/2 cup yogurt into a cereal bowl and top with frozen berries, almond butter, chia jam, goji berries, unsweetened coconut flakes, and a drizzle of honey.

The A-B-C (Apple-Almond Butter-Cinnamon): for apple pie lovers.

1/2 cup yogurt of choice.
1/2 cup stewed, chopped apple (see page 153)
1/2 tablespoon ground cinnamon
1/2 tablespoon coconut oil
1 tablespoon almond butter
1 tablespoon maple coconut granola (see page 44)

Add 1/2 cup yogurt into a cereal bowl and top with the stewed apple, almond butter, and granola.

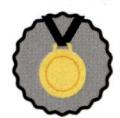

How to make homemade mixed berry chia jam:

1. Add **2 cups of berries** (frozen berries are actually even better than fresh) to a blender or food processor and process until smooth.
2. Heat the berry purée in a saucepan over medium heat until it begins to bubble. Remove from heat and mix in **1/4 cup chia seeds, 3 tablespoons of organic raw honey,** and **2 tablespoons of lemon juice.** Let it cool.
3. Store in an airtight glass container in the fridge for up to 1 week.

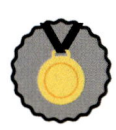

How to make stewed apples:

1. Heat **1 tablespoon coconut oil** in a saucepan.
2. Add in **1 chopped apple** and mix thoroughly with **1/2 tablespoon ground cinnamon.**
3. Keep stirring and cook until the apples soften and caramelize.

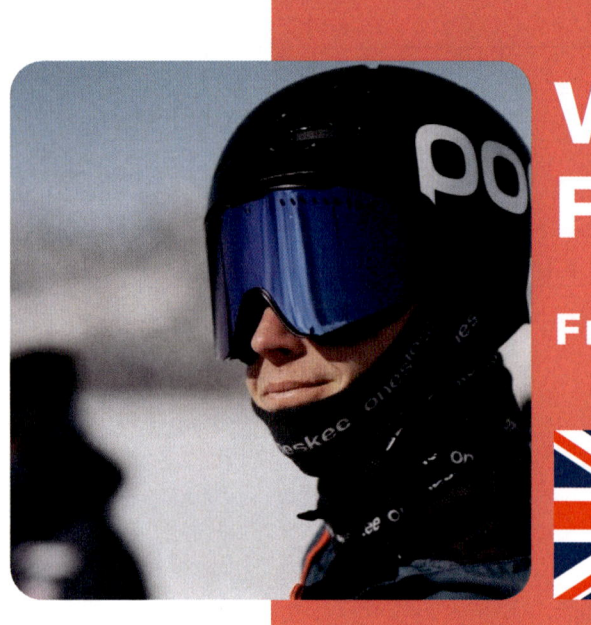

WILL FENELY

Freestyle Skiing

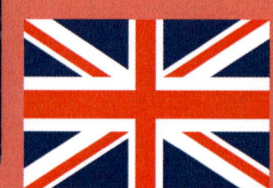

Sleep Habits:
"I get around 6-7 hours of sleep. It works for me, but some people want more. I find that if I'm struggling to sleep, getting out of bed for 10 minutes can help."

Olympic Memory:
The feeling of finally completing my run and knowing I was officially an Olympian was a very special moment. The result wasn't what I wanted, but I'd put it all on the line, and competed the hardest run I could possibly do. I left nothing on the table, and I'm really proud of myself for that."

Recovery Tip:
"I love my Theragun! It's great during or after a stretch. I also like to get out and about, exploring the places I'm training at, hiking, biking, and general walkabouts."

Mental Prep Tip:
"This can be really challenging. Especially during Olympic qualification and the Olympics itself. If I am really nervous, I remind myself that I'm choosing to put myself here, and I'm doing that because I love skiing. All you can do is control the 'controllable'. What other people have done, what score the judges will give you, what if my equipment breaks...these things are uncontrollable, so ignore them and focus on what you CAN control."

Morning Routine:
"I wake up and head down to breakfast. Usually, I prefer to have a small breakfast and take snacks for the day of training. After breakfast, I like to have a bit of time to relax and then get into my 40-minute warm-up. Then we get ready to go training for the day!"

Image by Makayla Gerken Schofield

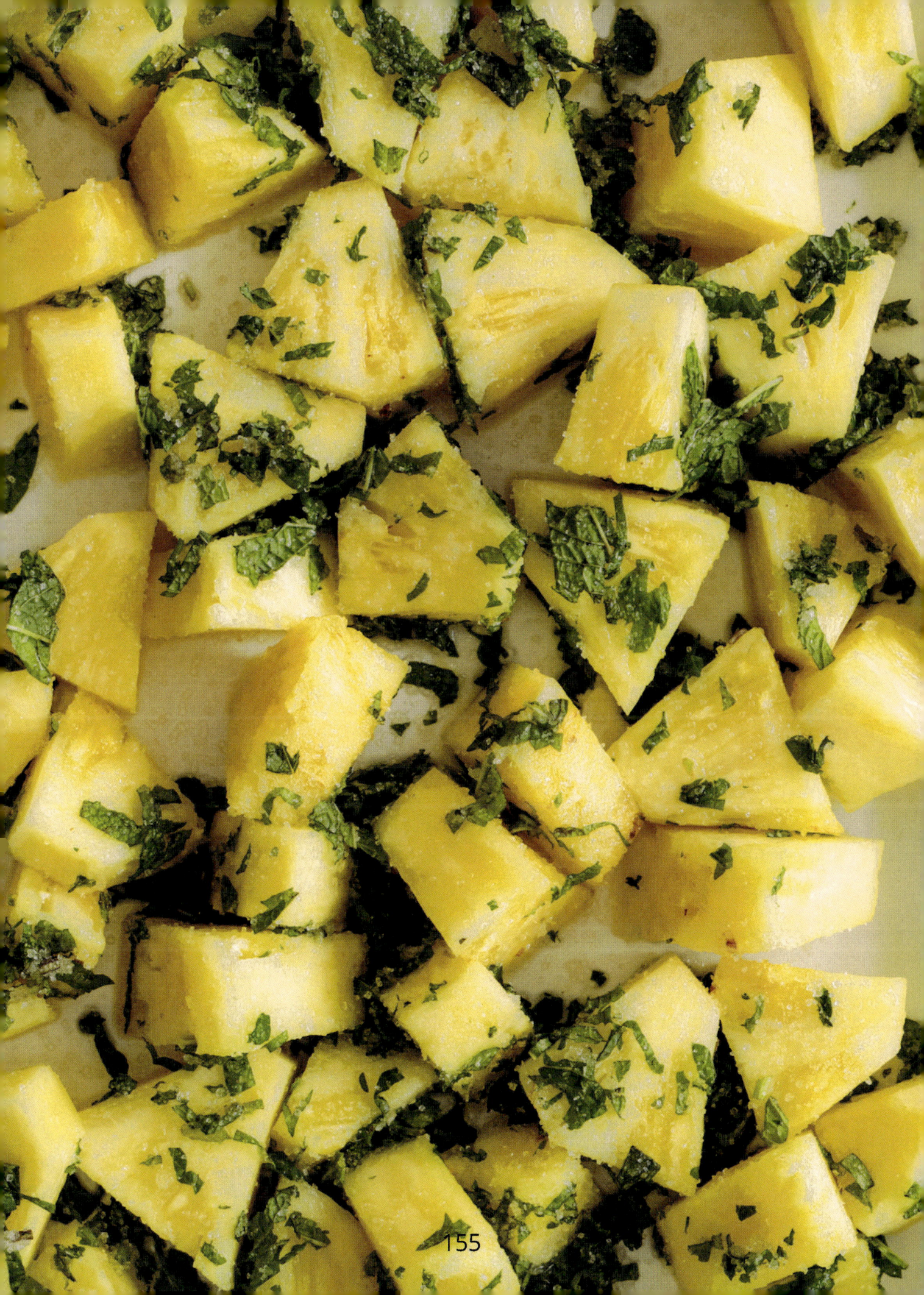

Sugar mint pineapple

for a sweet and sour treat

nf gf v df

Will Feneley is a freestyle skier who represented Great Britain at the Beijing 2022 Olympics. Originally from Norfolk, Will started skiing at 6 years old when he visiting Tremblant on a family vacation. He was the youngest British mogul skier to compete in the Junior World Championships in 2014 and now competes on the World Cup circuit.

Here Will shares his simple sugary mint pineapple recipe. The sour pineapple, with refreshing mint, and sweet sugar is the full trifecta! Enjoy this anytime, but it is particularly delicious on a hot summer day.

Makes 4 servings

1 pineapple, peeled and cored
1/2 cup mint leaves, finely chopped
3 tablespoons caster sugar
1 squeeze of lemon juice (about 1 tablespoon)

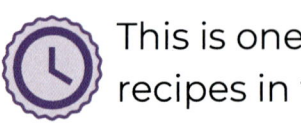

1. Peel, core, and chop the pineapple into large chunks.
2. In a small bowl, mix the mint leaves and caster sugar.
3. Arrange the pineapple on a plate, drizzle lemon juice on it, then evenly coat it with the minty sugar mix.

This is one of the fastest recipes in the cookbook, is easy to pack, and is great for those of you on the go.

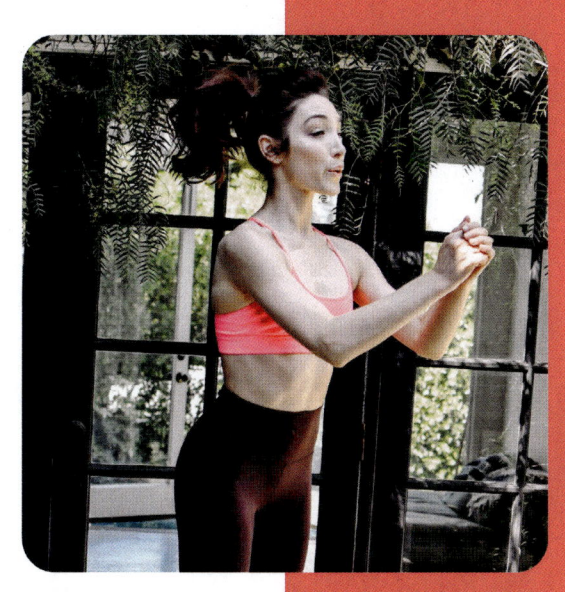

MERYL DAVIS

Ice Dance

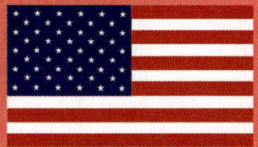

Sleep Habits:

"I sleep around eight hours a night these days. I actually sleep more now than I did when I was training. I find winding down sans technology really helpful and like charging my phone in a different part of the house so that I'm not tempted to scroll aimlessly before bed."

Olympic Memory:

"Some of my favorite Olympic memories are from the practice sessions between the team and individual events in Sochi. So much work went into preparing for the Games that I distinctly remember what it felt like to lean into that deep sense of readiness."

Recovery Tip:

"When I was training, I loved winding down with an episode of my favorite TV show before diving into schoolwork for the evening."

Mental Prep Tip:

"Before a competition, I tried to keep things in perspective by reminding myself that it was the love of my family that meant the most to me. Because what did or did not happen on the ice never had any bearing on that, it was easier to remember to simply enjoy the process."

Morning Routine:

"My morning routine when training was usually a mad dash to get out the door as quickly, and efficiently, as possible in order to maximize sleep. I loved showering, preparing my breakfast, and picking out my training clothes the night before so that a tap or two of the snooze button didn't set me back."

Image by Meryl Davis

158

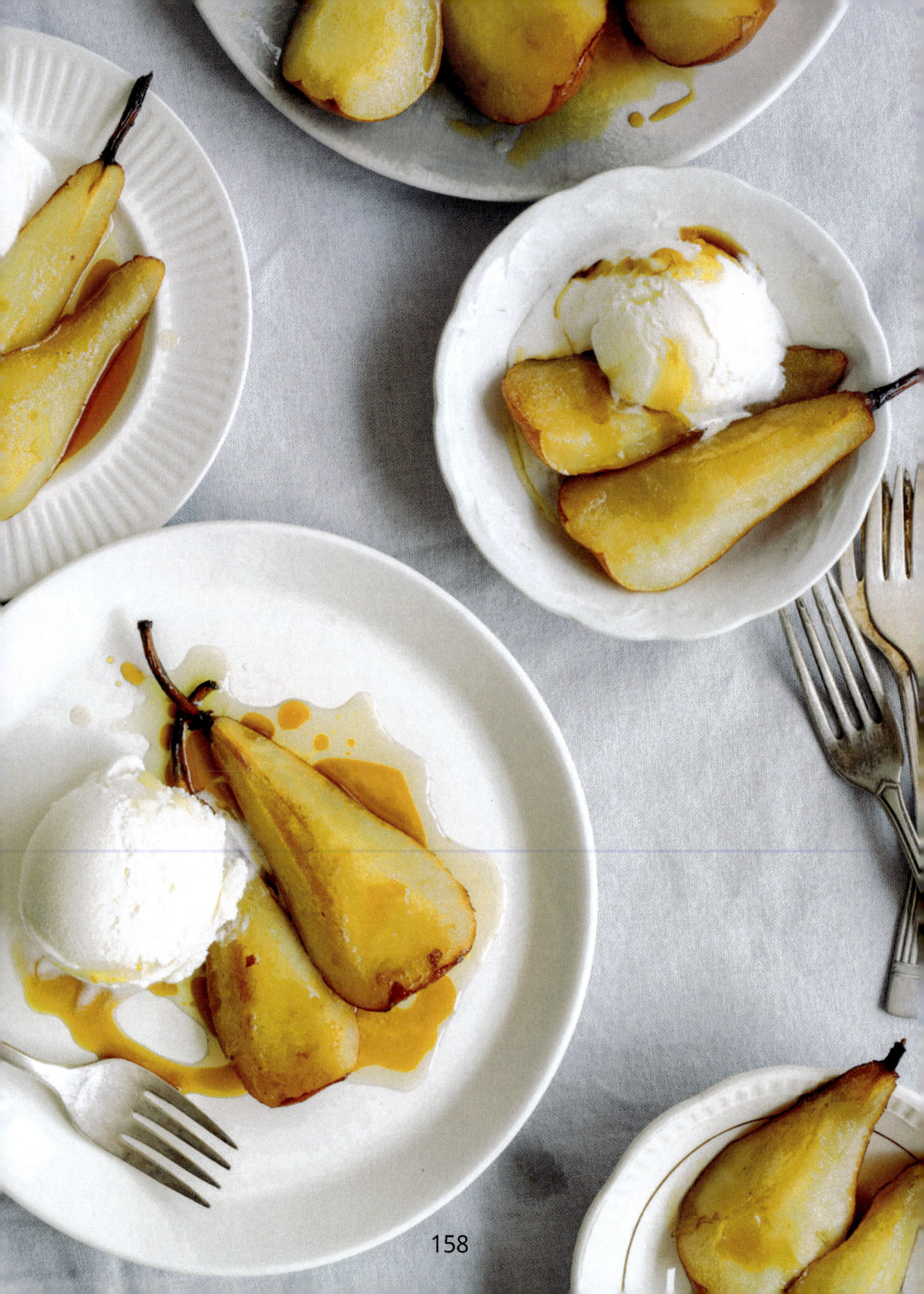

Caramelized Pears
for holiday celebrations

gf

Meryl Davis is an ice dancer who represented the USA alongside her partner Charlie White at the Vancouver 2010 Olympics, where they won silver, and the Sochi 2014 Olympics, where they won gold. She is a 2x World Champion, 6x National Champion, and 5x Grand Prix Final Champion. Meryl and Charlie are the longest-lasting American ice dance team (they started in 1997) and were the first American ice dance team to win the World and Olympic Championships. Outside of skating, Meryl won *Dancing With the Stars* in 2014. Her presence on and off the ice is so special and magical, and she has been such an inspiration to me throughout my skating career.

For Christmas, Meryl's family makes caramelized pears served with vanilla ice cream. This recipe is simple yet festive and cozy, making it perfect for Christmas Eve nights curled up by the fire or for larger gatherings.

Makes 12 servings

6 tablespoons unsalted butter
6 medium pears quartered and cored
1/2 cup packed light-brown sugar
2 tablespoons water
2 teaspoons pure vanilla extract
Salt
Vanilla ice cream, for serving

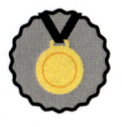

🏅 Use Anjou or Bartlett pears for the best result as they hold their shape when cooked and are sweet and juicy.

1. Melt the butter in a large pan on medium-high heat. Add the pears and cook one side of the pears until browned. Reduce heat to medium and cook for 3 more minutes.
2. Flip the pears and cook the other side for 3-4 minutes. Stir in the brown sugar and water.
3. Turn the pears skin side down, and allow the sauce to thicken slightly (about 2 minutes). Stir in the vanilla extract and a pinch of salt. Serve with vanilla ice cream.

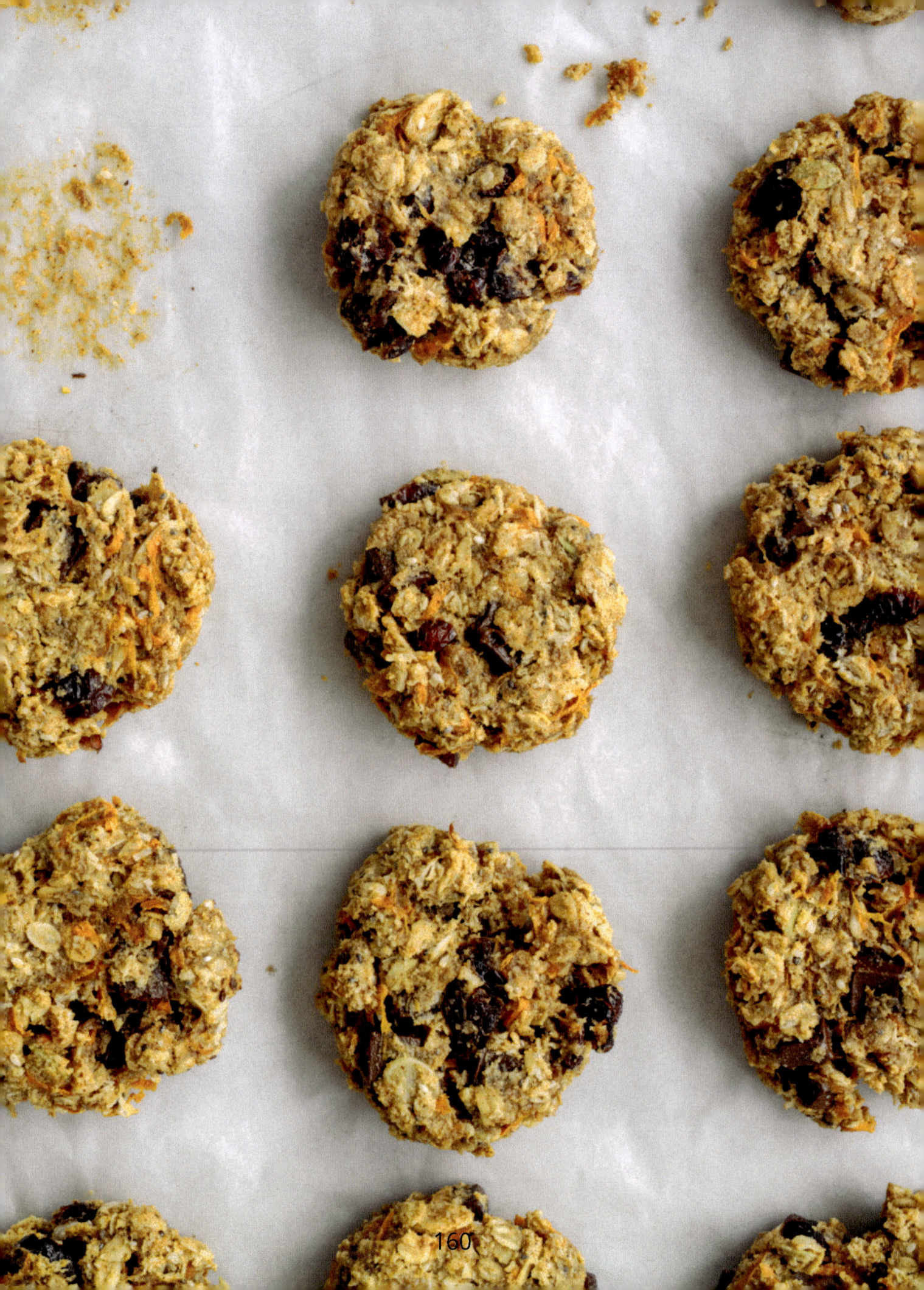

Ultimate Power Cookies
for a bite of energy

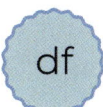

v df gf

I whip up a batch of power cookies each week as they make great fuel pre or post-workout. This cookie contains a variety of protein and fiber-packed seeds, nuts for healthy fats and sustenance, sneaky veggies that you cannot taste, and cranberries and dark chocolate for sweetness.

You can switch up the ingredients for the cookie to make any flavor you want (see ideas below)!

Makes 12 large cookies

Wet:
1/2 cup flax meal mixed with 1/2 cup water
2/3 cup almond butter
1/2 cup maple syrup
2 teaspoons vanilla extract
1 cup grated carrot

Dry:
2 cups rolled oats (or GF if sensitive)
1 cup almond flour
1 tablespoon chia seeds
1 tablespoon pumpkin seeds
1 tablespoon sunflower seeds
1 teaspoon sesame seeds
1/4 cup cranberries
1/4 cup slivered almonds
1/4 cup unsweetened desiccated coconut
1/2 cup dark chocolate chips
1/2 teaspoon sea salt

1. Preheat oven 350°F.
2. In a medium bowl, mix the wet ingredients until combined.
3. In a large bowl, mix the dry ingredients. Then add the wet ingredients to the dry and stir to combine completely.
4. Use an ice cream scoop or a large spoon to portion 12 large cookies onto 2 baking trays lined with parchment paper. Flatten each cookie to about 1/2-3/4" thickness.
5. Bake for 18-20 minutes. Let cool and store in the fridge for up to a week, or in the freezer for up to 2 months in an airtight container.

Want to mix it up?
- Swap the almond butter for peanut butter or cashew butter.
- Use 1/2 cup grated carrot and 1/2 cup zucchini.
- Swap cranberries, and almonds with 1 mashed banana.
- Swap flax meal + water, for 1 egg.

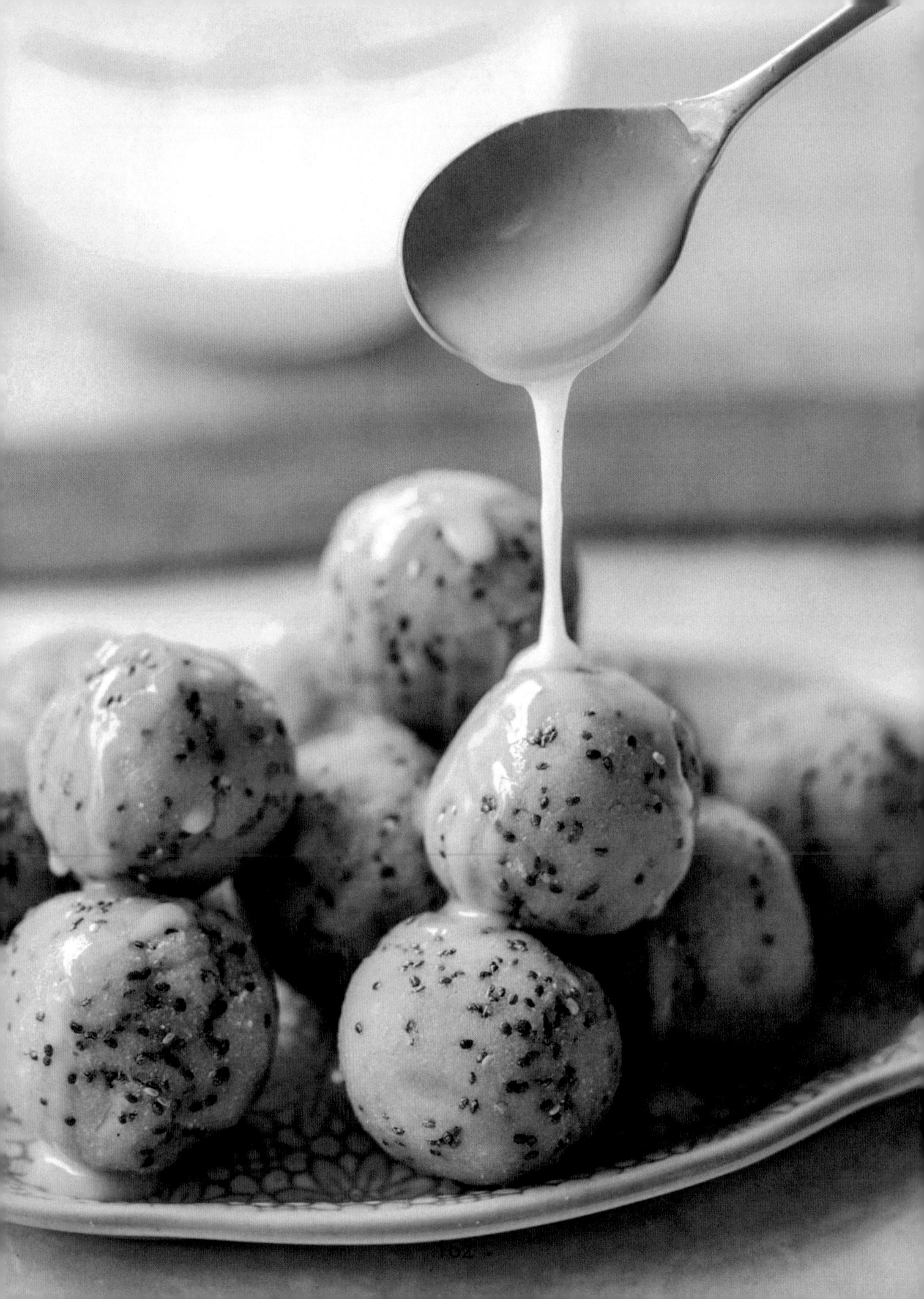

Lemon Chia Energy Balls

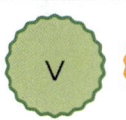

BONUS RECIPE

Meghan Tierney is a snowboarder who represented the USA at the Pyeongchang 2018 and the Beijing 2022 Olympics in the snowboard cross. She is the first-ever USA athlete to win both the NORAM and the Europa Cup Championships.

Here Meghan shares her lemon chia energy ball recipe, which uses chia seeds instead of the classic lemon poppyseed combination because they are packed with fiber and antioxidants. The tangy lemon is refreshing, especially in the summer, and it tastes better than lemon cake (in my biased opinion).

Makes 12 Balls

3/4 cup almond flour
3/4 cup coconut flour
2 tablespoons vegan protein powder
Pinch of salt
1/4 cup maple syrup
2 tablespoons cashew butter
1-2 tablespoons coconut oil
1 teaspoon vanilla extract
Juice and zest of 1 lemon
2 tablespoons chia seeds
1 tablespoon coconut butter

Optional lemon icing:
The juice of 1 lemon
3/4 cup confectioner's sugar
1/2 teaspoon lemon extract

1. In a food processor or high-speed blender, blend all of the ingredients except the chia seeds and pulse until a thick dough forms.
2. Add in the chia seeds and pulse until evenly combined.
3. Spoon out 1-2 tablespoons of the dough per ball and use your hands to roll it up into an even circle. If desired, mix the lemon icing ingredients and drizzle onto each ball.
4. Store the balls in an airtight container in the fridge for up to 10 days or in the freezer for up to a month.
5. If you opt for the freezer option, allow the balls to thaw for 5-10 minutes before consuming.

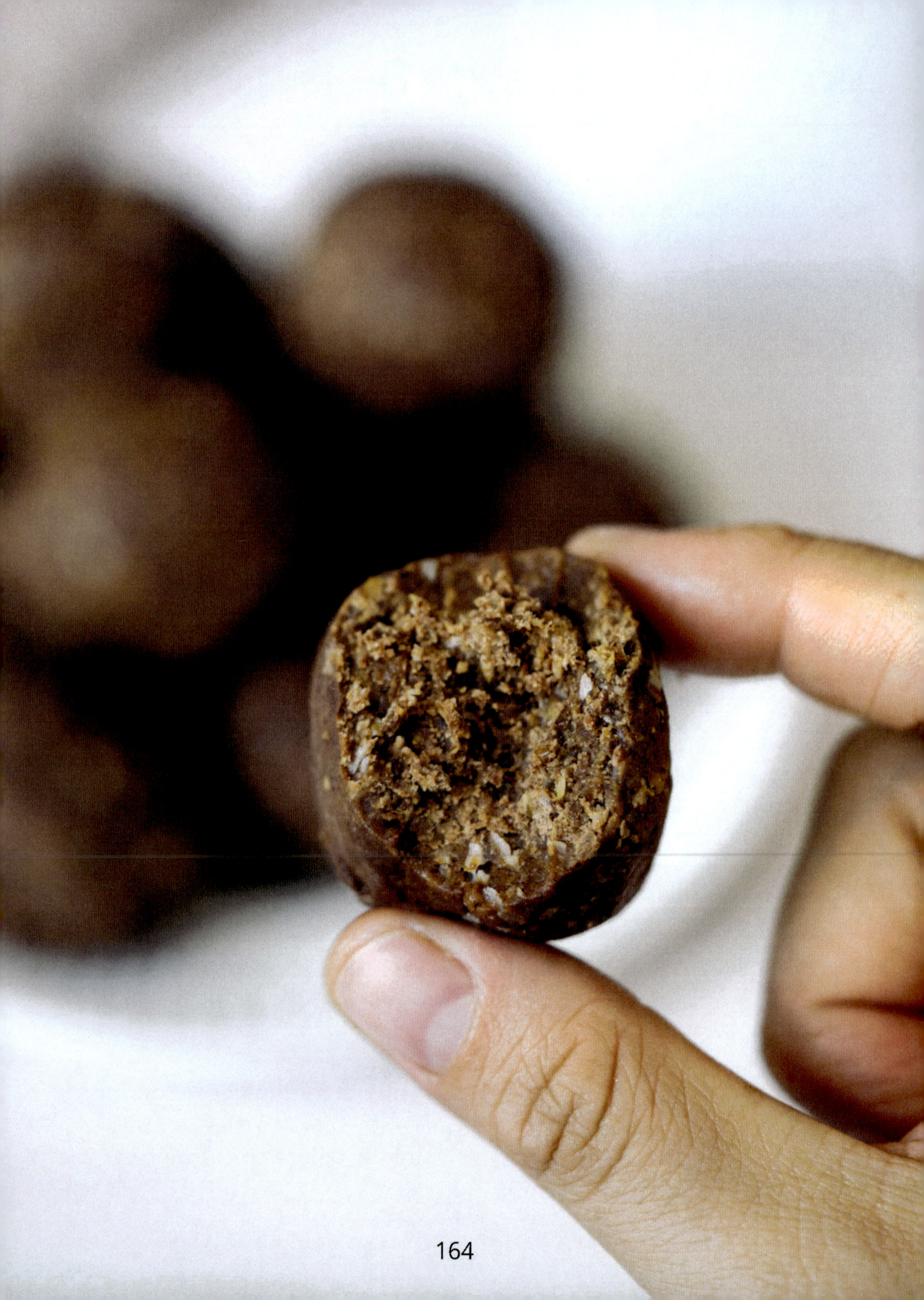

Cookie-dough Power Balls

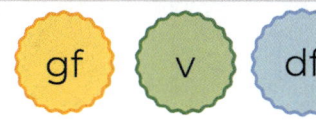

BONUS RECIPE

gf v df

Brian Orser is a former figure skater representing Canada. He won two Olympic silver medals at the 1984 and 1988 games, and is a 6x World Championship medalist and 8x Canadian National Champion. He is now a successful coach based at the Toronto Cricket Skating and Curling Club where he has trained Olympic champions and medalists Yuna Kim, Yuzuru Hanyu, and Javier Fernandez, as well as dozens of World Championship medalists.

Here Brian will share his favorite power ball recipe for on-the-go fuel between on-ice training or a workout. These energy balls are high in protein and healthy fats, keeping you sustained and fueled for any adventure. And a bonus is that they taste like cookie dough!!

Makes 12 Balls

1 cup oat flour (gluten-free if sensitive)
1/4 cup flax meal
1/4 cup shredded coconut
1 scoop of protein powder (vanilla is best)
1/4 cup almond butter
1/3 cup maple syrup
Dark chocolate chips (measure with your heart)

Make oat flour: blend oats in a food processor or blender and pulse until the oats are broken up into a fine flour.

nf **Make it nut-free:** sub almond butter for tahini or sunflower butter.

1. Mix the oat flour, flax meal, shredded coconut, protein powder, and chocolate chips in a bowl.
2. In a saucepan, stir in the almond butter and maple syrup on low heat. Once it bubbles, remove from heat and add the almond butter and maple syrup to the dry ingredients. Combine until the mixture is rollable and dough-like.
3. Use your hands to roll the mixture into bite-sized balls.
4. Store in a glass storage container and chill for at least 30 minutes before eating. Keep leftovers in the fridge for up to 10 days.

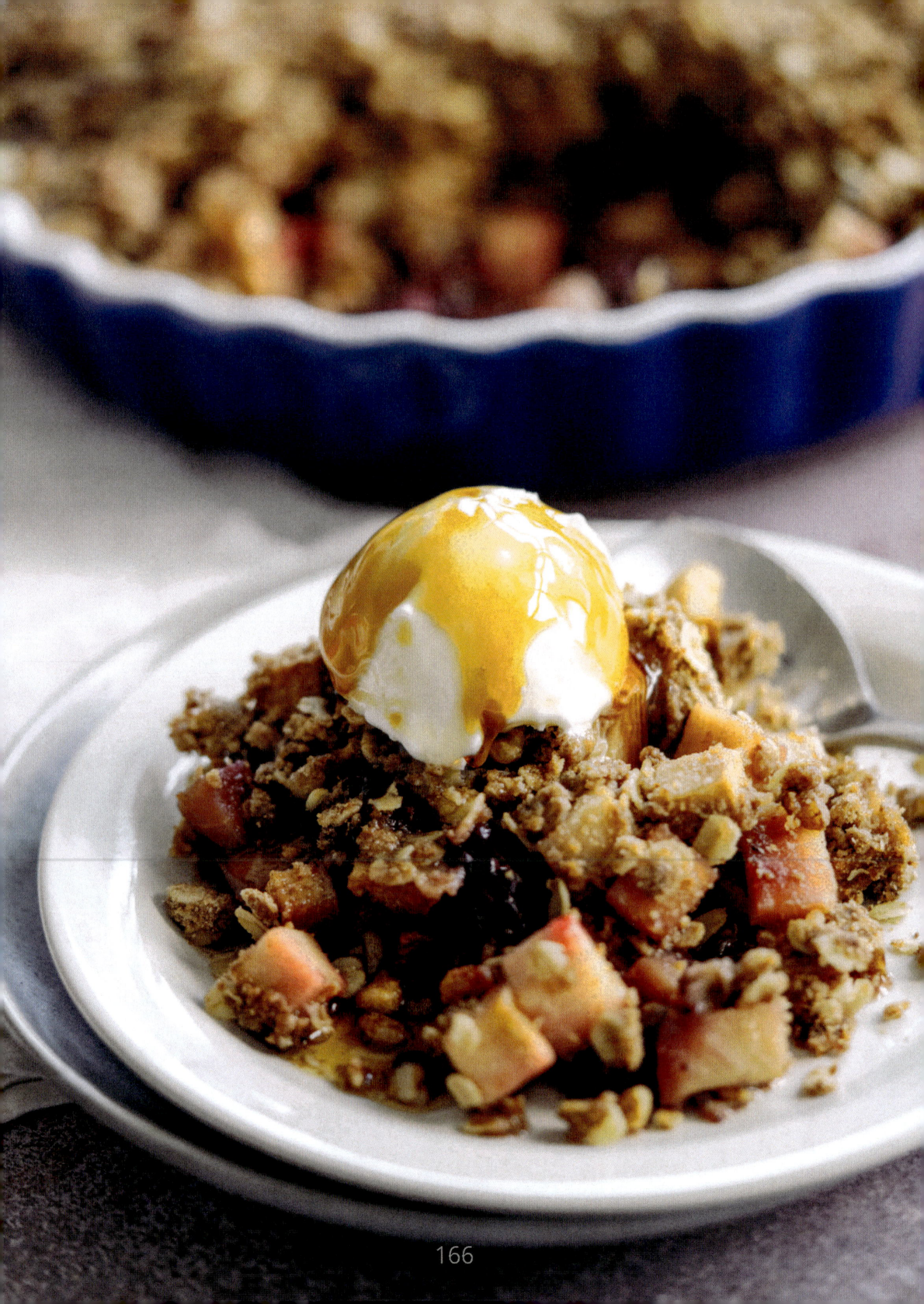

Apple and Blackberry Crumble
BONUS RECIPE

Amy Williams, MBE (Member of the Order of the British Empire) is a skeleton racer who represented Great Britain at the Vancouver 2010 Olympics. She was the first British individual gold medalist at a Winter Olympics for 30 years and was the only British medalist at that games! Amy is also a World silver medalist and a European bronze medalist; she now commentates and presents for high-level sporting events.

Here Amy shares her apple and blackberry crumble. Although Amy was strict about what she put into her body, she loved making this dessert on special occasions. This crumble uses coconut sugar which is lower on the glycemic index, therefore giving you less of a sugar spike and crash. This recipe is timeless and can be made at any time of year as you can use whatever fruit is in season! I particularly love using peaches, cherries, and berries in the summer, but apples will always have my heart.

Makes 8-10 servings

Apple base:
7 cups honey crisp apples, cored, peeled, and sliced.
3 cups blackberries
1/3 cup coconut sugar
1 tablespoon white whole wheat flour (or GF if sensitive)

Crumble topping:
1 cup rolled oats
1 cup white whole wheat flour
1/3 cup coconut sugar
1/4 teaspoon baking powder
1/4 teaspoon baking soda
1 teaspoon cinnamon
1/2 cup melted butter or coconut oil
1/2 cup finely chopped walnuts or pecans

1. Preheat oven 350°F. Spray a large baking dish with non-stick spray.
2. In a large mixing bowl, combine the apples, blackberries, coconut sugar, and flour. Pour into the baking pan.
3. In another bowl make the crumble by combining the ingredients under "Crumble topping."
4. Sprinkle the crumble evenly over the apple and blackberry mixture.
5. Bake for 40-45 minutes, or until the crumble is golden and the apples are bubbling.
6. Let it cool 10 minutes. Serve with vanilla ice cream, yogurt, and a drizzle of maple syrup or honey.

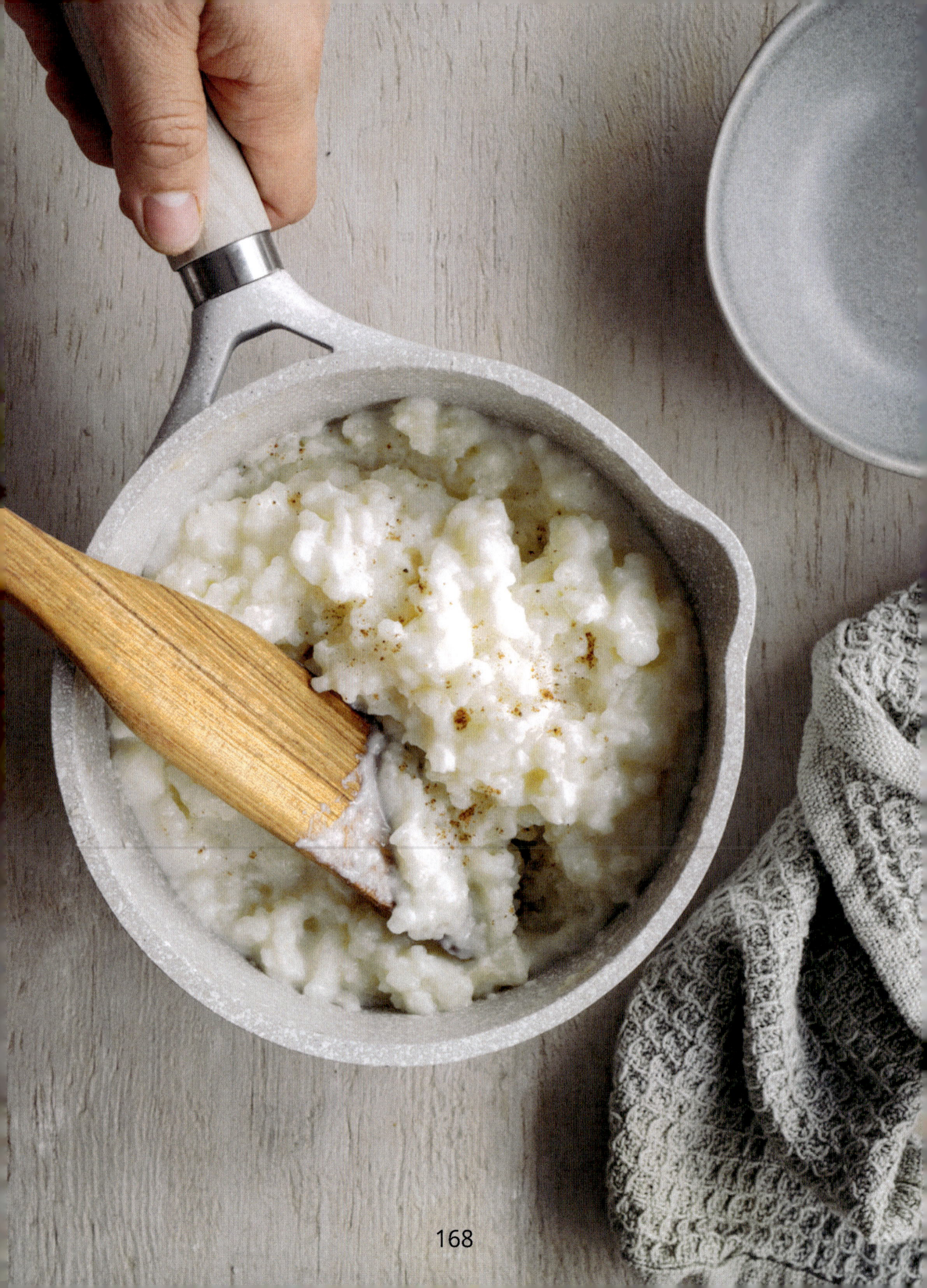

Race-Ready Rice Pudding

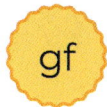

BONUS RECIPE

gf nf

Emily Brydon is a 3x Olympic Alpine Skier who represented Canada at the Salt Lake 2002, Turin 2006, and Vancouver 2010 Olympic Games. She also competed in multiple World Championships, is a 9x World Cup medalist, and was a member of the Canadian National Team for 13 years. In 2006, Emily started The Emily Brydon Youth Foundation as a way to give funding to children in the Elk Valley so that they could pursue their dreams, whether they were in sport, education, or the arts. Emily was born and raised in Fernie, BC (which is where my mom is from!) and is a true inspiration and legend in our town. She is also fearless, funny, and definitely knows how to make a mean rice pudding.

Here Emily will share her easy rice pudding recipe, which she describes as "the soul food of all soul foods." The creamy texture of the rice with a sprinkle of sugar is the perfect comfort food after a tough training day. When Emily needs a little soul put back into her life, she makes a good hearty portion of rice pudding. I mean, food is medicine, right?

Makes 1 serving

2 tablespoons margarine or butter
1/2 cup short-grain rice
2 tablespoons sugar
2 1/2 cups milk

df v — Want to make it dairy-free and vegan?
Swap the margarine or butter for vegan butter.
Swap the milk for 1 1/2 cups of non-dairy milk (soy or almond), and 1 cup of full-fat canned coconut milk.

1. Melt the margarine or butter in a saucepan.
2. Stir in the rice to coat, and mix in the milk and sugar.
3. Cover saucepan and bring to a boil.
4. Reduce the heat and simmer for 25-30 minutes, or until the milk is absorbed and the rice is tender.
5. Keep stirring frequently. You may need more milk if the pudding is too stiff.
6. Serve warm or chilled. Store in an airtight container in the fridge for 3-4 days.

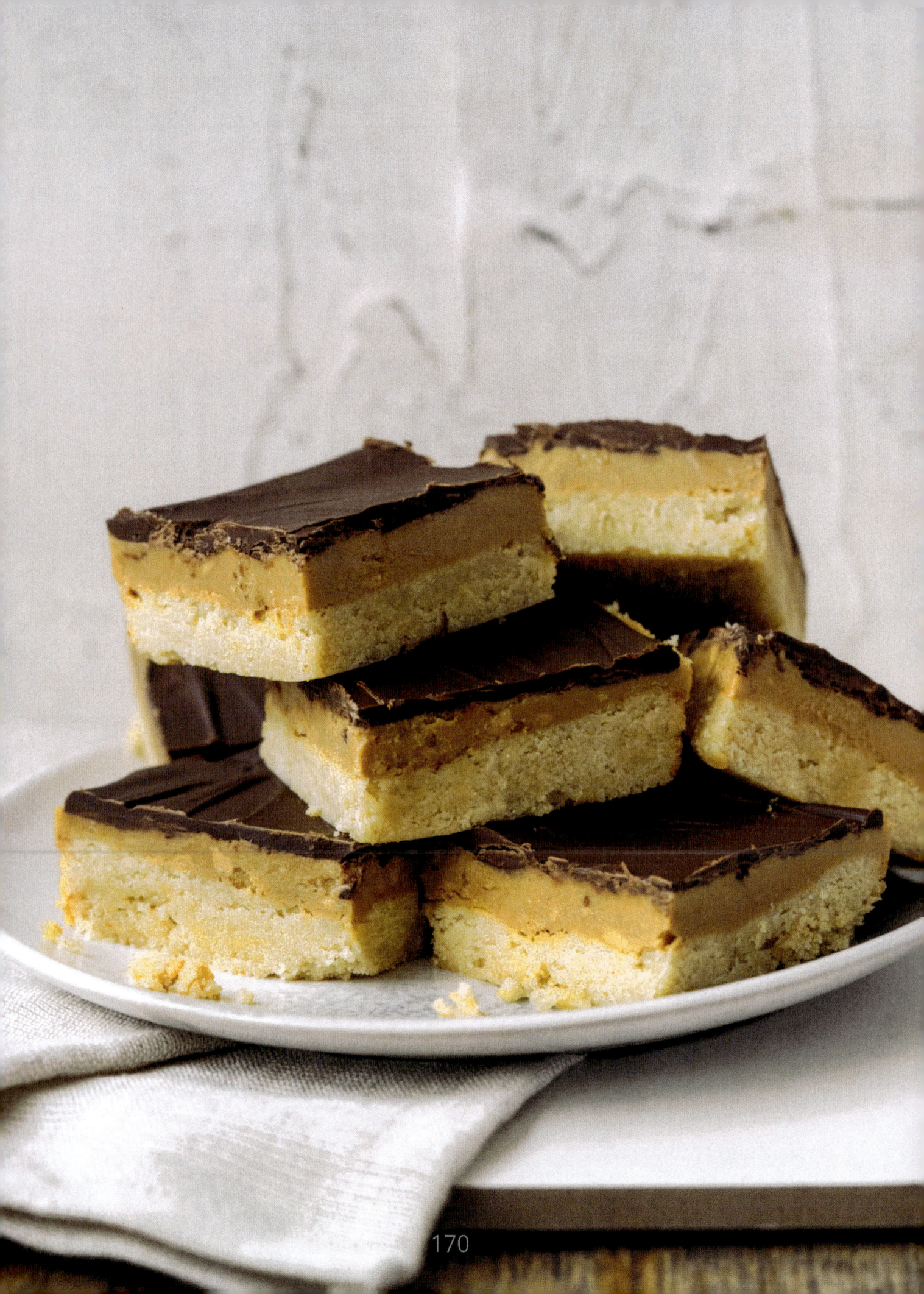

Millionaire Shortbread

BONUS RECIPE

df gf v

Lewis Gibson is an ice dancer who represented Great Britain at the Bejing 2022 Olympics alongside my sister, Lilah! The pair placed 10th in Beijing and most recently finished 2nd at the European Championships and 4th at the World Championships in 2023. Lewis is like the big brother I never had (no offense Georgia and Lilah), a fellow cookie addict, and a home decor aficionado.

Here Lewis shares his homemade treat recipe: the one and only millionaire shortbread bars. Think Twix bar, but with better-for-you ingredients. For anyone who loves caramel, chocolate, and a almond-based crust, this one is for you! Let's just say, when I make these I certainly do not share. Tip: try freezing these for 15 minutes before consuming for a fudgey caramel texture.

Makes 12 Bars

Crust:
1 1/2 cups almond flour
1/4 cup coconut flour
1/2 cup maple syrup
1/3 cup coconut oil
1 teaspoon vanilla
1/4 teaspoon salt

Caramel layer:
3/4 cup cashew butter (or sub for almond, peanut, sunflower butter)
1/3 cup coconut oil, melted
1/4 cup maple syrup
1 teaspoon vanilla
Pinch of salt

Chocolate Topping:
3/4 cup dark chocolate, melted

1. Preheat oven 350°F and line an 8x8 inch pan with parchment paper.
2. In a mixing bowl, combine the ingredients under "Crust" until a dough forms. Press the dough into the pan and bake for 15 minutes. Let it cool for 15 minutes.
3. While the crust is cooling, mix the cashew butter, coconut oil, and maple syrup in a saucepan on medium heat until fully combined. Remove from heat and stir in the vanilla and salt.
4. Spread the caramel evenly on top of the crust layer and freeze for 30 minutes.
5. In a microwave-safe bowl, melt the dark chocolate. Pour the chocolate over the caramel layer. Refrigerate for 1 hour and store in the fridge.

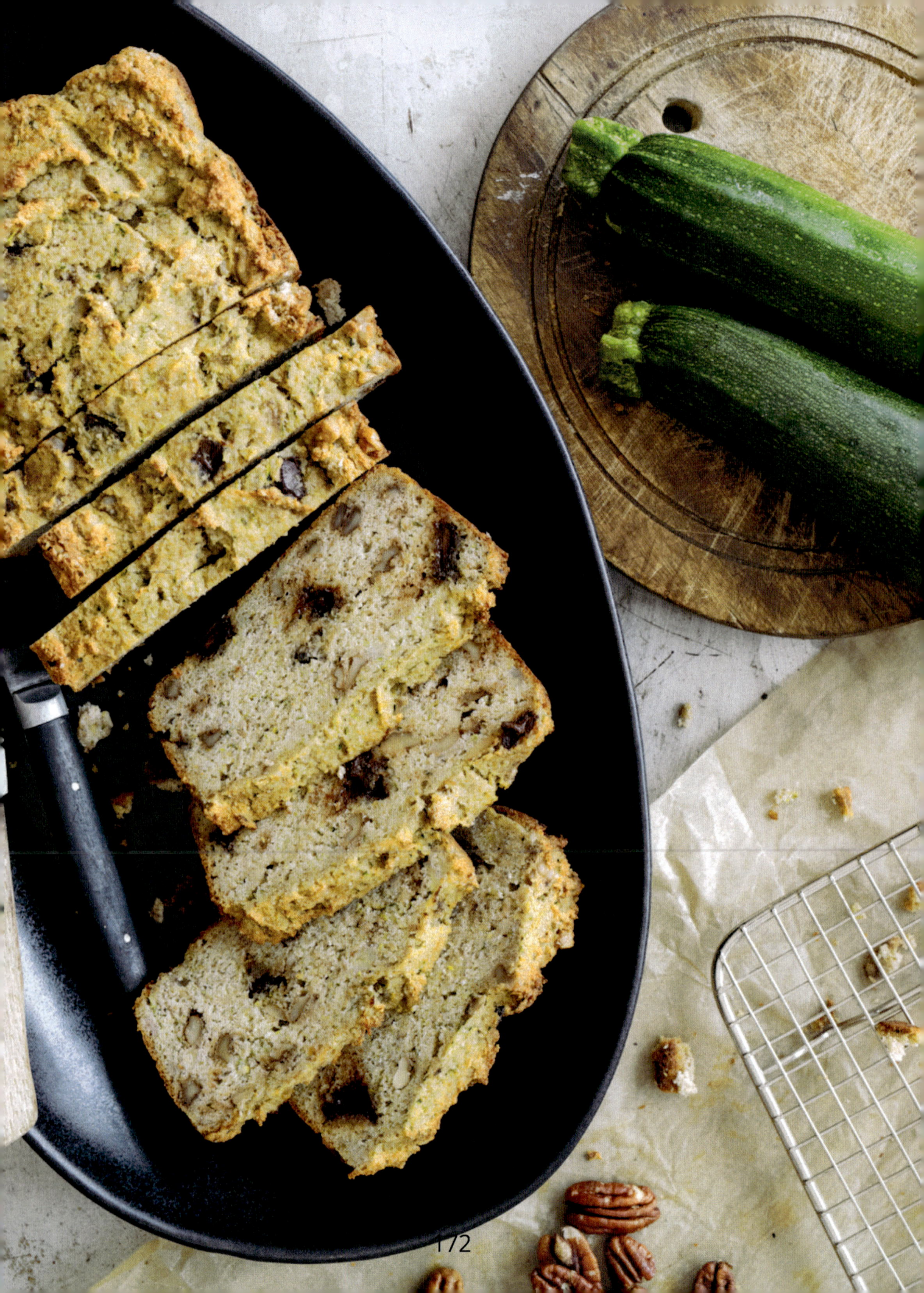

Zucchini Banana Bread
BONUS RECIPE

df gf

There is nothing like the smell of banana bread. During the pandemic, Lilah Fear jumped on the banana bread baking bandwagon and made this zucchini banana bread weekly. If you are looking to put a twist on classic banana bread, this recipe is for you. It is only sweetened by banana and has a sneaky portion of vegetables that you cannot even taste. Although the zucchini makes it look a little green, I promise it tastes AMAZING!

If you prefer, make this into muffins!

Makes 8-10 servings

1 cup mashed banana
1 cup shredded zucchini (squeeze out excess moisture)
3 eggs
2 cups almond flour
1/2 cup flax meal
1 teaspoon baking powder
1/2 teaspoon cinnamon
1/4 teaspoon nutmeg
1/3 cup dark chocolate chips (optional, but you're missing out)

Optional: 1/3 cup chopped nuts like walnuts or pecans.

1. Preheat oven 350°F.
2. In a medium bowl, mix the banana, zucchini, and egg until smooth. Mix in the almond flour, flax meal, baking powder, cinnamon, nutmeg, and chocolate and nuts if desired.
3. Line a loaf pan with parchment paper and grease the top of the paper with some coconut oil to prevent sticking.
4. Bake for 45-50 minutes and or until a toothpick comes out clean. Let cool and store in the fridge for up to a week or in the freezer for up to 2 months in an airtight container.

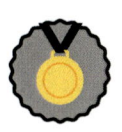

Best served warm with some greek yogurt, a drizzle of nut butter, and a sprinkle of granola.

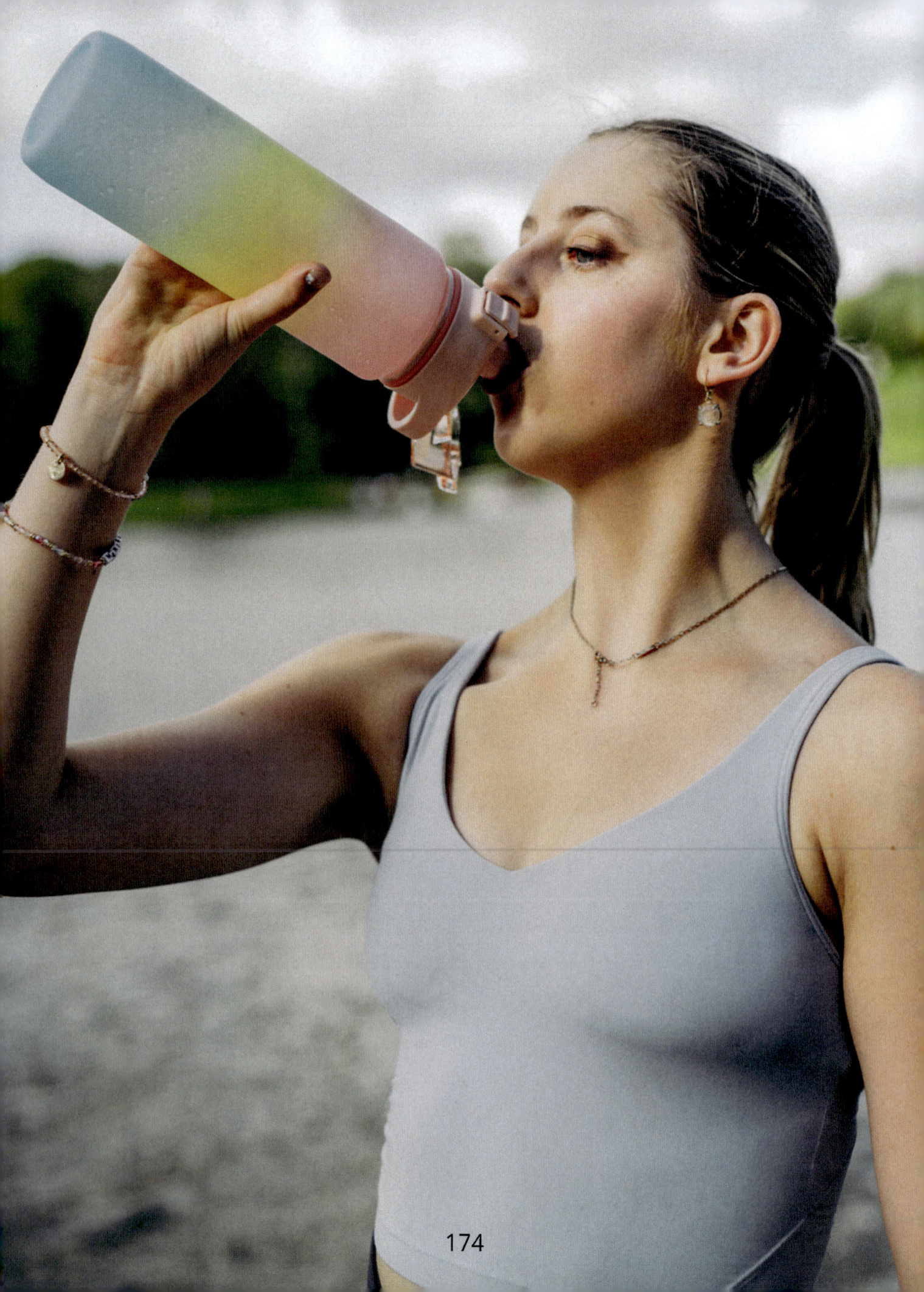

HYDRATION STATION

Alkalizing Smoothie   176

Chocolate Peanut Butter + Banana "Milkshake"   179

Electrolyte Lemon Limeade   182

Vanilla Nut + Seed Milk   184

The Immunity Booster   186

Anti-inflammatory Golden Milk   188

Tranquility Tea   190

BONUS RECIPE: Cool as a Cucumber Water   192

BONUS RECIPE: Sunrise Smoothie   194

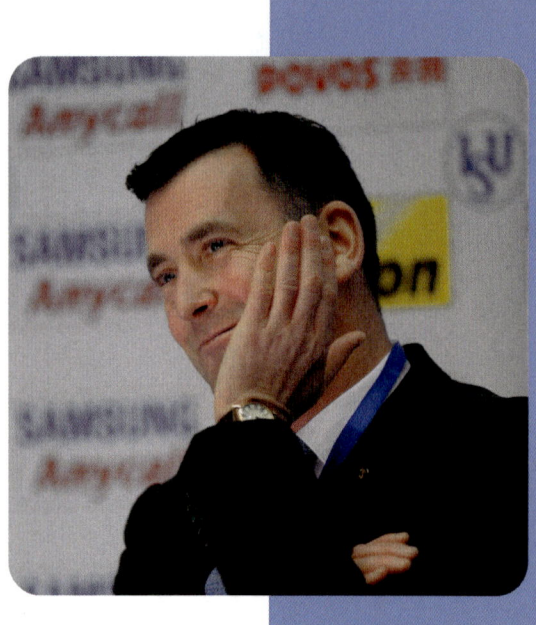

BRIAN ORSER

Figure Skating

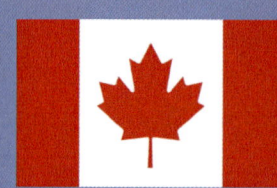

Mental Prep Tip:

"I would literally tell myself, just before they would call my name "imagine yourself at a late stage in your life, say 90 years old, and know just how tiny this moment is in the big picture of your life." I would feel my shoulders drop, and my heartbeat slow down. It is putting your life and this moment into perspective. Another great tool for mental preparation was to be physically prepared. I hated going to a competition "hoping" to compete well. And finally, you can always count on your average. Train to increase your average. Pay attention to it. If my average was 98% going into a competition, that's a good thing. I just say "do your average."

Recovery Tip:

"Light jog and stretching"

Olympic Memory:

"Carrying the Canadian flag into the opening ceremonies in a home country games."

Morning Routine:

"Each season was different. The schedule, the training hours, and the balance of on-ice vs off-ice was different. In the summer we started at 6:20 am on the ice, so before my 30 min run or bike ride, I'd have just juice. Getting home after the run, I would have a piece of toast and a boiled egg. Shower, change my clothes, and then off to the rink."

Sleep Habits:

"8 hours is perfect for me."

Image by Brian Orser

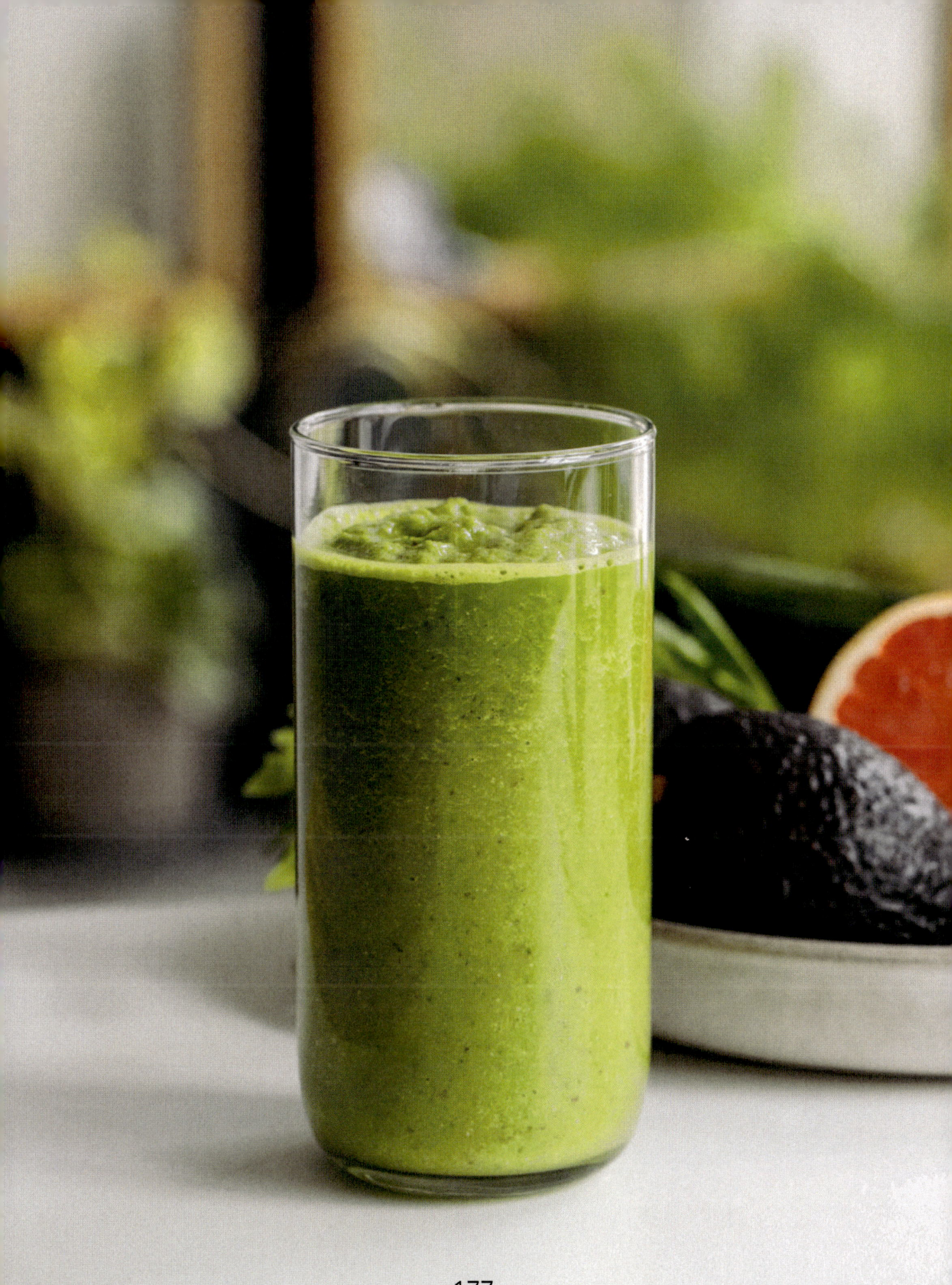

Alkalizing Smoothie

nf gf v df

For a gut-healing start to the day

Brian Orser is a former figure skater representing Canada. He won two Olympic silver medals at the 1984 and 1988 games, and is a 6x World Championship medalist and 8x Canadian National Champion. He is now a successful coach based at the Toronto Cricket Skating and Curling Club where he has trained Olympic champions and medalists Yuna Kim, Yuzuru Hanyu, and Javier Fernandez, as well as dozens of World Championship medalists.

Here, Brian shares his favorite refreshing green smoothie recipe to start his day before on-ice training or a workout. He drinks this before his morning coffee to alkalize his body. This gut-healing smoothie is packed with greens and fruit which are great sources of fiber and antioxidants, as well as ginger—which reduces inflammation. The avocado is full of healthy fats that provide energy for digestion, metabolizing, and burning fat.

Makes 1 Serving

1 cup filtered water
2 handfuls of spinach
4 inch cucumber (with skin on)
1/2 medium size fruit: peeled grapefruit, apple, or frozen banana.
1/2 inch diameter fresh peeled ginger
1 or 2 sticks of celery
1 teaspoon apple cider vinegar
1 tablespoon chia seeds
1/2 an avocado

In a high-speed blender, combine all of the ingredients and blend until smooth. If the smoothie is too thick to blend, add a splash of water.

> Brian's tips:
> 1. Shop for all of the ingredients on Sunday and prepare them the night before. This makes it easy and quick in the morning.
> 2. If you choose banana for the smoothie, peel and freeze it to make the smoothie cool and thick without ice. You can still add ice if you like.

MARCUS WYATT

Skeleton

🇬🇧

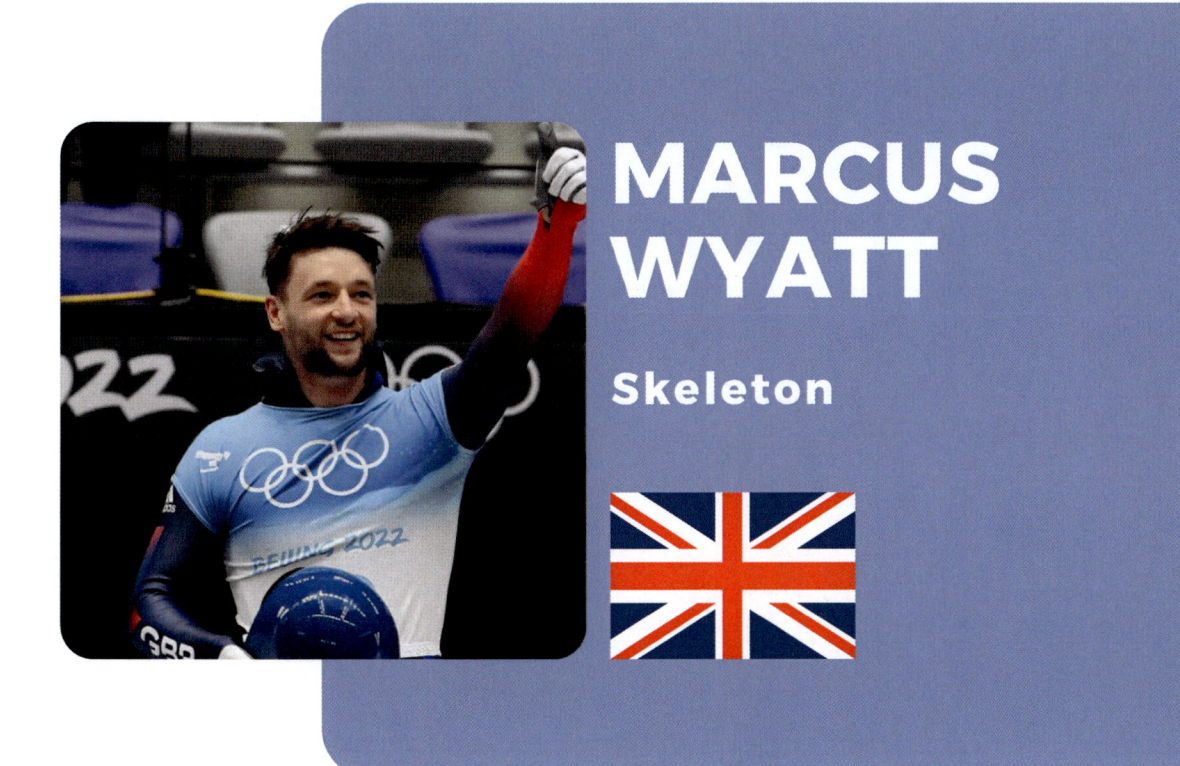

Mental Prep Tip:
"For me, it's about being in a state of 'soft focus' just before I race. This means I'm focused on myself and what I need to do, but I'm not focused on one thing specifically. I'm just trying to take it all in, be in the moment, and react to what I am seeing and feeling on the track. This helps me make the best decisions when going 80mph headfirst on ice!"

Recovery Tip:
"Walking into the stadium for the Opening Ceremony was utterly mind-blowing. Being there with my friends—with whom I've trained side by side for seven years—is something I will never forget, and it will undoubtedly be one of the most special things I'll ever do."

Recovery Tip:
"I really enjoy cooking and learning new recipes: taking ingredients and turning them into a nice meal gives me a lot of pride when it goes well. I also like a bit of gaming—either online or board games with friends."

Morning Routine:
"Wake up with plenty of time before training. Feed our pet rabbits first, then get my breakfast ready. I usually eat porridge with protein and fruit. After that, I get in some mobility/stretching/rolling before driving to training and starting our first session of the day."

Sleep Habits:
"I tend to get close to 8 hours every night. The tip I always say is to find a pillow you love and take it with you wherever you're going to sleep. I spend 6 months away per year, and my pillow goes everywhere with me."

Image by *Robert Michael (Getty)*

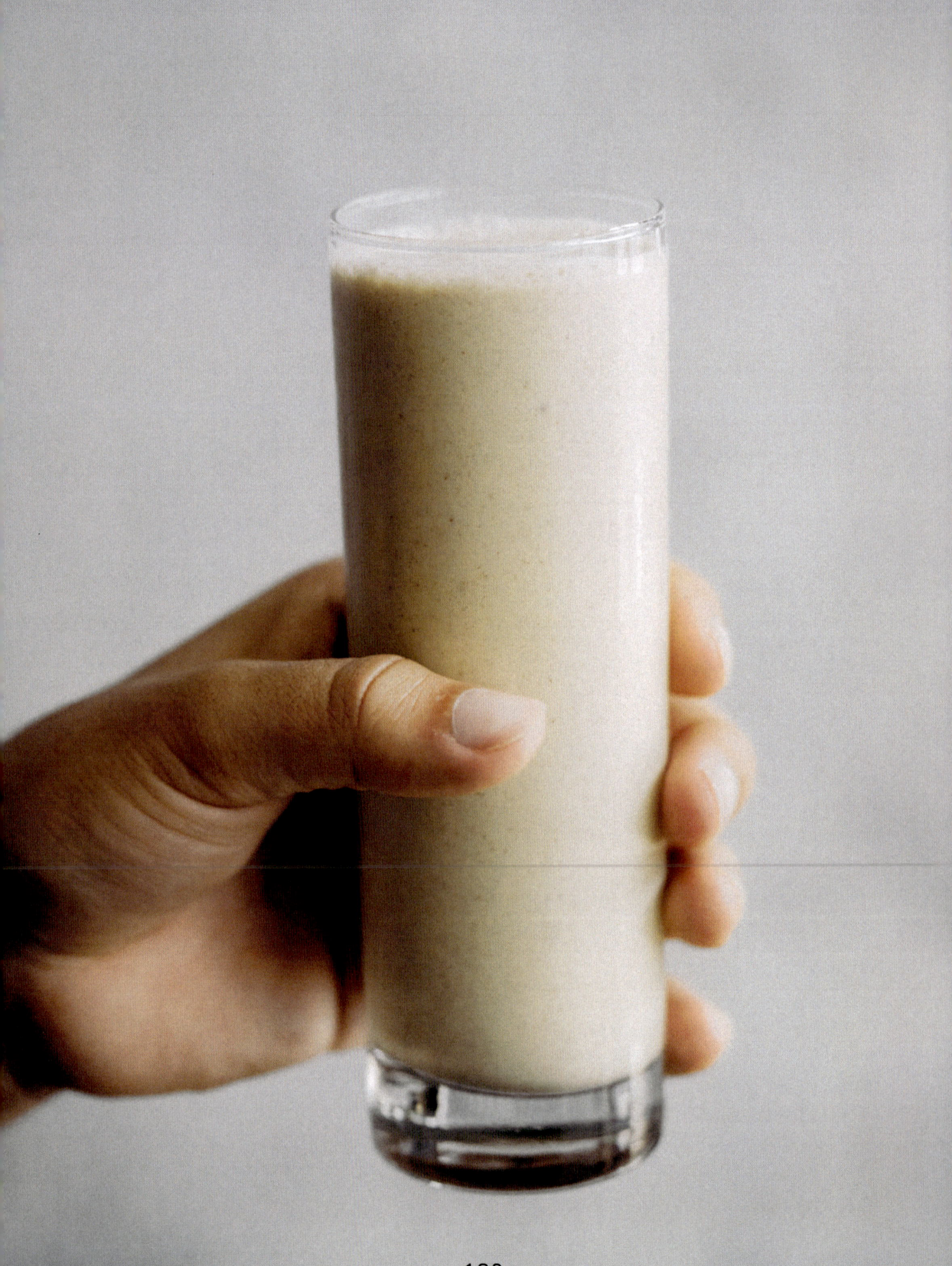

Chocolate Peanut Butter + Banana "Milkshake"
For a tasty post-workout recovery

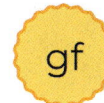

Marcus Wyatt is a skeleton racer who represented Great Britain at the Beijing 2022 Olympics, and he is also the first British Men's World Cup Medalist since 2013.

Marcus's go-to post-workout snack is this chocolate peanut butter and banana "milkshake." If this "milkshake" isn't an incentive to workout, I don't know what is. This delicious recipe is perfect for those on the go because it only uses 5 ingredients!

Makes 1 serving

2.5 cups of milk (dairy-free if sensitive)
1 scoop of chocolate protein powder
1 medium banana (frozen for a creamier texture)
3 tablespoons smooth peanut butter
1 handful of ice cubes

1. Add the milk, protein powder, banana, peanut butter, and ice into a blender and blend on a high speed until smooth.
2. Pour into a large glass and enjoy! If you are saving it for later, store it in an airtight glass jar in the fridge for up to 4 days. Shake before drinking.

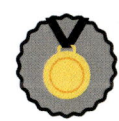

Don't have chocolate protein powder?
Simply use plain flavored protein powder and add 1.5 tablespoons cocoa powder.

V To make this recipe vegan, use non-dairy milk and vegan protein powder.

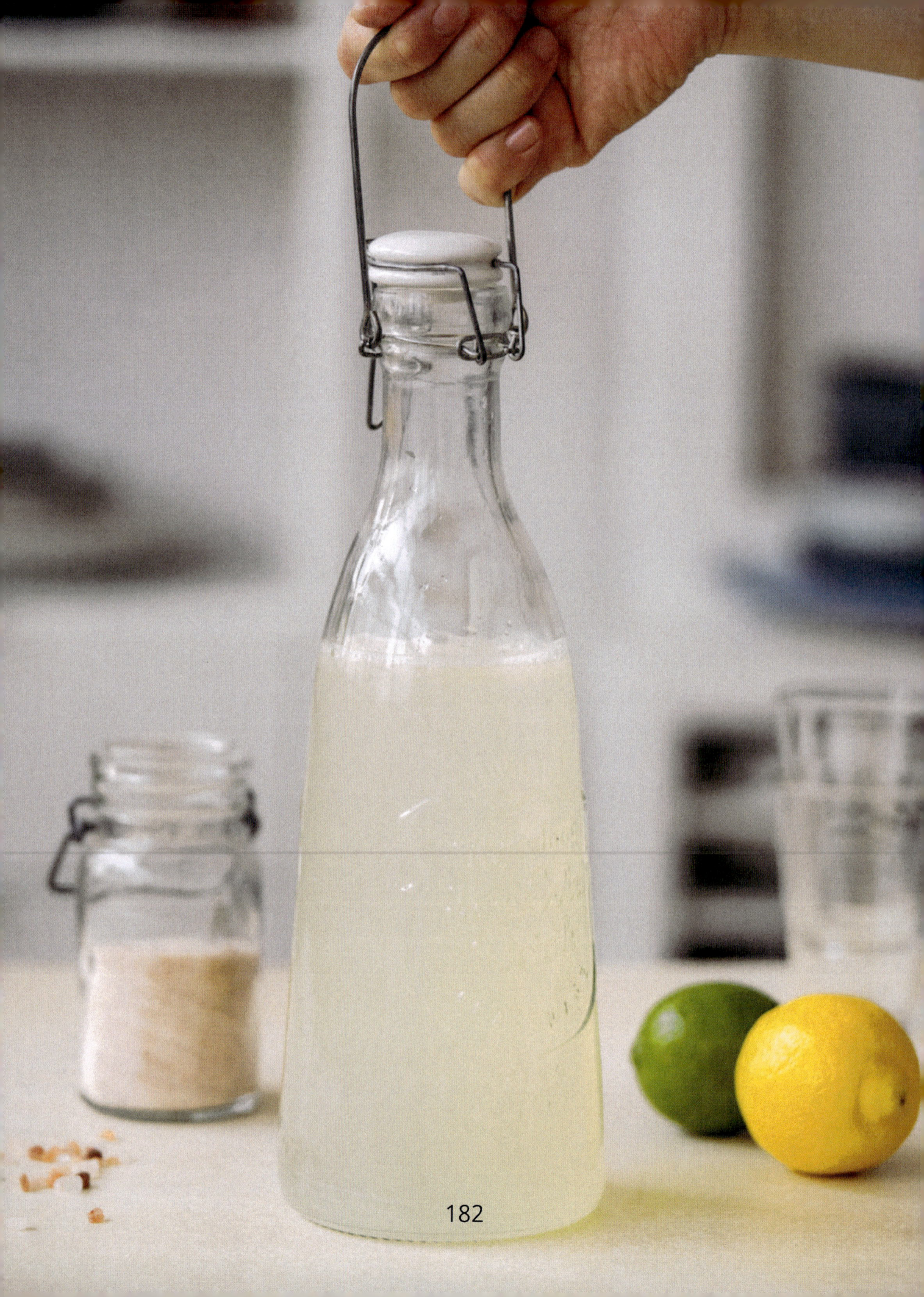

Electrolyte Lemon Limeade

For refreshing hydration

v df gf

Chugging lots of plain water is not always enough when hydrating. This is because water doesn't contain all of the electrolytes, salts, and minerals necessary for restoring our body's fluid balance. Most electrolyte sports drinks are advantageous, but they contain high levels of sugar and additives, meaning they are not great to have every day.

This lemon limeade recipe is simple, delicious, and covers all of the bases to ensure proper hydration, especially before and after a sweaty workout.

Makes 4 1/2 cups

2 cups coconut water
2 cups filtered water
1/4 cup fresh lemon juice (about 1 lemon)
1/4 cup fresh lime juice (about 1 lime)
1/4 teaspoon Himalayan pink salt
2 tablespoons raw honey (optional)

1. In a pitcher or glass jar, combine the coconut water, filtered water, lemon juice, lime juice, salt, and honey (if using).
2. Stir the mixture, and cover the pitcher or jar in the fridge for up to a week.

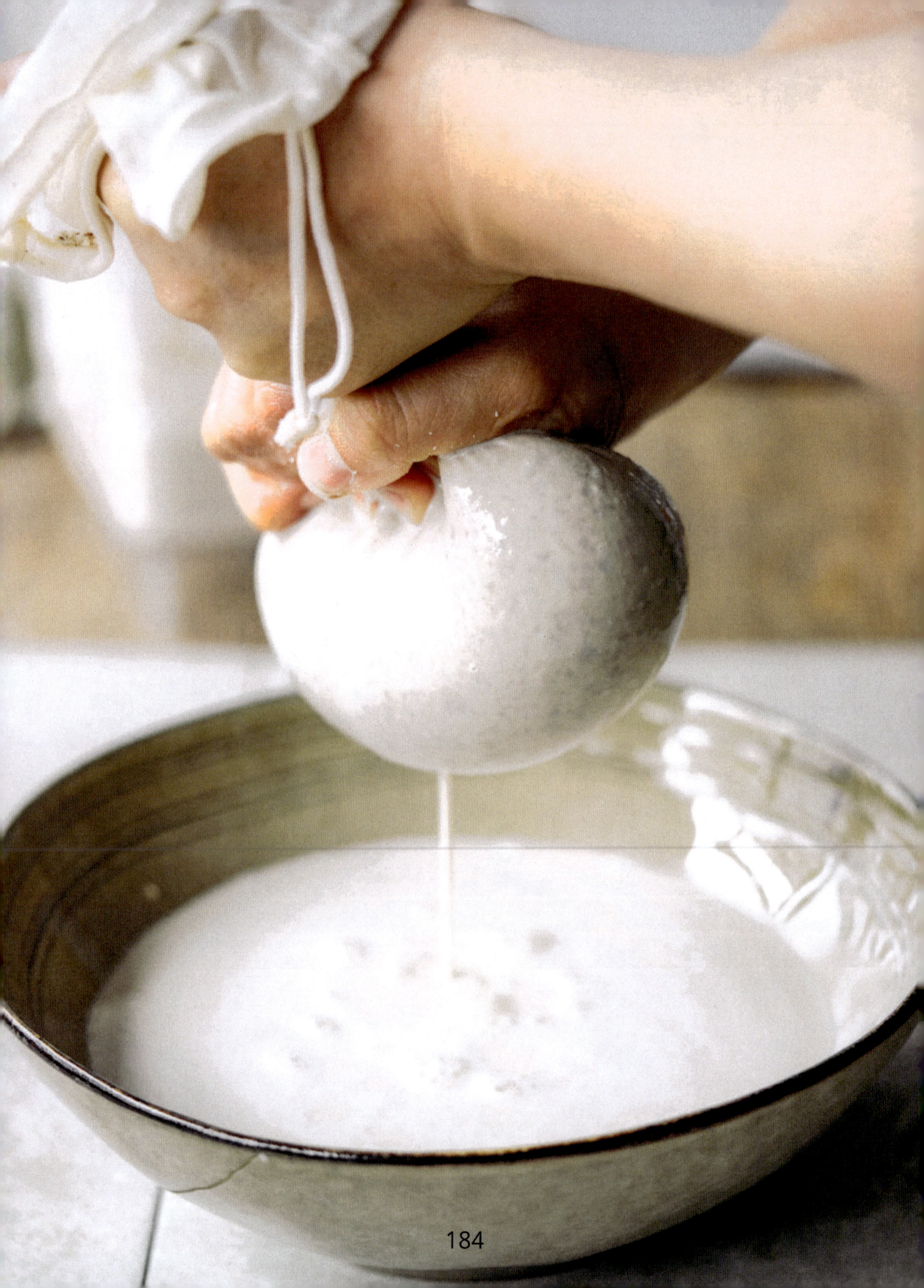

Vanilla Nut + Seed Milk
For a sweet sip

v • df • gf

I have a slight obsession with Vanilla Almond Butter, so this recipe is a staple in my house! Not only does it taste like birthday cake (especially when using cashews or almonds as the base), but it can be added to oatmeal, overnight oats, pancakes, or a morning coffee for extra sweetness and flavor. Or, like me, you can just drink it straight from the jar post-workout. Soaking the nuts overnight makes the milk extra creamy and increases their nutrient bioavailability and digestibility. Kate Hansen loves making sesame milk (blend 1/4 cup sesame seeds into a powder, then blend in 2 cups warm water, 5 dates, and cinnamon!).

Don't want to wait all night for the nuts to soak? No problem! Simply use 4 tablespoons of your favorite nut or seed butter instead of 2 cups of nuts.

Makes 5 cups

2 cups nuts or seeds, soaked if desired
4 cups cold filtered water
4 Medjool dates, pitted
1/2 teaspoon vanilla extract
Pinch of salt

Extras:
1/4 teaspoon cinnamon (or any spice)
1 tablespoon maple syrup (or any other liquid sweetener)

1. Add the nuts, water, dates, vanilla, and salt into a blender and blend on high speed for about 90 seconds or until the mixture is smooth and frothy.
2. Place a nut-milk bag over a bowl and pour the mixture into the bag. Twist and squeeze the top of the bag to ensure all of the milk is collected.
3. Pour the nut milk into a pitcher or large glass jar and cover with a lid. Store in the fridge for up to 5 days. Shake before serving as the milk is likely to separate.

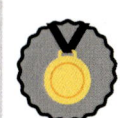

Creaminess tips:

- Soak the nuts for 4-12 hours (overnight is best). Drain and rinse the nuts well before blending.
- Strain all kinds of milk for the smoothest texture; apart from cashew milk, hemp milk, and pumpkin seed milk.

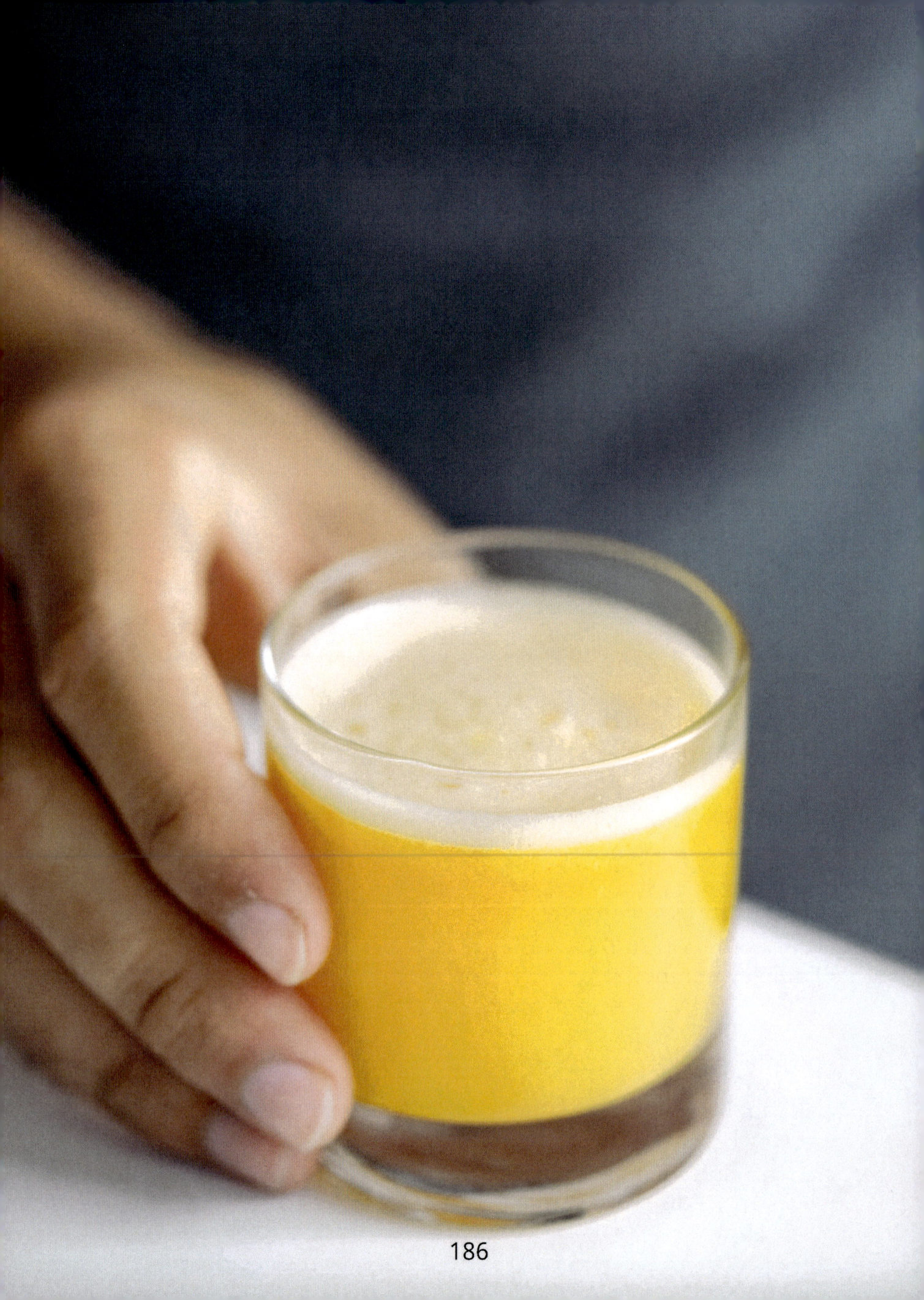

The Immunity Booster

For a fiery kick to wake up all of your systems

v df nf gf

This immunity-boosting tonic fires up your digestive and immune systems and is best to take first thing in the morning so that the body can quickly absorb all of the beneficial nutrients and compounds. Immune-boosting foods work best when you start to feel symptoms of a virus coming on before it has had a chance to settle in your body.

Here is a quick breakdown of each ingredient:
- Apple cider vinegar balances PH levels in the body, adds good bacteria for the gut and immune function, and aids digestion.
- The citrusy lemon and orange juices improve digestion and are full of vitamin C, which strengthens immunity.
- Spices like ginger, turmeric, and cayenne pepper are anti-inflammatory and rich in antioxidants, which protect our cells and promote health.
- Raw honey is full of antioxidants, is antibacterial, and soothes a sore throat or cough.

Be warned, this drink is incredible for immunity, but its overpowering (and fiery) taste is not for the faint of heart. I confess that I struggled to find the bravery to recipe test this one!

Makes 2 1/2 cups

1 cup unfiltered orange juice
1 cup water
1 tablespoon apple cider vinegar
1 (2 inch) piece fresh ginger, peeled
1/8 teaspoon of cayenne pepper
1/4 teaspoon ground turmeric
1 lemon, peeled, sliced, and seeded
1 tablespoon honey

1. In a high-speed blender, combine the orange juice, water, apple cider vinegar, ginger, cayenne pepper, turmeric, lemon, and honey. Blend on a high speed until smooth.
2. Pour into a glass jar or bottle, then store in the fridge for up to 4 days; freeze in ice cube trays for up to 3 months.
3. Drink a shot-glass-size amount first thing in the morning, or 15-30 minutes before a meal. Chase with water.

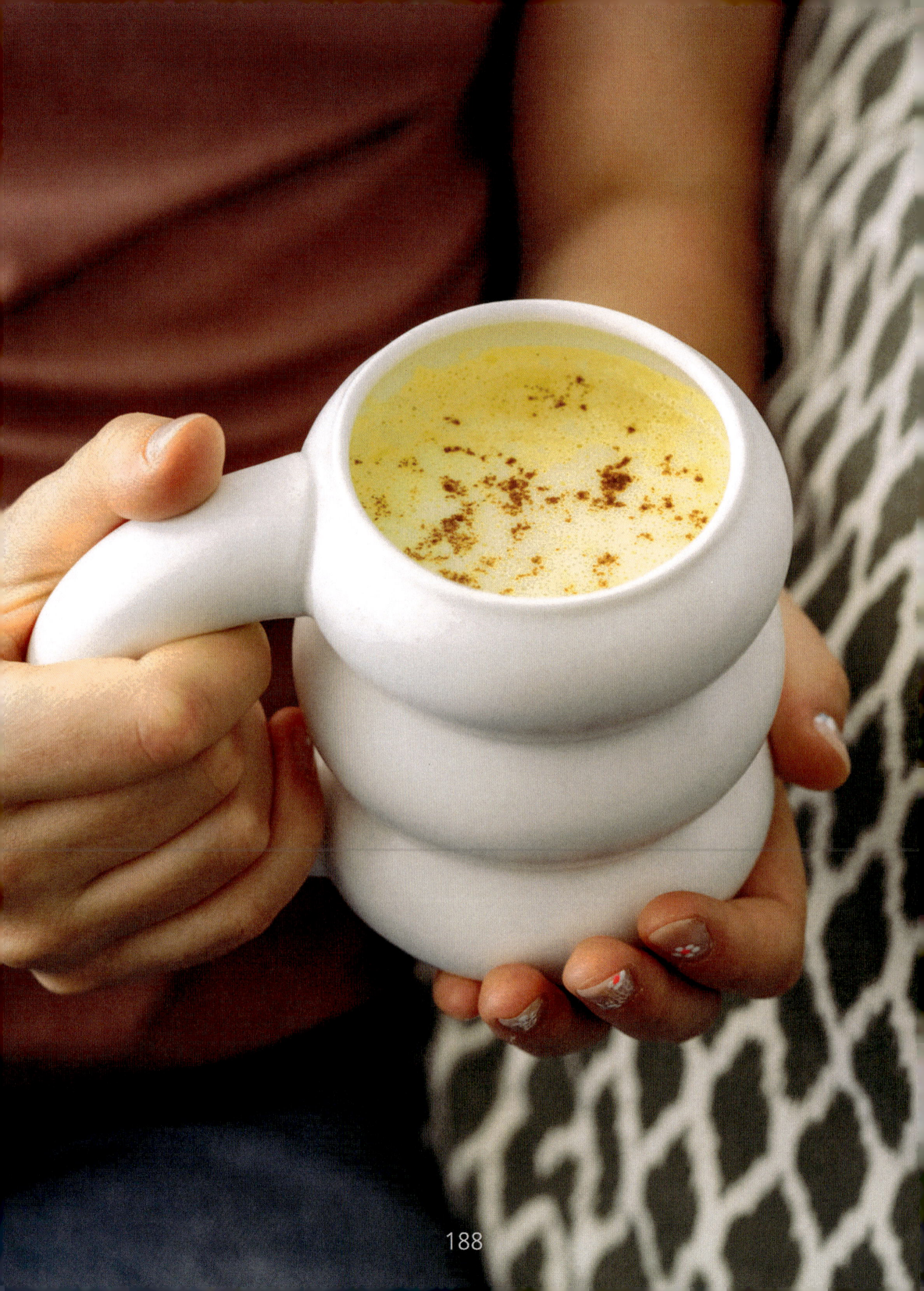

Anti-Inflammatory Golden Milk

For a golden start to the day

v · df · gf

This golden drink has so many health benefits, it's sure to get you closer to your gold medal. The flavorful anti-inflammatory spices such as ginger, turmeric, cinnamon, and cardamom—all paired with nut milk—are comforting for early mornings or even for an afternoon pick-me-up.

Most store-bought nut milks have a lot of additives which means they are less nutritious and can be difficult to digest. Making your own nut milk not only tastes better, but it is more nourishing as the simple ingredients ensure that every nutrient is available.

This milk can be heated on the stove for a cozy drink, or used in our G.O.A.T.meal (page 39), our Champion Chia Overnight Oats (page 51), any of our smoothies (pages 178, 195), or added to coffee and tea for an extra nutrient boost.

Makes 1 serving

3/4 cup cashews
3 cups filtered water
1/4 teaspoon raw honey OR 3 Medjool dates
1-inch ginger root, peeled
1/2 teaspoon ground turmeric
Pinch of ground cinnamon
Pinch of ground cardamom

Note: unlike other nut milks, cashew milk doesn't need to be strained as cashews become very soft after soaking.

1. Mix all of the ingredients in a glass jar or container and seal. Allow the nuts to soak by storing the jar in the fridge overnight.
2. In the morning, use a high-speed blender to combine all of the ingredients and blend until smooth or creamy. If the milk is too thick, add a splash of water for a lighter result.
3. Store in a jar in the fridge for up to 4 days.

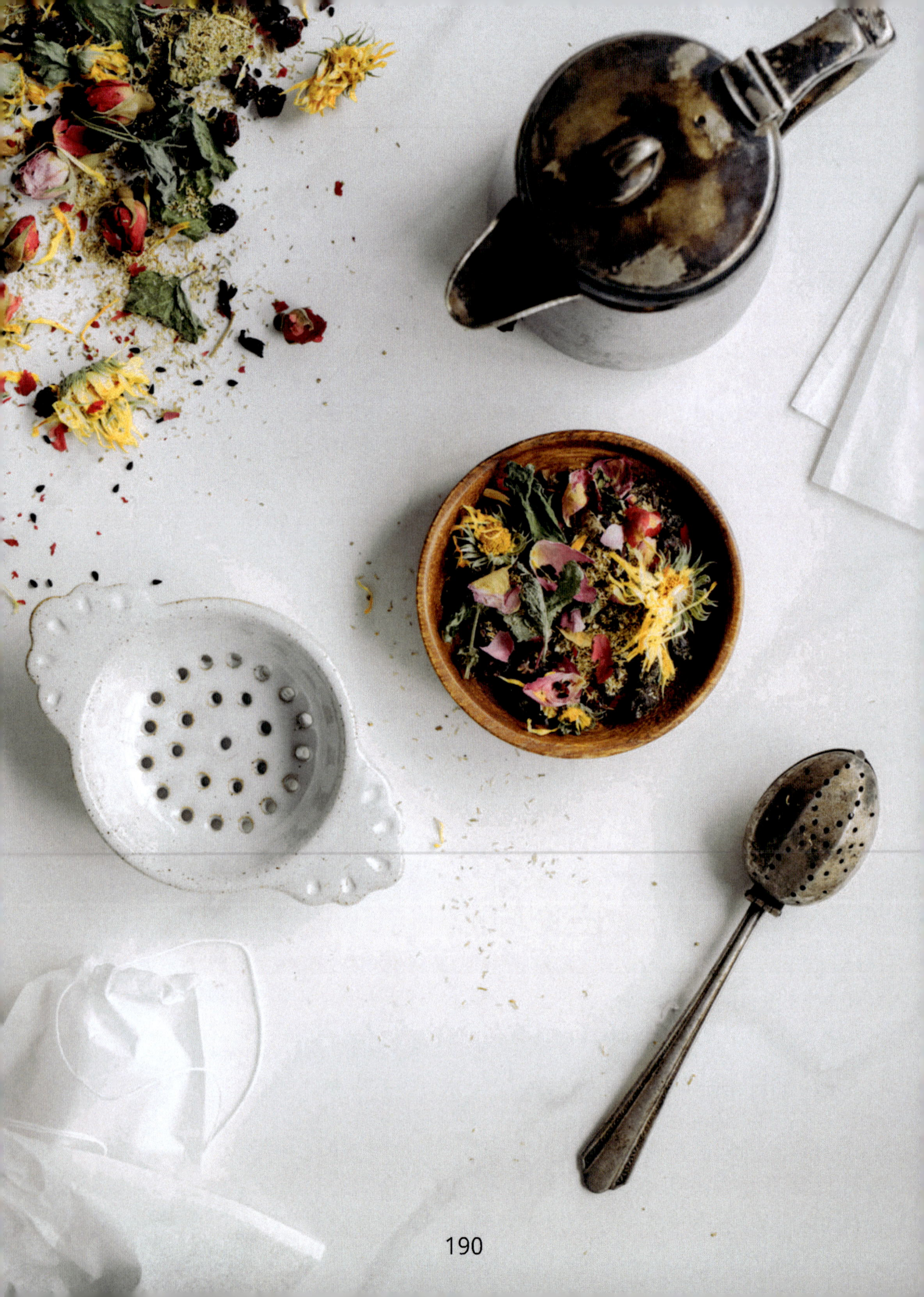

Tranquility Tea
For a deep sleep

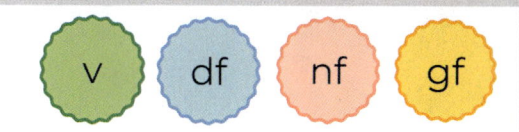

v · df · nf · gf

This calming tea includes organic botanicals that encourage restful sleep, relaxation, and help the body wind down before bed.

Here is some more information about the benefits of each ingredient:
- **Chamomile:** has a gentle sedative effect that calms the nervous system.
- **Rose:** is for muscle tension and reduces inflammation in the body.
- **Lemon balm:** aids indigestion, muscle cramps, and alleviates stress.
- **Red currants:** improve digestion, immunity, and are full of antioxidants.
- **Holy basil:** a miracle herb for the mind and body. It's rich in antioxidants and anti-inflammatory. As an adaptogen, it restores balance in the body, mind, and spirit. It eases the nervous system to decrease stress and promotes repair and recovery in an overworked body.
- **Hibiscus:** is packed with antioxidants and is extremely flavorful.
- **Calendula:** a medicinal flower rich in antioxidants that promotes tissue repair and is anti-inflammatory.

Makes 25 cups of tea

0.4 ounce organic chamomile
0.5 ounce organic dried rose petals
0.25 ounce organic dried lemon balm
0.4 ounce organic dried red currants
0.4 ounce organic holy basil
0.4 ounce dried hibiscus
0.1 ounce organic calendula
Boiling water, for brewing
Optional: honey, for serving

1. Combine the chamomile, rose petals, lemon balm, red currant, holy basil, hibiscus, and calendula in a glass jar or tea tin and shake until all the ingredients are mixed evenly. Store in the pantry for up to 3 months.
2. To brew the tea, simply place 2-3 tablespoons of the blend in a tea bag or tea infuser and pour 1 cup of boiling water over the top. Cover and let it steep for 5-7 minutes. Remove the infuser and add honey if desired.

NOTE: while this blend is generally regarded as very safe, we can all react differently to herbal teas. If you have any medical concerns or are pregnant, consult with a doctor before consuming.

192

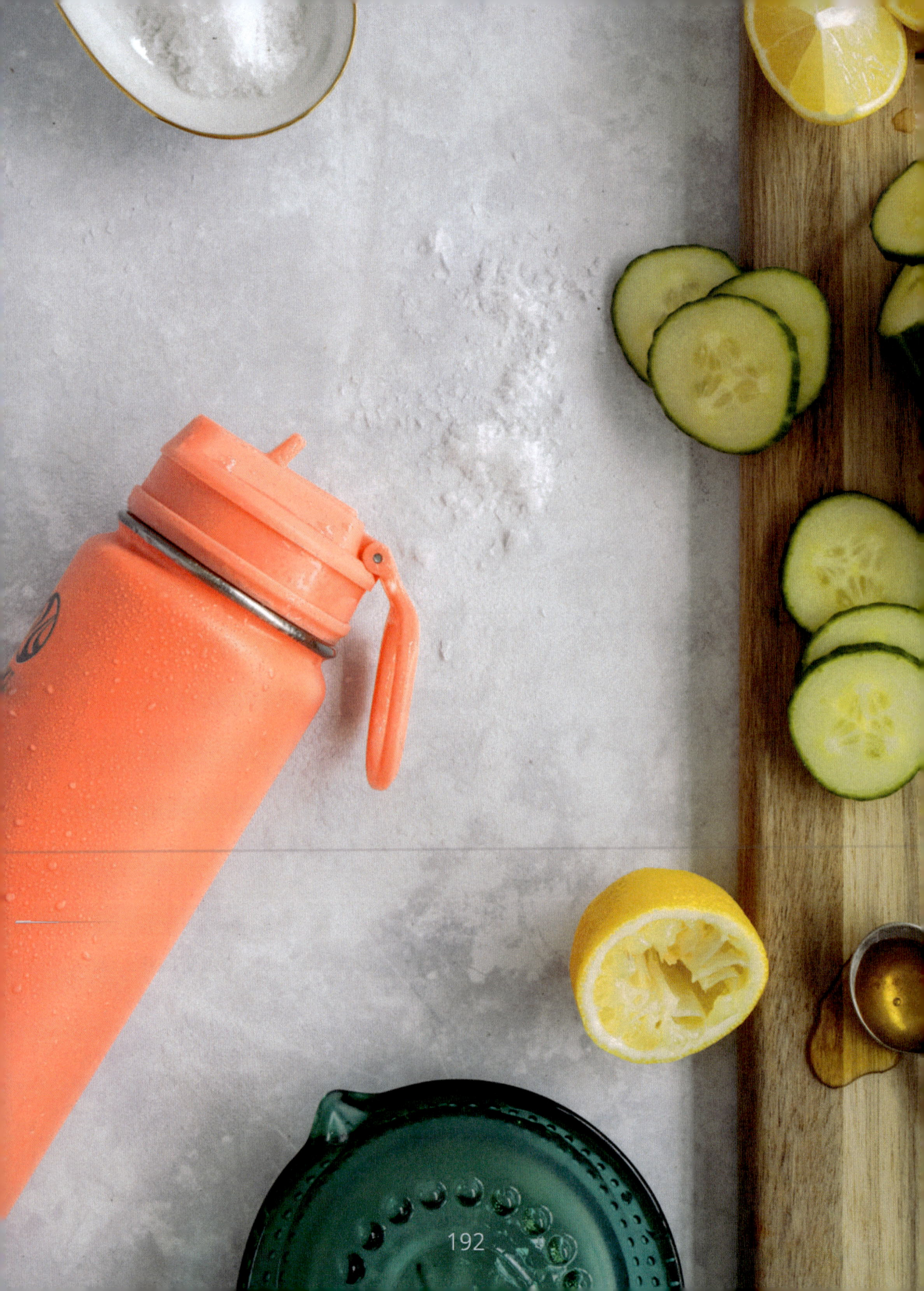

Cool as a Cucumber Water

BONUS RECIPE

Guillaume Cizeron is a French ice dancer who won silver in Pyeongchang 2018 and gold in Beijing 2022 alongside his partner Gabriella Papadakis. Not only is he an Olympic Champion, but he is also a 5x World Champion, 5x consecutive European Champion, 7x National Champion—and he has broken world records 28 times. Guillaume and Gabriella are known for their lyrical and modern movements, and the quality of their skating skills is unparalleled. It is a privilege to train with G&G, and they are some of the best ice dancers of all time. Check out Guillame's book *Ma Plus Belle Victoire* where he opens up about his homosexuality and becoming his truest self.

Here Guillaume shares his post-training recovery drink. The lemon juice provides phytonutrients and aids digestion, and the cucumber provides antioxidants and is a naturally hydrating food (they are made of 95% water!). The sprinkle of salt restores electrolytes, and the honey allows your muscles to absorb glucose after intense training.

Makes 1 serving

16 ounce bottle of water
Juice of 1/2 a lemon
6 slices of cucumber
1 teaspoon honey
Pinch of salt

1. Add the lemon juice, cucumber slices, honey, and salt to the bottle of water. Close the lid and shake until fully combined. Store in fridge to keep cool.

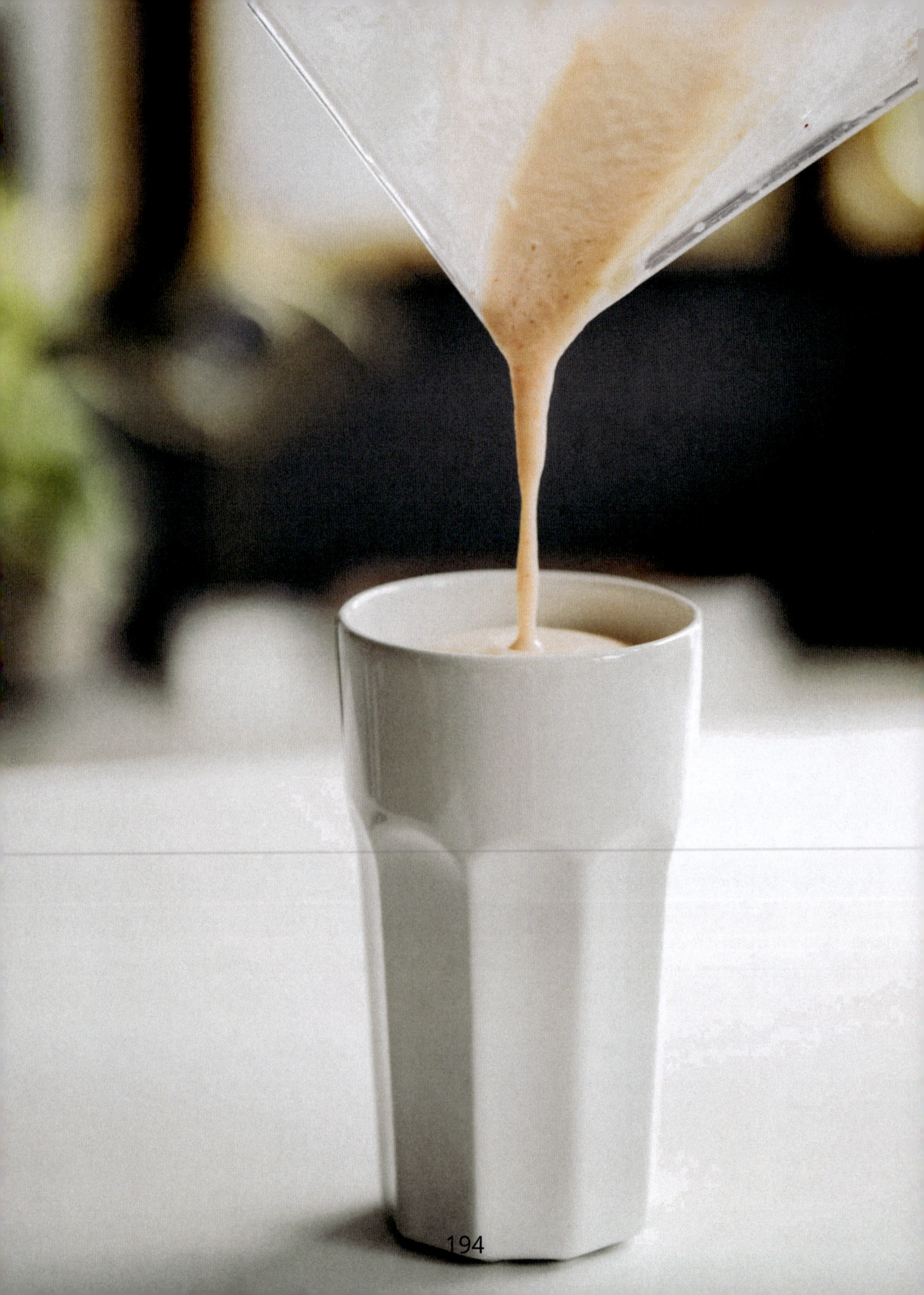

Sunrise Smoothie
BONUS RECIPE

gf

Bruce Mouat is a Scottish curler who represented Great Britain at the Beijing 2022 Olympic Games. Not only did he carry the team to an Olympic Silver Medal, but he is also a 3x World Championship medalist.

Here, Bruce will shares his favorite smoothie recipe that he makes as a snack, but it can be a great breakfast option, too. The frozen fruit paired with the greek yogurt makes a creamy, dreamy smoothie that tastes like a tropical paradise.

Makes 1 serving

1 frozen banana
1/2 cup frozen strawberries
1/2 cup frozen mango
1/2 cup of Greek yogurt
Splash of almond milk or milk of choice
Optional: 1 tablespoon honey for sweetness

In a high-speed blender, combine all of the ingredients and blend until smooth. If the smoothie is too thick to blend, add a splash of water or extra milk.

df **Want to make it dairy-free?**
Swap out the Greek yogurt for 2 tablespoons of collagen peptides, hemp protein, or hemp seeds for a protein boost.

Try to avoid pea protein and whey protein powders as they tend to be high in additives and toxins, and are difficult to digest.

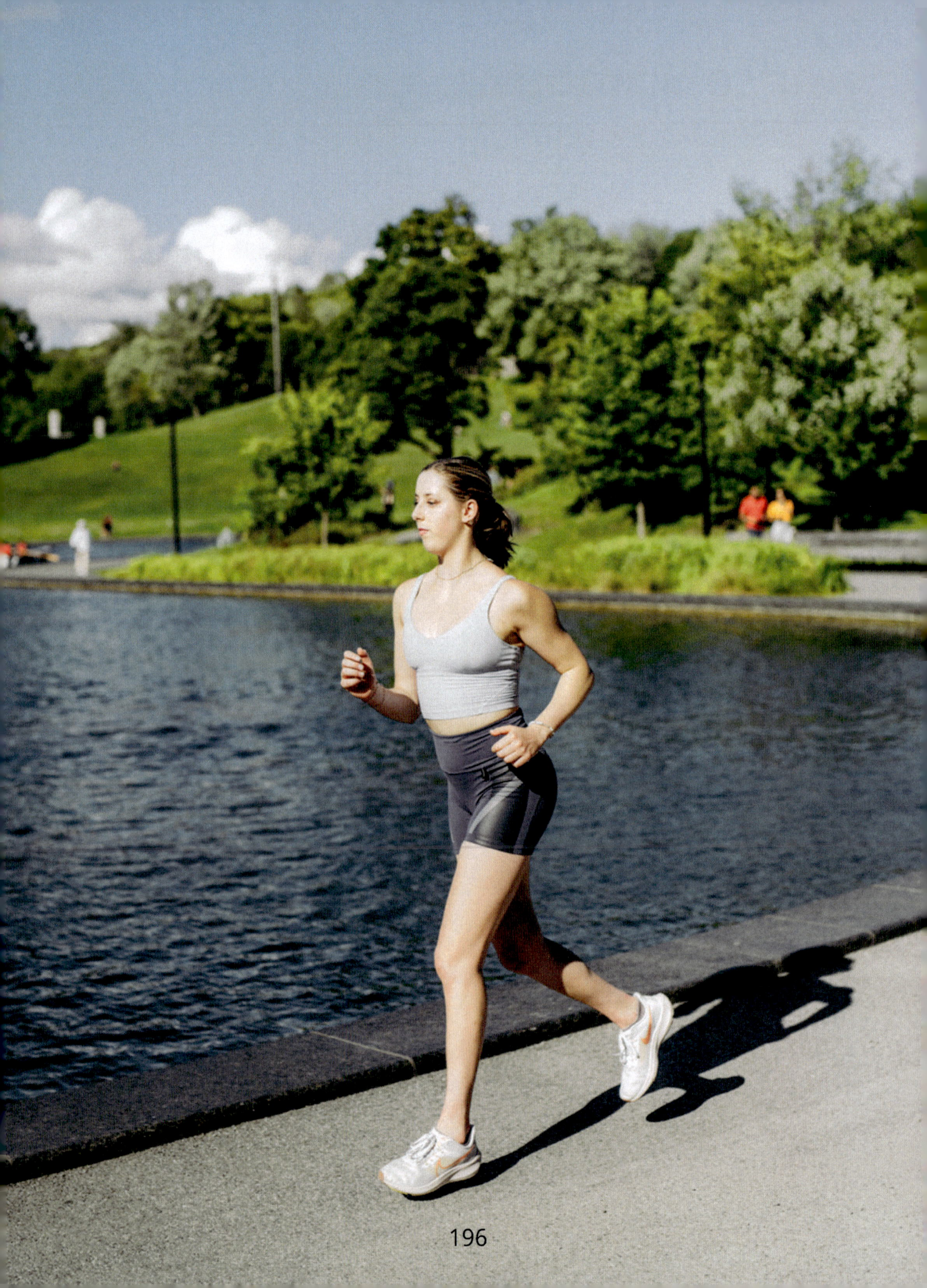

TRAIN TO GAIN

Exercise inspiration
a training exercise each Olympian swears by

Athlete	Exercise
Lilah Fear (Ice Dance)	Romanian Deadlifts (see page 205) ☑ Strengthens the posterior chain
Brian Orser (Figure Skating)	Running, hopping, and grapevine 30 seconds on 30 seconds off ☑ For building stamina
Bruce Mouat (Curling)	Power Cleans (see page 205) ☑ High intensity and works upper and lower body
Hailey Duff (Curling)	Rowing Intervals: • 30 seconds on 30 seconds off sprint OR 500m sprint Cycling or stationary bike intervals: • 30 seconds on 30 seconds off sprint OR prolonged cycle
Emily Brydon (Alpine Skiing)	Cross-Training: Mountain Biking ☑ "There is speed, fear, lines, jumps, tactics, fun."

Benjamin Alexander (Alpine Skiing)	Quick Spin Class: "I love crushing 20-minute Peloton classes." ☑ Shorter high-intensity rides allow you to maintain a high resistance and cadence versus long-distance rides
Jason Brown (Figure Skating)	Swimming laps and treading water ☑ Low impact cardio (great for injuries) Step-ups with weight (see page 207) ☑ Improves power and lower body conditioning
Shaolin Liu and Shaoang Liu (Short-Track Speed Skating)	Cardio favorites: bike and running ☑ Running strengthens joints and bones
Charlotte Kalla (Cross-Country Skiing)	Cardio favorites: Roller skating, running, strength on the bike, and cross country skiing ☑ "I do a few hours of distance training, and 15% of it is at a higher pace." Olympic barbell and free weights
Marcus Wyatt (Skeleton)	Cardio favorite: 80m sprints (2 sets x 10 reps). Sprint 80m at 80-90% intensity, then walk back to the start and go again

Kai Owens (Mogul Skiing)	Cardio favorites: Mountain biking, stationary bike sprints, and swimming laps Strength: Single leg explosive leg press and straight leg deadlifts (see page 205)
Bree Walker (Bobsled)	Rear-foot Elevated Split Squats (see page 207) ☑ Targets lower body: "the main emphasis is on our legs being in a quarter squat for most of our sessions on the snow"
Jaelin Kauf (Freestyle Skiing)	Daily core and back squats (see page 205-206) ☑ Stabilizing weights on back squats improve lower body, lower back, and core strength
Jon Eley (Short-Track Speed Skating)	Plyometric drills or muscle lab testing in the gym: ☑ Explosive movements where your muscles exert maximum force in a short interval of time to increase power
Kate Hansen (Luge)	Strength training favorite: Pull-Ups ☑ Best for targeting upper body strength
Bree Walker (Bobsled)	Power Cleans (see page 205) ☑ Focuses on explosive power

Francesco Costa (Bobsled)	Trains twice a day:
	  1. Sprints on a running track to target fast-twitch fibers, increase speed, and improve stamina
	  2. Gym: squats, bench press, clean, and deadlift for full-body strength (see page 205)

Anna Fernstädt (Skeleton)	"I do a lot of functional and dynamic strength. I love Romanian deadlifts with kettlebells and burpees!"
Neville Wright (Bobsled)	Trap Bar Deadlifts: ☑ To develop the glutes, hamstrings, and back Box Jumps: ☑ For explosive vertical jumping power
Meryl Davis (Ice Dance)	Oblique Crunches ☑ Sculpt waist and abdominals Lunge Walks with Weights ☑ For lower body strength and stability Y-T-Ws (see page 206) ☑ For full upper body strength
Michelle Uhrig (Speed Skating)	Inline Skating ☑ Helps develop power, strength, and helps train the fundamentals needed on the ice
Josh Williamson (Bobsled)	Strength: Power cleans and squats Cardio: Sprints with plenty of rest between reps to allow the body to recharge

Lewis Gibson (Ice Dance)	"I love stability training and finding imbalances in my body as it's so connected to my sport. I feel a sense of accomplishment when I get beyond the real thinking stage and find myself flowing and moving evenly on both sides of my body." Favorite Cardio: Beat Spin Classes ☑ Low impact: riding to the beat of the music is important as ice dance is a performance sport
Dawn Richardson Wilson (Bobsled)	Snatches: "I love the technical aspects that go into snatches, and how—when done correctly—it just flows."
Amy Williams, MBE (Skeleton)	"For skeleton, you need to be powerful, fast and explosive, so we do very specific exercises to help us get strong in the bent-over position as we push the skeleton sled" Gym: "Powerlifting like squats, cleans, snatch, leg press, bench press, and then more specific, single leg work, stability, and core for balance as we push the sled with one arm"
	Favorite Exercise: Cleans "I feel so much speed and power when I get it right and the bar flies up. Seeing my performance improve, even if it's tiny weight increases each week or two, is always a great feeling."
Gabriella Papadakis (Ice Dance)	"I love taking my roller skates to the Formula 1 circuit in Montréal and just doing laps and laps until I'm dead. It trains a lot of the same muscles that I need for skating, but it's nice to go as fast as I can, and the view is wonderful."

Guillame Cizeron (Ice Dance)	Cardio: Stationary Bike 4 x 20 seconds full out on gear 20, rest 20 seconds (4 rounds total) Strength: Abs on a Swiss Ball (see page 205) ☑ Extends the range of motion when you do a crunch, activating more abdominal muscles
Adrian Fässler (Bobsled)	Cardio: Wattbike Intervals: 4-second sprint, 3 reps, air resistance 6, rest 4 min 4-second sprint, 3 reps, air resistance 5, rest 4 min 4-second sprint, 3 reps, air resistance 4, rest 4 min
Will Finely (Mogul Skiing)	Strength: Back Squat ☑ It's necessary to have strong legs, not just for power, but also for protection Strength: Calisthenics exercises "I think it's important to be able to move your bodyweight any way you need, having as much control and grace as possible."
Britt Cox (Mogul Skiing)	Cardio: "I fell in love with cycling while recovering from an upper-body injury. I used a virtual cycling platform called Zwift where you use smart training to race people around the world. This scratched my competitive itch while I was unable to compete on snow, but has since become a regular part of my training." Strength: Anything Single Leg: "There is so much value in bilateral lower limb training for mogul skiing—it's also a useful way to load the lower body without requiring extra weight/equipment."

Ryan Harden (Curling)	Strength: For sweepers: anti-rotation trunk work For shoulders: single-arm plank hold For shooting: walking lunge or step-ups Full body: Dead Bug is "the king of all movements" (see page 205)
Mercedes Nicoll (Snowboarder)	Strength: Clock Lunges (see page 207) ☑ Build strength in knees and ankles, and improve agility and balance

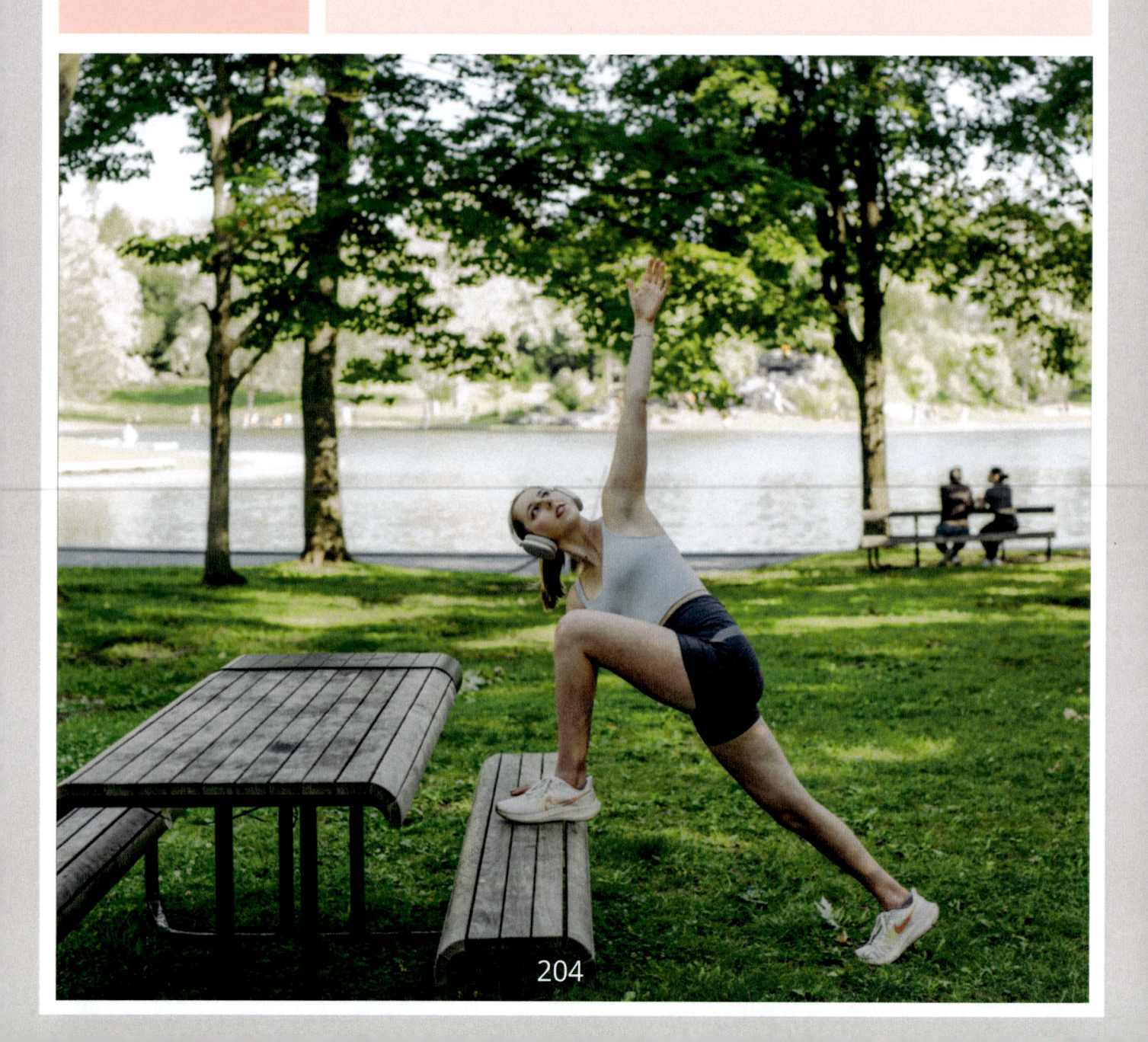

Single-Leg RDL

With or without a weight, reach your hands towards the ground while lifting and lengthening one leg behind you.

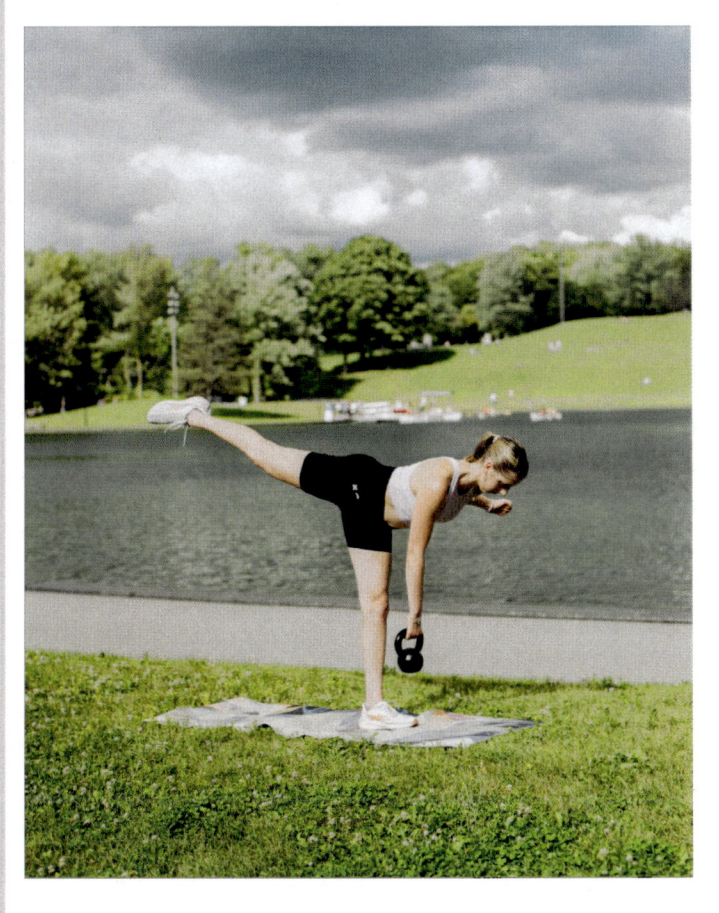

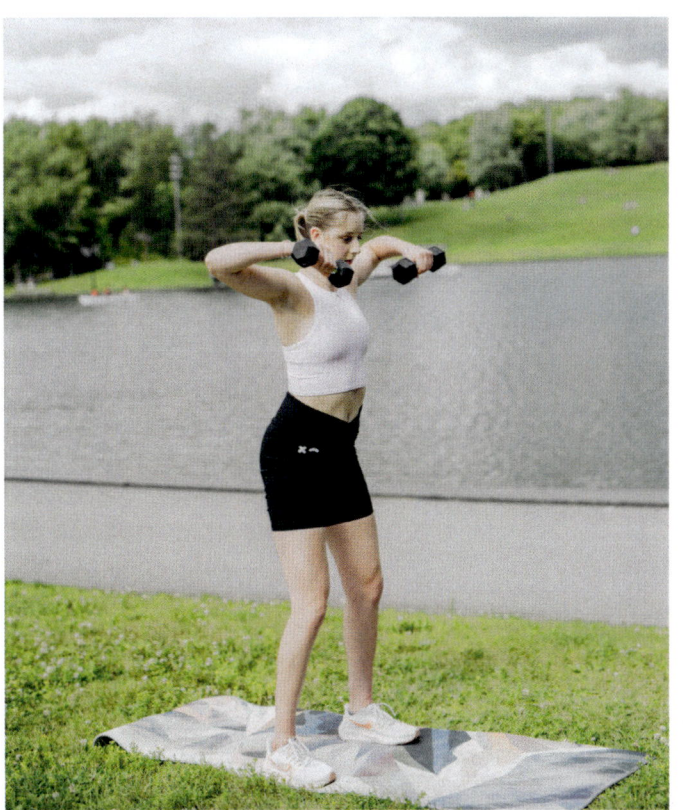

Power Clean

Start in a squat, feet hip distance apart, with a flat back and engaged core. As you stand, pull the weights or barbell up and thrust your hips forward. Shrug your elbows and feel your shoulder blades pulling down your back as you catch the weight on the front of your shoulders.

Crush Your Core

Use a pilates ball or Swiss ball. Press lower back into the ball to engage the core. Crunch up, reach one hand to the opposite knee, and slowly come down.

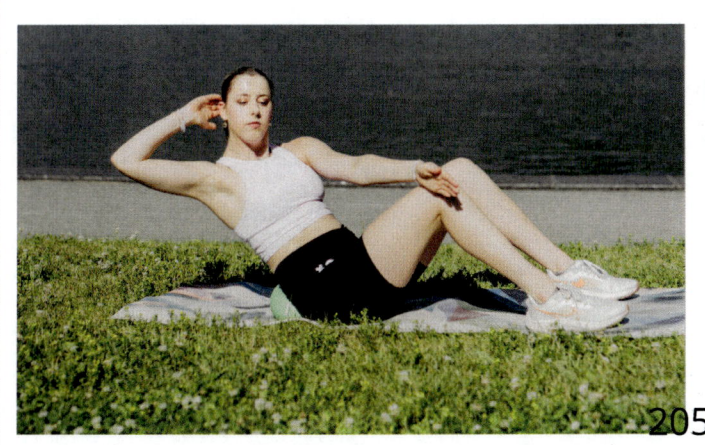

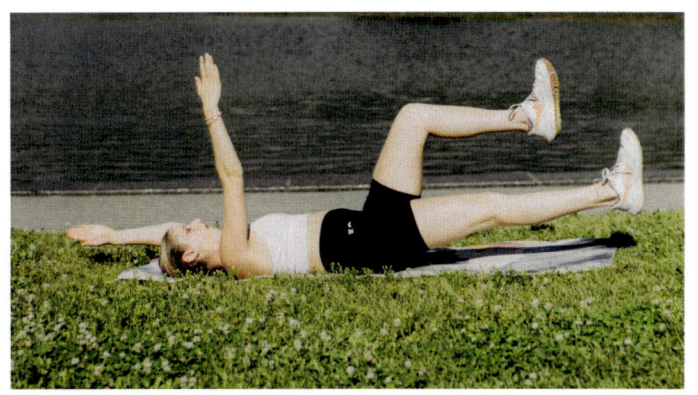

Deadbug

Reach one arm and leg in opposite directions pressing your lower back into the mat. Alternate sides.

TRX T-W-Y's

Lean back on an incline with your arms straight in front of you. Engage your lats, and reach your arms to the side into a T position. Slowly come back down, keeping tension in your shoulders and lats, and the TRX straps. Then bend your elbows and pull your knuckles back in a W position. Come down slowly. Finally, lift your arms above your head into a Y position.

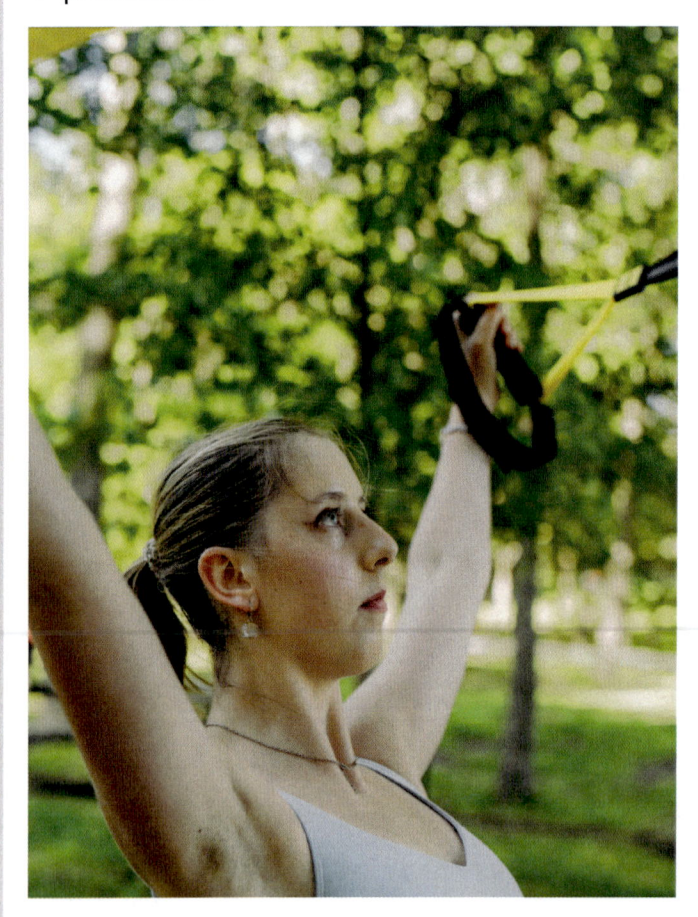

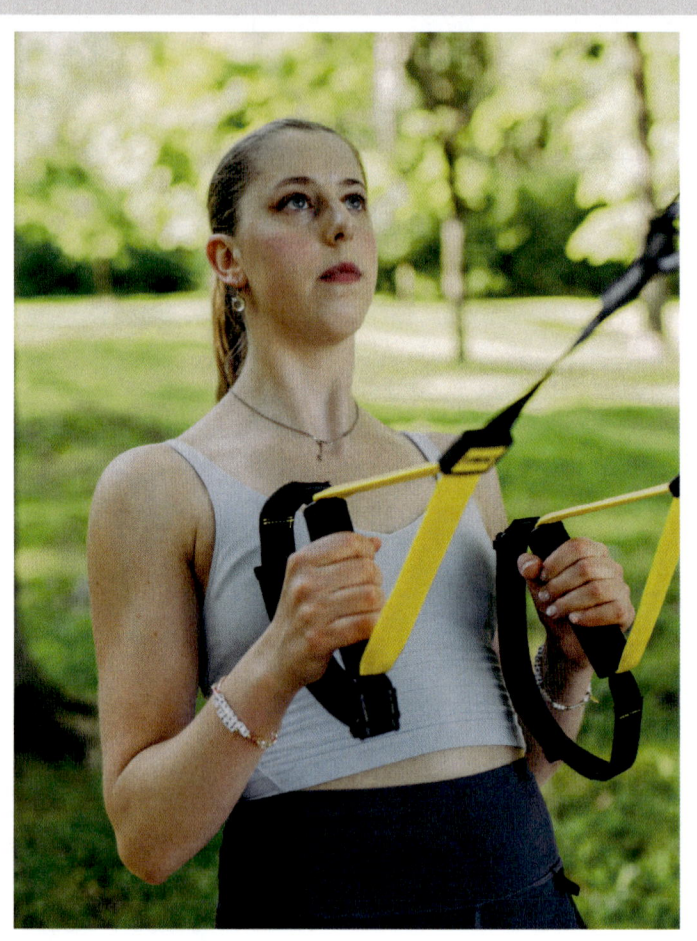

TRX Rows

Lean back on an incline to create an upright plant position with your arms straight in front of you. Pull your elbows tight into the side of your body with your palms facing in. Lower down slowly while still keeping your shoulders and lats engaged.

Planks

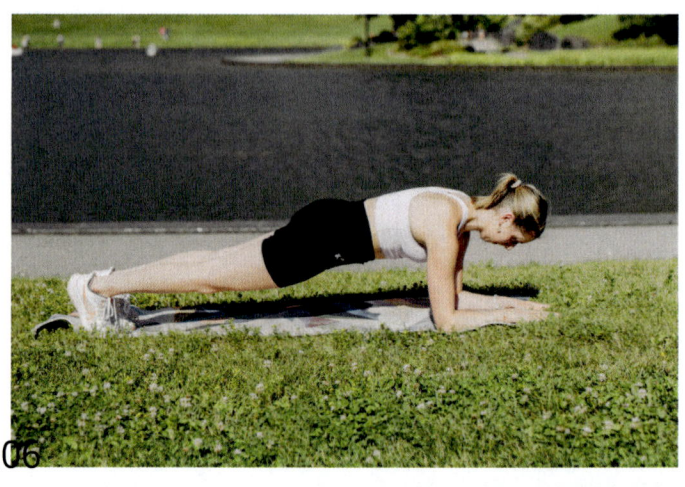

Challenge: One-arm planks. One arm is parallel to your chest and the other is behind your back.

Want to work those obliques? Hold a side plank for 45 seconds on each side. Add hip dips to take it to the next level.

Clock-Lunges

On one leg, lunge to the front, side, back, and across. Add ankle weights for difficulty.

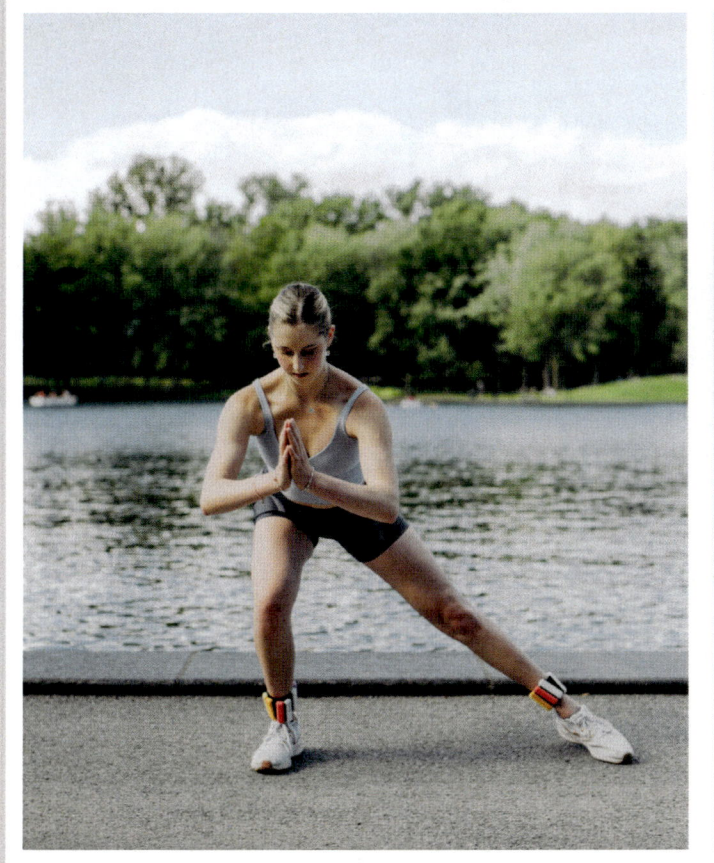

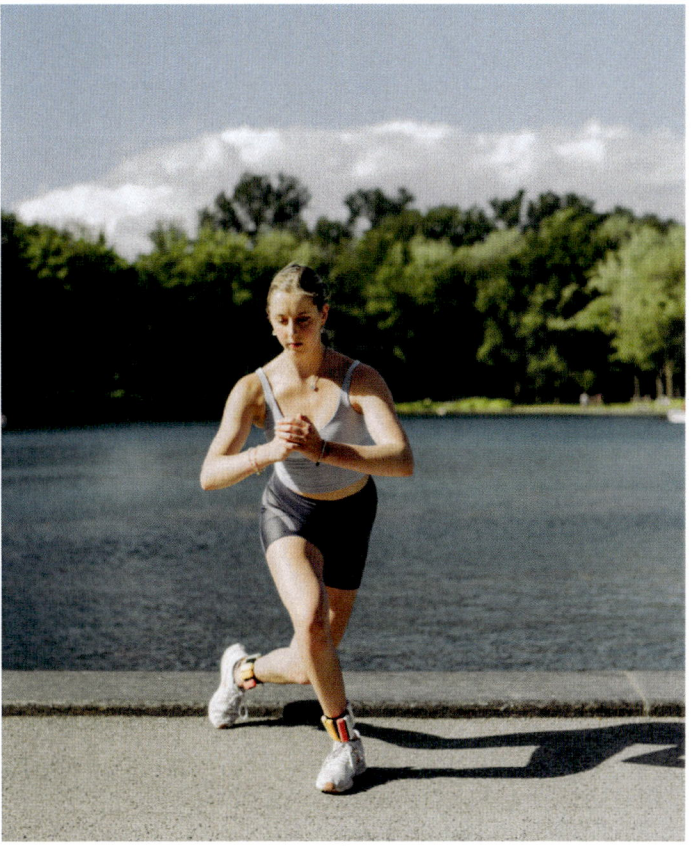

Elevated Split Squat

Step Ups

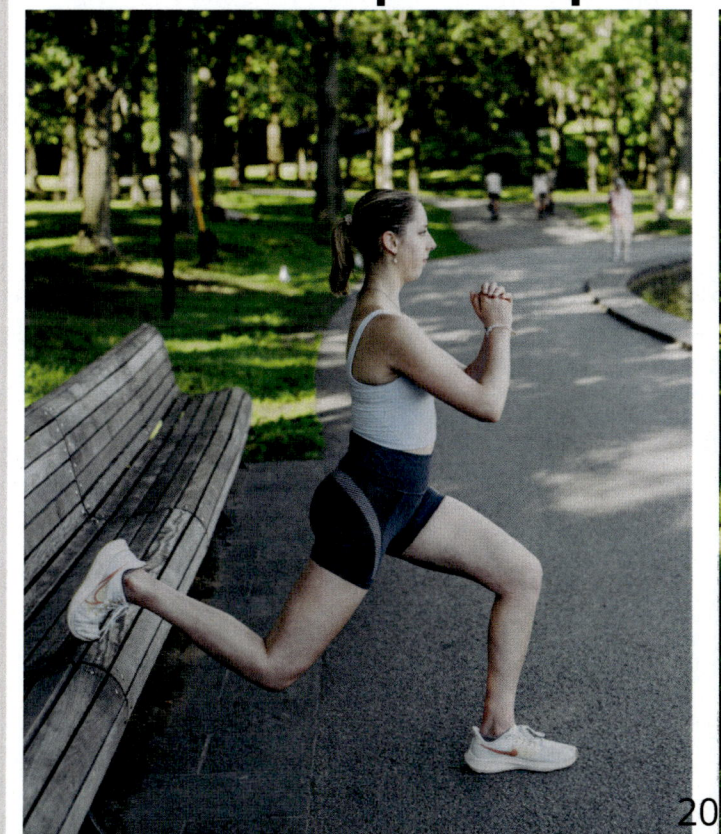

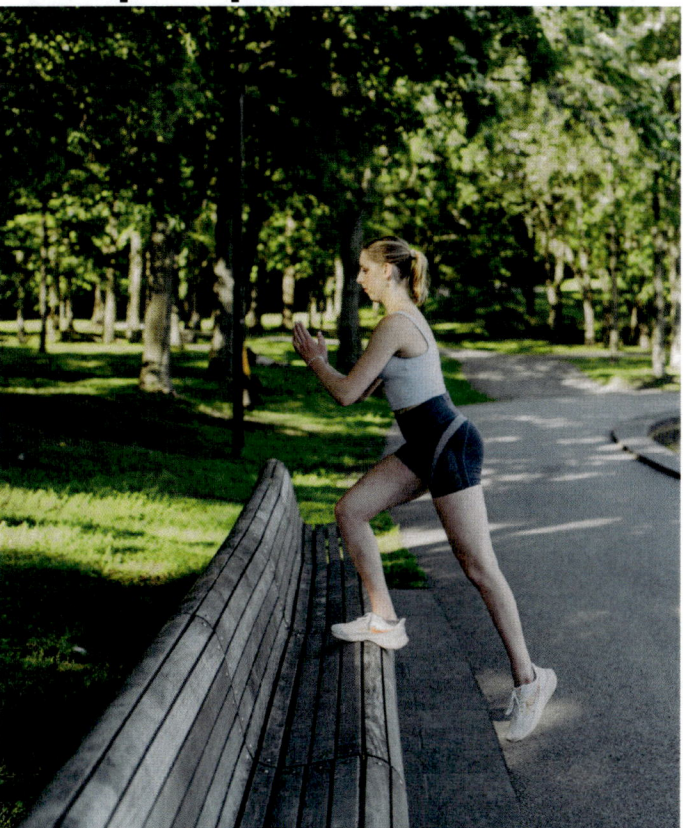

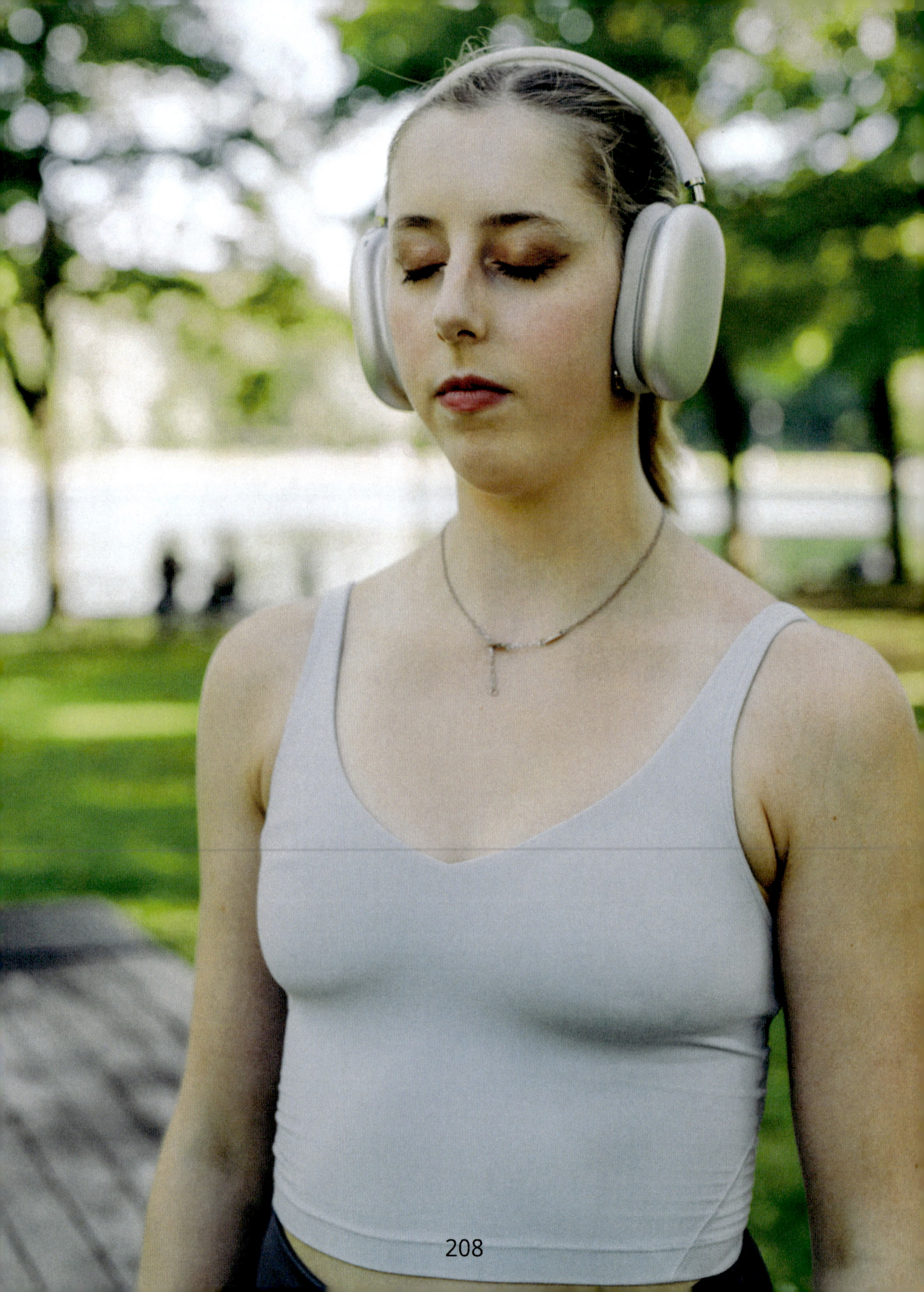

MENTAL PREPARATION

"Excellence can be achieved only today—not yesterday or tomorrow, because they do not exist in the present moment. Today is the only day you have to flex your talents and maximize your enjoyment. Your challenge is to win in all aspects of life. To reach that goal, you need to set yourself up for success by winning one day at a time. Procrastination is no match for a champion...think gold and never settle for silver."

— Jim Afremow, *The Champion's Mind: How Great Athletes Think, Train, and Thrive*

MENTAL TOOLS
how to get grounded and focused for competition

Mental preparation is equally important to physical preparation. Like any other muscle, it needs to be trained and strengthened. The way you perform all stems from how you think, your self-talk, and your mental resilience. If you decide you are going to fail, lose, or find something hard, guess what? You will. Your thoughts create feelings, and feelings create actions, and those actions create results. By shifting any destructive inner thoughts, finding self-belief, and staying present in your journey, you will have the mental freedom to grow, learn, and enjoy the process fully. Psychological skills such as visualization, goal-setting, concentration, mindfulness, positive self-talk, and developing a consistent routine, are all tools that elite athletes use to succeed. It takes years of practice to develop these skills in competition—to be at a place where you can truly trust your training and be present.

Most athletes are similar in their physical preparation, so being mentally prepared will really set you apart from the competition. The Olympics is every 4 years, making it rare, and this adds more pressure. Athletes who succeed set effective goals, learn from and accept criticism, are team players, and are extremely determined. Building champion-like habits and thoughts requires discipline, and you may feel resistant at first. You don't need to be perfect, but moments where you need to dig deep and hold yourself accountable will require more focus. For example: you may be lacking motivation at the gym or tempted by a plate of cookies. In those moments, come back to your WHY—what is your goal and ultimate dream? What drives your purpose? This will give you a surge of motivation and the ability to overcome any obstacle so that you can win the day.

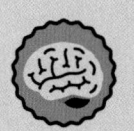

Mental Preparation Tools from Winter Olympians:

1. Lilah Fear's pre-competition mental ritual: Breath Work

- Close your eyes, take 5 slow deep breaths. Inhale through the nose, exhale through the mouth.
- Repeat a daily positive affirmation: for example "I am present, I am joyful, and I trust the process."
- The repetition of saying "I am..." rewires your brain, strengthens your self-belief, and changes your self-talk for good.

Tip: Personalize your self-talk to boost its effectiveness. For example, Lilah would say "you've got this, Lilah!"

2. Jason Brown's pre-competition mental ritual: Mantras

"On competition days, I always try to take an hour nap or even just set aside 10 minutes (depending on how tight the schedule is) to breathe, slow down my heart rate, and calm my mind. I remind myself that I am prepared, repeating the mantra **"preparation beats fear."** Before I step onto the ice, I clear my head as best as possible, telling myself how lucky I am to have this opportunity to perform and get to show people what I have been working so hard on. Then, I take one big, deep breath right before the music starts to ground myself in the present moment."

What would your pre-competition mantra be? Write it below:

3. Francesco Costa's pre-competition mental ritual: Music

How does music help before competition?
- **Staying in the zone:** it allows an athlete to put aside distraction and focus on the task-at-hand, envisioning what they want to accomplish.

- **Getting in the mood:** music alters emotional and physiological arousal and so can be used before competition as a stimulant. Upbeat music can increase your energy, focus, and "psych" you up, while low tempo, calm music can "psych" you down.

- **Moving to the rhythm:** the beat of music can increase the efficiency of performance, build endurance, and boost output during repetitive training exercises as your body synchronizes with the rhythm of a song. This is especially true for running, cross country skiing, rowing, or cycling.

4. Jaelin Kauf's pre-competition mental ritual: Reflection

Reflection, and why it is important:
Reflecting on what went well and what didn't go well in a training session, competition, conversation with a coach, or something else is a crucial part of the feedback loop of improvement. Without looking back on what worked and didn't, you will not be able to make the necessary adjustments to your training plan, your support team, or your competition approach.

Use a training journal to keep track of progress made, how to consistently produce that result, and what you need to do to bring that forward. Do the same for what did not work, why it did not work, and use that knowledge to find a better solution.

5. Hailey Duff's pre-competition mental ritual: Visualization

What is visualization?
It's using all of your senses to create a mental image or intention of what you want to happen, feel, or achieve in reality.

Visualization is a powerful mental tool because it:
- Boosts your confidence
- Offers you an opportunity to mentally rehearse
- Improves the quality of athletic movement
- Increases the power of concentration

Put it into practice:
1. **Close your eyes** and choose a scenario or outcome you want to achieve.
2. **Imagine the detail** and the way it will feel to achieve the desired outcome.
3. **Use the senses:** kinesthetic (what do you feel?), visual (what do you see?), or auditory (what do you hear?).
4. **Don't speed through the process.** For example, if you are visualizing a 400m sprint, then the visualization should take over 50 seconds.
5. **Repeat daily** to familiarize yourself with a mental run-through, especially before, during, and after training.

6. Benjamin Alexander's pre-competition mental ritual: Power Poses

"I smash my chest a few times to get the adrenaline flowing; you really need to be mentally prepared to fight for every single turn to succeed."

Like Benjamin's chest smashes, proud posture and high-power poses can positively affect our emotional and psychological states before competition. The more we make ourselves feel large and take up space, the more powerful we feel.

High-power poses to try:
- **Basic Beautiful Posture:** stand tall, lift the crown of your head to the ceiling, elongate your spine, and pull your shoulders down your back.
- **The Wonder Woman:** stand up tall and put your hands on your hips.
- **Morning Stretch:** Stand tall with your feet close together, clasp your hands overhead, and stretch your body up to the sky.

7. Kai Owens's pre-competition mental ritual: Journaling

A lot of athletes want to feel that perfect balance of being grounded but also fired up and alert. Some days you might feel more nervous and unsettled or have doubts, and some days you might feel totally confident, calm, and present.

Whatever feeling you're working with, don't fight it or try to change it. What you resist, persists. There is no "right" or "wrong" way to feel, but how you use that energy and channel it into your performance is where the magic happens.

Your journal is your friend:
Journaling is seriously underrated. It is a wondrous tool to get all of the thoughts, ideas, intentions, and worries out of your head.

Here are 5 journaling prompts to ask yourself before training and/or competition to get you grounded and in a great headspace:

1. What can I see, hear, smell, feel, and taste? (try this one in the arena or racecourse to get familiar with and settled into your environment).
2. What is my intention for the day?
3. How do I want to show up and how do I want to feel?
4. Are there any limiting beliefs holding me back? If so, how can I reframe them into something powerful?
5. Three things I am grateful for:

---

8. Josh Williamson's pre-competition mental ritual: Building Confidence

What makes you feel empowered and confident?
Write out a list below and apply it to training and competition:

Music that empowers me: ....
Clothes that empower me: ....
People that empower me: ....
Hairstyle/Makeup that empowers me: ....
Self-Talk that empowers me ....
Anything Else that empowers me: ....

9. Jon Eley's pre-competition mental ritual: Self-Talk

What is your self talk like?
The minute you say "I can't do this," or "this won't work for me," your brain shuts down and your mind and body will follow.

Choose one **core belief** and write it down daily, say it, or sing it out loud. Beliefs you have are a *choice*, and choices can be changed and rewired. Here are some examples of how you can turn those negative, limiting beliefs into positive and empowering affirmations:

LIMITING BELIEF EXAMPLE	→	POSITIVE AFFIRMATION
"This won't work for me"	→	"How can I make this work for me?"
"I am so bad at this"	→	"I am learning and growing from this experience"
"I am not good enough"	→	"I am enough just the way I am, and I'm exactly where I need to be."

10. Kate Hansen's pre-competition mental ritual: Tapping

What is tapping?
Tapping is an Emotional Freedom Technique (EFT) that uses a combination of acupuncture and psychology to reduce stress, anxiety, and pain.

How it works:
- **Identify the issue:** name one issue or distress you're feeling and that will be the focus.
- **Test the intensity:** on a scale of 0-10 (10 being the worst or most difficult), assess the initial emotional or physical discomfort you feel

from your focal issue. This sets a benchmark level to see if there were any improvements after performing the EFT.
- **Find your comforting phrase:** before beginning, choose a phrase that describes what the issue is and how you will accept yourself and feel safe no matter what: "Even though I have this [fear or problem], I deeply and completely accept myself and choose to relax." Even if your fear or pain is about someone else, the mantra must be phrased about *you* in order to feel any relief.
- **The tapping sequence:** tap each of these points 8 times consecutively, while reciting your comforting phrase 3 times. Continue tapping and repeating the phrase as you move down your body in the order below.

1. Start by tapping the karate chop point of your hand
2. Next, the eyebrow
3. Then, the side of the eye
4. Then, under the eye
5. Next, the chin
6. Then, the top of the collarbone
7. Then, under the arm or armpit
8. Finish at the top of the head.
9. Repeat the sequence three times through, then rate the intensity on a scale of 0-10 and notice if your anxiety and fears lessened. Continue the process until you are at 0.

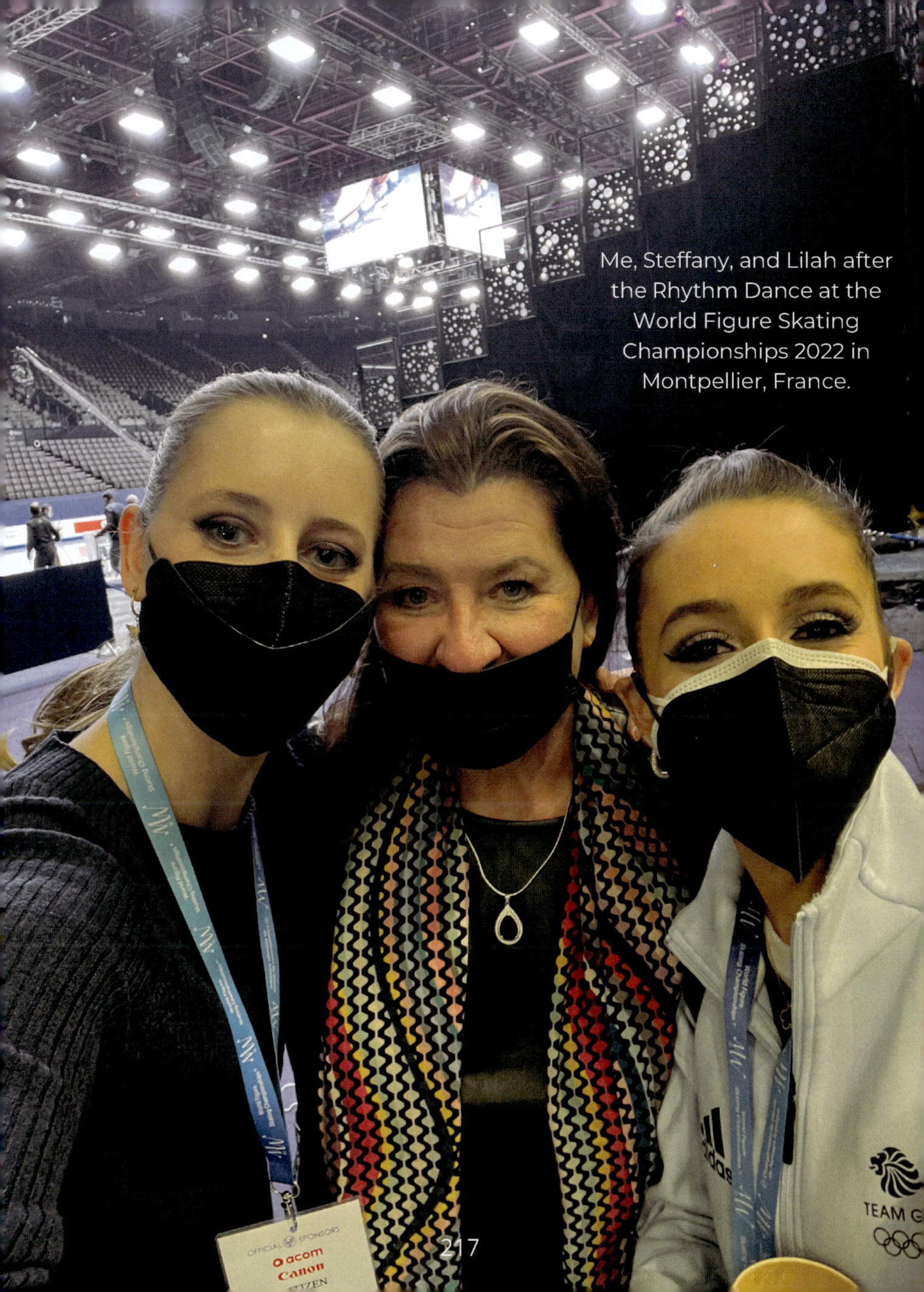

Me, Steffany, and Lilah after the Rhythm Dance at the World Figure Skating Championships 2022 in Montpellier, France.

Interview with Performance Coach, Steffany Hanlen:

On setting intentions, what it takes to be a Champion, and how to get out of emotional trenches.

Q: What does your morning routine look like?
Before I go to bed, I set an intention to sleep well and wake up refreshed with an open mind. Once I wake up, I meditate before I get out of bed. I quiet my mind and focus on how I want my day to feel.

Q: How can athletes use the morning to get grounded for training or competition?
Not all athletes are naturally 'morning' people, so it depends on how they approach it, how they set themselves up, and how they organize themselves. Many will plan for the morning by preparing their food, putting out the training gear, and pre-setting their coffee or their morning shake. It's important they understand what works for them to take advantage of what they feel is 'easy.'

Q: What traits do you see in Olympians? How do they get ready for the day and prepare for training?
Again, learning about themselves and what works for their energy and focus management. Being organized is one of the top traits of being a Champion. There is a difference in being organized and trying to control one's environment, and this requires an ability to differentiate between the things they can control and the things they cannot. Weather, traffic jams, for example, are uncontrollables that can throw off a morning routine, so having a time buffer when setting alarms or reminders is something they can control. Having a plan to follow allows for most athletes to work within a framework that is a foundation of confidence.

Q: If an athlete hits a roadblock or falls into an emotional trench, what is the best way to get out of that state and back into performance mode?
The best way through a rut is to slooooowwww down and remind themselves of the basics. Roadblocks always have clues in them. Digging into it and circling back to the basics like journaling, reading, and

checking if sleep, hydration, or nutrition need to be adjusted—these are all things they can control. Emotional ruts, or what I call "Energy Leaks," provide feedback and clues to what may be happening. Any heaviness or darkness can be shifted by being brought around to "WHAT is." Energy leaks are generally a sign someone is frustrated by having unmet expectations, fear, or anxiety by looking too far into the future, or slipping into a depression or guilt phase by living or thinking too much about the past.

Q: How do you set an intention, and why are they important?
An intention is a personal or expressed statement, written or spoken, or a focus point that gives clarity to action. Once an intention is set, one can then take the next, right action in the direction of their goals. Without an intention, actions can be unorganized and unclear.

Q: What are the traits of a Champion?
There are 2 traits I see in ALL of the Champions I work with:

1. They are ORGANIZED (in a way that serves them in the area of life that is most important to them in the moment—it may not make sense to others).
2. They DECIDE. They stick to a plan. If the plan isn't giving the result they want in the time it's needed, they quickly move on. The GOALS don't change, the plan can. Letting go of something that isn't working takes courage and communication.
If there is a powerful intention set about WHO they are, WHAT they want and WHY they want it, then it is a much simpler way to make changes in real time. The how and the where become clear. The athlete's coachability and environment support the goals, and this supports the plan.

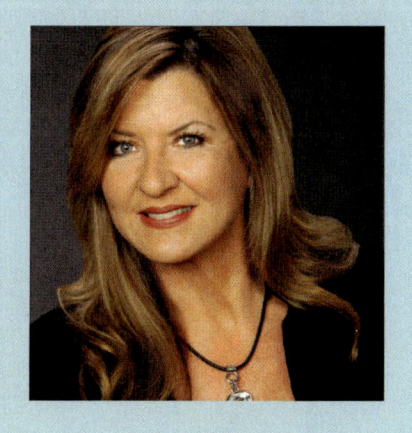

For more from Steffany, visit steffanyhanlen.com and quantumspeed.ca

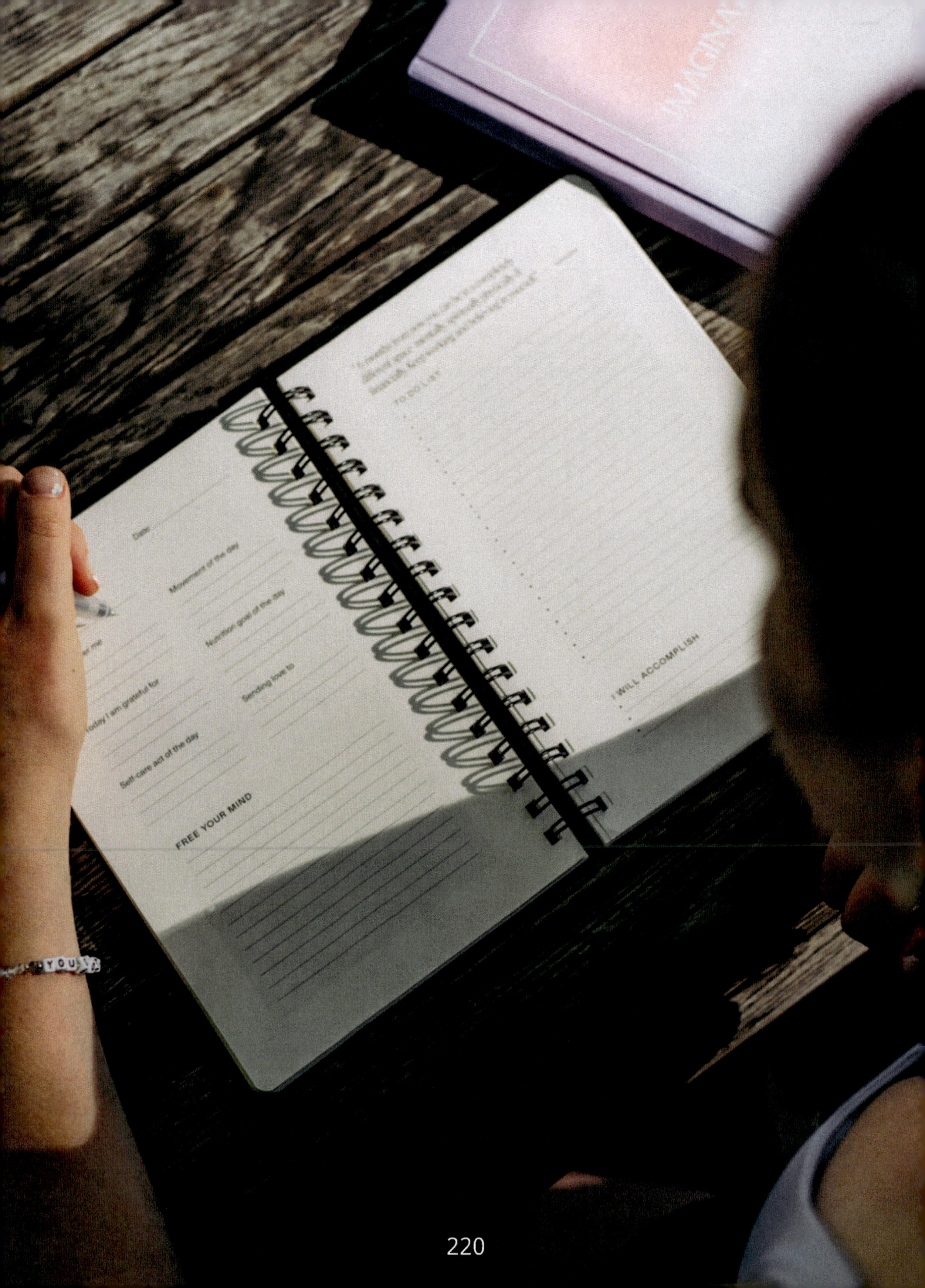
Date:
Movement of the day
Nutrition goal of the day
Sending love to
Self-care act of the day
FREE YOUR MIND
I WILL ACCOMPLISH

SLEEP AND RECOVERY

SLEEP
how to optimize sleep and catch some zzzz's

Sleep is just as important as training and nutrition. It's a key factor in an athlete's recovery and muscle memory. Increased quantity and quality of sleep improves athletic performance and focus, therefore decreasing the risk of injury. It also boosts an athlete's mental performance because when we sleep we form and consolidate memories. By getting more sleep, therefore, any skills or practices we learn during training are more likely to be maintained long-term.

11 tips to improve sleep:

1. Stick to your sleep schedule:
Establish your wake and sleep times and try not to deviate from them during the weekends. Irregular sleep patterns can affect your circadian rhythm and melatonin production levels, which let the brain know it's time to sleep. It also affects REM sleep which plays a big role in repairing the body.

2. Optimize your environment:
The best environment for sleep is cool, dark, and quiet. Try to get blackout blinds or an eye mask to eliminate any excess light.

3. Set app limits:
Just one more episode of "The Bachelor?" I can relate. Set limits so that apps are locked after a certain amount of time using them. This will help to remind you that it is time to sleep.

4. Turn off your screens:
Blue light from our devices confuses the brain (it thinks it's daytime and therefore reduces the production of hormones that promote deep sleep). It's recommended to turn off screens 1 hour before bed and focus on calming activities to do instead like reading (nothing too juicy!), stretching, and meditation.

Can't avoid your screens? Here are some tips:
- Try setting a timer 1 hour before bed to remind yourself that it is time to wind down.
- Buy 100% blue light-blocking glasses. A study found that people who wore these glasses fell asleep and woke up 2 hours earlier than those who didn't!

5. Use lavender:
This scent activates the parasym-

pathetic nervous system and helps us feel calmer. (Note: not suitable if you are pregnant, trying to conceive, or breastfeeding).

6. Steer clear of caffeine 6 hours before bedtime:
Consuming caffeinated substances like coffees, teas, energy drinks, and sodas 6 hours before bed lowers the quality of sleep. This is because caffeine stimulates the nervous system, making it hard to relax. As a substitute for an afternoon coffee, try our "sleep tea" to get the body ready for deep sleep.

7. Go to bed feeling satisfied:
Waking up in the middle of the night with hunger pangs means you didn't fuel enough during the day. If you are hungry before bed, have a snack with healthy fats to keep you satisfied throughout the night. If you aren't hungry, it's best not to eat right before bed because the muscles that metabolize and digest our food start working when they should be resting, and this can impact the efficiency of sleep.

8. Write down your worries:
Put pen to paper and write down any negative thoughts, worries, or to-do list stresses before bed. This helps to get the thoughts out of your head so you can focus on a relaxing sleep.

9. Track your hours of sleep:
Elite and endurance athletes require 8-10 hours of sleep a night.

10. Learn to power nap:
If you didn't get adequate sleep or have jet lag, take a 20 minute power nap. These are great because they are short enough to give you a quick boost in energy, and not long enough for you to go into REM sleep. Reaching REM sleep puts you at risk of not being fully awake in time before a competition, and this could hinder athletic performance. The optimal window to nap is earlier in the day, before 3:30pm.

11. Foods that aid sleep:
- Melatonin and serotonin rich foods: poultry, fatty fish, low-fat dairy and eggs.
- Vitamin C rich foods: citrus fruit, leafy greens, and sweet potato.
- Magnesium-rich foods: bananas, avocados, leafy greens, whole grains like oats, and legumes.
- Recipes for sleep: Miso Salmon Bowl (page 95), Anti-Inflammatory Golden Milk (page 189), BYOYP (page 150).
- Drinks for sleep: tart cherry juice is naturally high in melatonin, chamomile tea, or our Tranquility Tea (page 191).

lavender

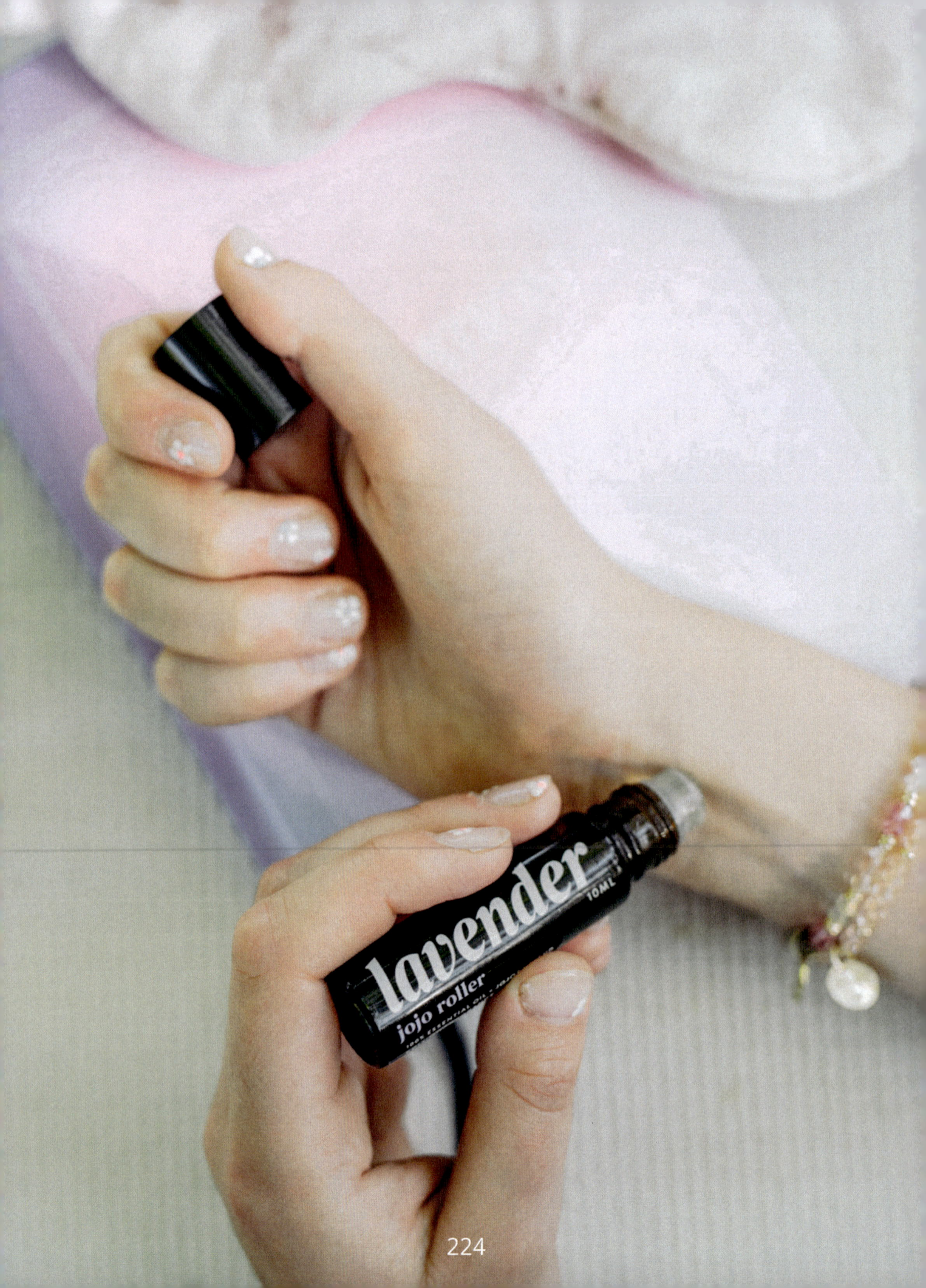

jojo roller

Jet Lag? We don't know her. But here are some ways to combat jet lag when traveling:

1. Shift your body clock a few days before you leave by sleeping and training as if you were in the country you are traveling to.
2. When you travel, adjust the times of meal and fluid intake to the new time zone.
3. Light exposure during training helps to re-align your circadian rhythm.
4. Take melatonin to preserve sleep if needed.

RECOVERY
how to recharge and come back even stronger

PART 1: TECHNIQUES

How do Olympians recover? Here is a list of all of the best ways to decompress after training and relieve tension.

1. Stretch it out: stretching before and after exercise is important to keep muscles flexible, strong, and mobile in order to maintain a good range of motion in the joints. Without it, our muscles shorten, tighten, and become weak when we need them to fully extend during performance.

2. Take a hot bath with Epsom salts: when you soak in an Epsom salt bath, the magnesium sulfate from the salts is absorbed by the skin and decreases muscle soreness.

3. Normatec air compression therapy: these air compression sleeves are the crème de la crème for improving muscle soreness and recovery because they improve blood circulation. Another great brand for compression recovery is Hyperice because they supply air, ice, and heat compression products for legs, hips, and arms.

4. Theragun: this handheld device gives a concentrated deep tissue

massage to one area. It helps to minimize muscle soreness and tightness. However, if injured be careful because the hammering motion of this percussion therapy can be damaging to any muscle or ligament sprains and can potentially bruise the muscle.

5. Foam rolling: this is a great way to relieve muscle tension and lengthen muscles. It also reduces inflammation and promotes muscle recovery. However, foam rolling can be harmful if not done properly.

Here are some common foam rolling mistakes:

- Attacking knots or the sore spot right away. Roll the fascia above and below the tightest spot first to loosen it up so that it will be easier for the tight spot to release later.
- Rolling a "cold" muscle. Unless your muscles are warmed up, start slow and with light pressure, to avoid bruising a muscle.
- Rolling in only one direction. Roll front to back, and side to side to cover all of the fasciae.
- Spending too much time in one area. Roll for approximately one minute per area. Start with static pressure on the muscle for about 30 seconds, then move up and down the muscle, applying a smooth constant pressure, for another 30 seconds.
- Applying too much pressure on sensitive areas. The pain should be mildly uncomfortable, but not excruciating. The goal of foam rolling is to find a "release" in the muscle. Breathe easily and relax the body.
- Rolling the IT band: The IT band is not a muscle, so it cannot be loosened like one. Focus on rolling areas around the knee, hamstrings, quads, and glutes to get relief in the IT band.
- Rolling slow and steady wins the race: if you rush and are not mindful when rolling, your muscles will not fully relax and release. The slower the better.

6. A lot of athletes love going on easy walks or watching a movie after training to decompress their muscles and mind.

227

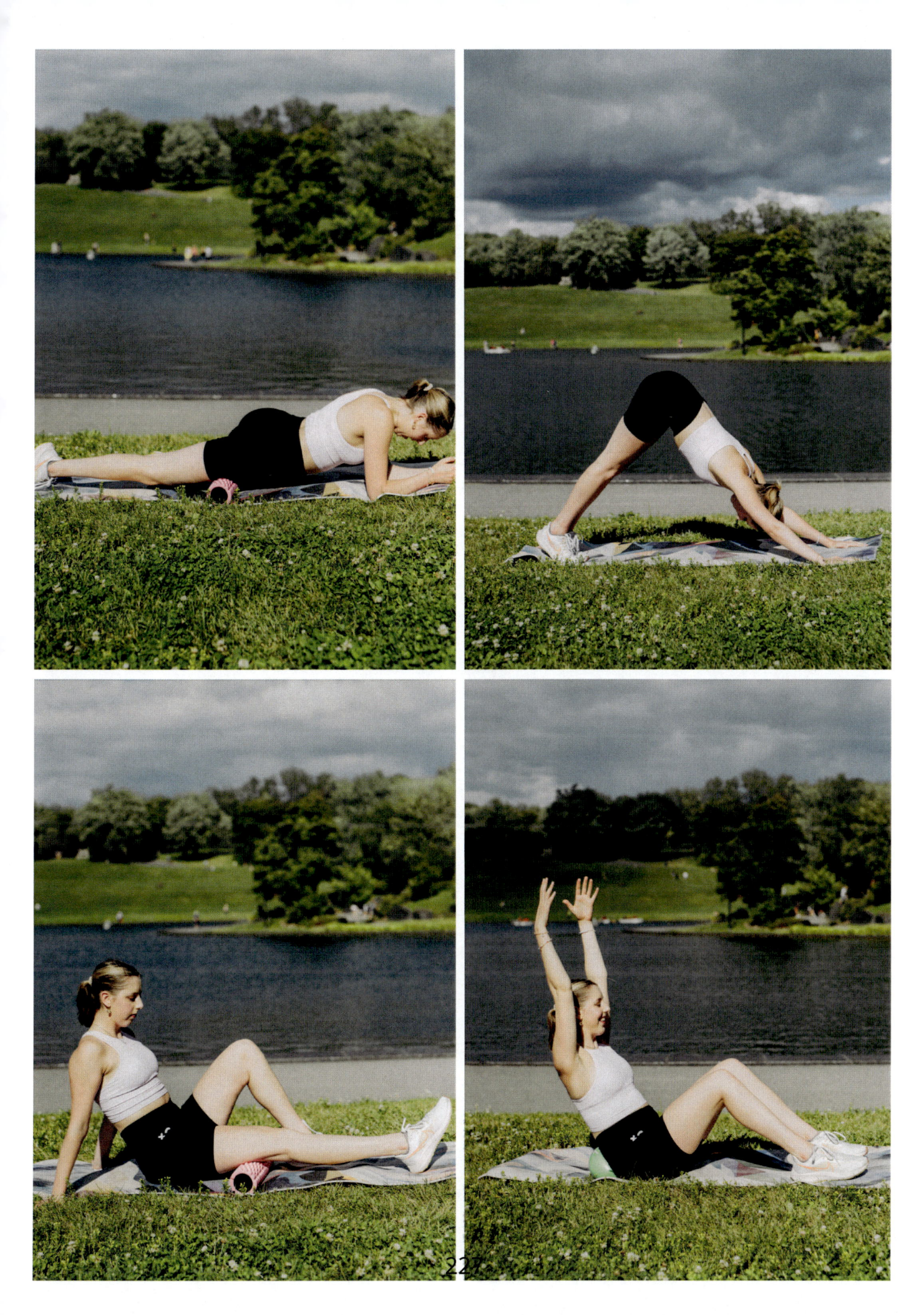

PART 2: FOOD IS MEDICINE

Food is medicine. When injured, reach for nutrient-dense foods instead of painkillers. You will be surprised at how healing food can be! Fueling your body properly pre and post-workout has a huge impact not only on your performance, but your muscle repair, bone health, energy levels, and hydration.

Restorative Recipes:

Dehydration:
Focus on three things post-workout: fluids, salt, and minerals. Not only is it important to drink lots of water before, during, and post-workout, but restoring electrolytes that are not found in water is crucial for restoring your body's fluid balance. Although energy drinks contain a lot of electrolytes, most energy drinks contain lots of sugar and artificial ingredients which are not beneficial for your health. Try swapping energy drinks out for natural drinks and whole foods that provide the proper hydration pre and post-sweat session. The best combinations for electrolytes include coconut water diluted with filtered water or freshly squeezed citrus juices (lemon, orange, or pure cranberry juice) diluted with filtered water. Post-workout, prioritize mineral-rich foods like bananas, citrus fruits, vegetables, soups, or high-quality sea salt to restore sodium, calcium, magnesium, and potassium levels.

Drink recipes for proper hydration and post-workout:
- Cool As A Cucumber Water (page 193)
- Electrolyte Lemon Limeade (page 183)

Muscle Recovery:

After a workout, your body needs nutrient-rich foods to replenish its glycogen stores and to repair and grow its muscle proteins. It is optimal to re-fuel within 30 minutes of working out. By fueling properly, your body will recover faster and you'll have fewer aches and pains.

The best proteins to have after training include eggs, fish, and poultry; or nuts, seeds, beans, and tempeh if you're plant-based. These proteins contain all 9 amino acids, making them optimal for muscle recovery. But don't forget carbs! Consuming carbohydrates like whole grains, fruit, or quinoa play a large role in reducing muscle soreness and getting you fired up for your next training session.

Recipes for muscle recovery:
- High Protein Toast (page 62)
- Miso Salmon Nourish Bowl (page 95)
- Wholesome Stir Fry (page 130)

Inflammation:

Chronic inflammation is the result of poor sleep habits, an unhealthy diet, and constant stress on an area without the proper recovery. Our favorite foods that contain natural anti-inflammatory properties include spices, herbs, berries, tomatoes, leafy greens, and omega-3 rich foods like fish, olive oil, nuts, apple cider vinegar, and seeds. I would much rather add extra olive oil or turmeric to my sweet potatoes than popping anti-inflammatory painkillers!

Recipes for inflammation:
- Anti-Inflammatory Golden Milk (page 189)
- Tranquility Tea (page 191)
- Alkalizing Smoothie (page 178)
- Matcha Smoothie Bowl (page 54)

Stress Fractures:
Stress fractures are caused by overuse and repetitive impact on a bone. The best way to recover from a stress fracture is to fill up on nutrient dense foods that are high in calcium, magnesium, vitamin C, vitamin D, and Omega-3 fatty acids. Refined sugar, trans fats, and other acid-forming foods draw out minerals from our bones and can make them weak and brittle in the long-term. The best foods to combat stress fractures and boost bone health include bone broths, leafy greens, nuts and seeds, seaweed, whole grains, whole-milk yogurt, and eggs.

Recipes for bone health:
- BYOYP (Build Your Own Yogurt Parfait) (page 150)
- Cypriot Grain Salad (page 100)
- Avocado Toast with Poached Eggs (page 58)

Tips for recovery:
- REST!
- Cold packs or ice baths to reduce inflammation and pain
- Lower impact cross training like swimming or biking if your doctor allows it

Athletic Amenorrhea:
This is the absence of menstruation because of low estrogen levels in female athletes as a result of both high-energy output and insufficient nutritional intake. This can be caused by disordered eating habits or poor food selection, which leads to a deficient intake of complex carbohydrates, protein, and fatty acids. This can be serious long-term as it could lead to infertility or osteoporosis. Not having enough of the right fuel can also result in stress fractures, low bone density, and other issues that can increase the risk of injury. Prioritizing high-quality calories is a game-changer to preventing athletic amenorrhea; healthy fats like nuts, seeds, beef, salmon, sardines, butter, eggs, olive oil, avocados, whole-milk yogurt, and coconut oil are all great calorie-dense whole foods. The most common micronutrients to be low in are iron, magnesium, calcium, B vitamins, and folic acid—all of which are crucial to supporting bone health and muscle tissue repair.

Recipes to prevent or conquer amenorrhea:
- Chicken Schnitzel (page 85)
- Chocolate Protein Pancakes (page 42)
- Mediterranean Roast Salad (page 89)

FUN FACT: Did you know that, as a woman, your sex hormones are at their lowest point during the week you are on your period? This means that your body can actually handle MORE stress and recover FASTER, making it a great time for high-intensity workouts or competition.

Low Energy and Burnout:

Do you feel "hangry" all the time? Stressed? Overworked? We've got you. When you are giving 100% and pushing your body to the limit, it is important to get enough nourishment to keep your body energized and its systems running optimally. It may be difficult to get enough nourishment throughout the day if you are relying on packaged foods, caffeine, or sugary snacks. If you are having crazy mood swings or your metabolism is out of whack, this is a sign that your hormones are not balanced or functioning properly. Consuming more complex carbohydrates and healthy fats is a great way to boost your calorie intake and combat burnout. If you are feeling tired, this can also be a sign of low iron stores (see "Anemia" page 232). Other important players in our diets are B Vitamins. These help break down our food and convert it into energy. Foods that are rich in B Vitamins include meat, vegetables, whole grains, legumes, and tempeh (for any plant-based or vegan athletes).

Need quick energy? Try adding dates or dark chocolate (at least 70% cocoa) to your meals as a source of glucose, or swap out caffeine for green tea; this will give you an energy boost instead of a crash.

Recipes for increasing energy and decreasing stress:
- G.O.A.T.meal (page 39)
- Almond Butter Banana Bites (page 140)
- Ultimate Power Cookies (page 161)

Anemia:

Anemia is caused by low iron levels, resulting in a deficiency of red blood cells. Red blood cells are important for athletes because they transfer oxygen to working muscles. The higher the level of red blood cells, the more oxygen in your body—more oxygen means higher athletic performance. Having mild anemia causes tiredness and therefore decreased levels of performance. To restore iron levels, incorporate foods like red meat, dark meat chicken, spinach and leafy greens, beans, dark chocolate, dried fruit (apricots, raisins, dates), seafood (like shellfish), and cumin. Tomatoes and citrus fruits like grapefruit, oranges, and lemons increase iron absorption; while calcium, tea, and coffee decrease iron absorption. It is also important to include the nutrient Vitamin B_{12} in your diet which helps the production of red blood cells.

Best way to take iron:
1. Take it a few hours before or after a workout
2. Take it 1-2 hours before or after a meal.
3. Take with vitamin C

Check with your doctor first whether an iron supplement is needed because it is possible to overdose.

Recipes to prevent anemia:
- The Immunity Booster (page 187)
- Chill Out Chili (page 127)
- Winner Winner Chicken Dinner (page 124)

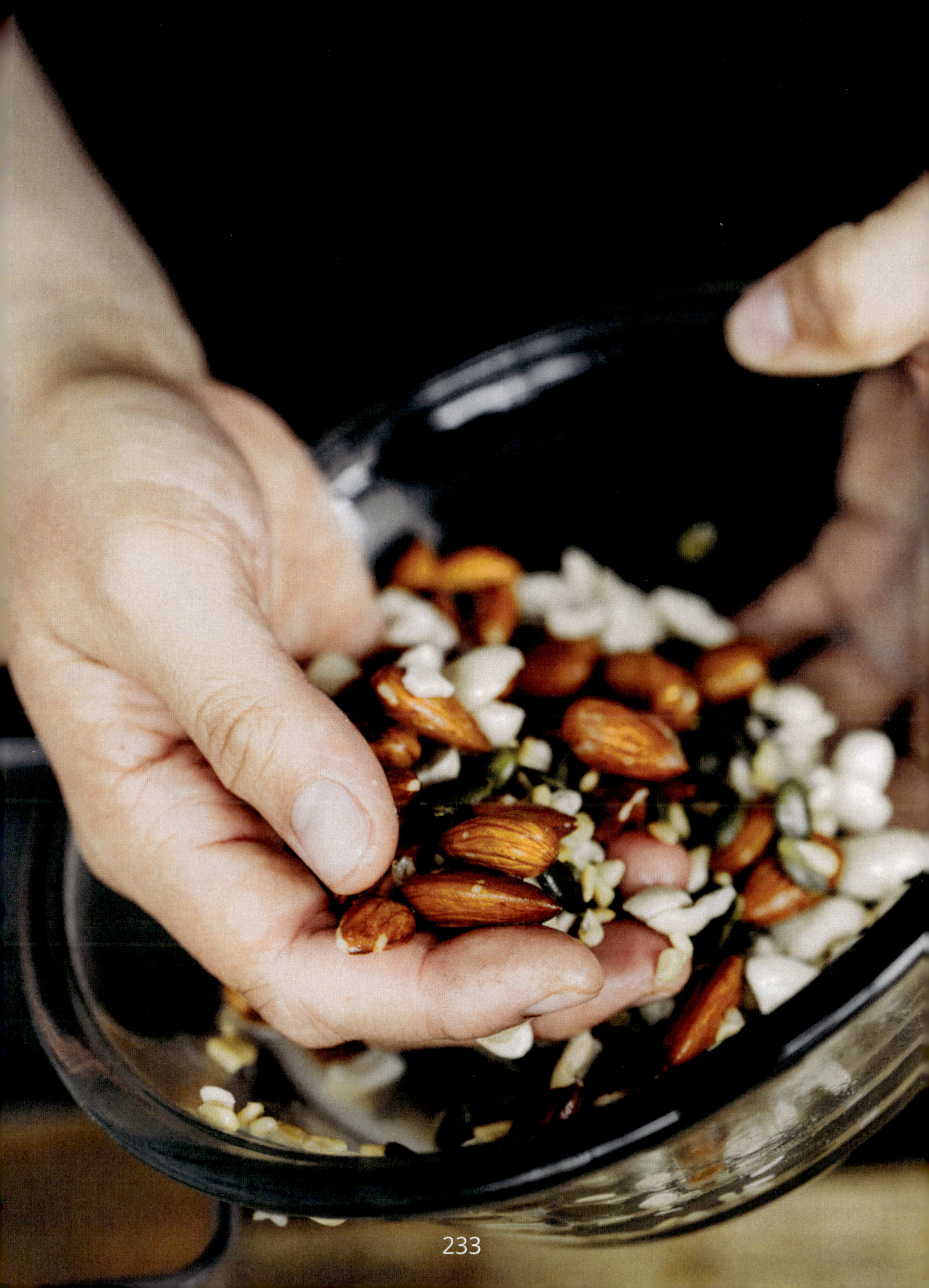

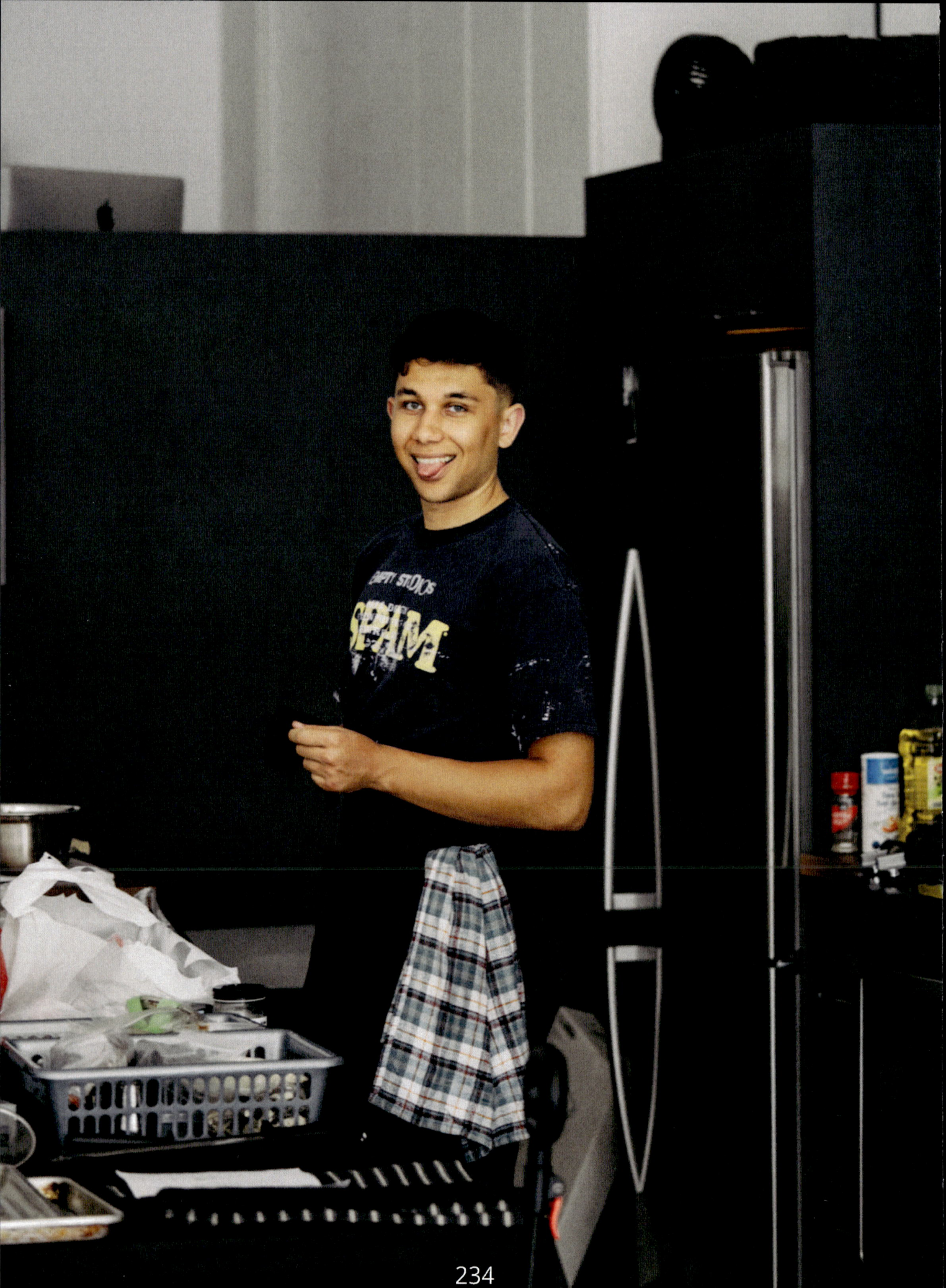

Acknowledgments

I would like to thank the amazing team behind *Plate to Podium*.

To every athlete who contributed, thank you for inspiring me, the next generation of athletes, and for your unwavering dedication to your craft. You are true superhumans.

To Cameron, the best editor and fellow spin class addict. Thank you for fixing my grammar and spelling all the way from Germany!

To Aimee, my incredible recipe tester. Thank you for being the most creative cook who goes above and beyond. These recipes probably would have been inedible if it wasn't for you.

To Alison, the best food photographer, for your beautiful photos, attention to detail, and laughs on set. You are truly one of a kind.

To Kerri, my extremely talented food stylist and recipe crafter, thank you for your organization, creative vision, and support along the way.

To Liam, thank you for being the best sous chef and friendly face on set.

To the photographers that allowed me to feature their incredible photos of the athletes: see page 2 for a full list of photographers.

To my family and friends who recipe tested, thank you for taking the time to help me perfect each recipe.

To my parents, thank you for holding me accountable, being my biggest cheerleaders, helping me get sh*t done, and for all the love throughout this project.

To my sisters, thank you for being both expert eaters and my bffs, and for not taking life too seriously.

Love to our partners, **KidSport Canada,** who are striving to make a difference for future athletes.

About the author

Sasha Fear is a Team GB ice dancer who grew up in London, England but now trains with the Ice Academy of Montreal. She is a European and World competitor, International Medalist, and a 3x National Champion. As an athlete, Sasha is inspired by the enriching power of food to fuel herself and the next generation. Outside of the rink and the kitchen, you can find Sasha exploring new cafés and areas in Montreal (or any new city where skating competitions and travel take her). If you need a city guide, she is your girl! Sasha also has a passion for business, wellness, and learning about becoming elite in all areas of life. She studies at Dartmouth College. Follow her on Instagram @sashadfear.

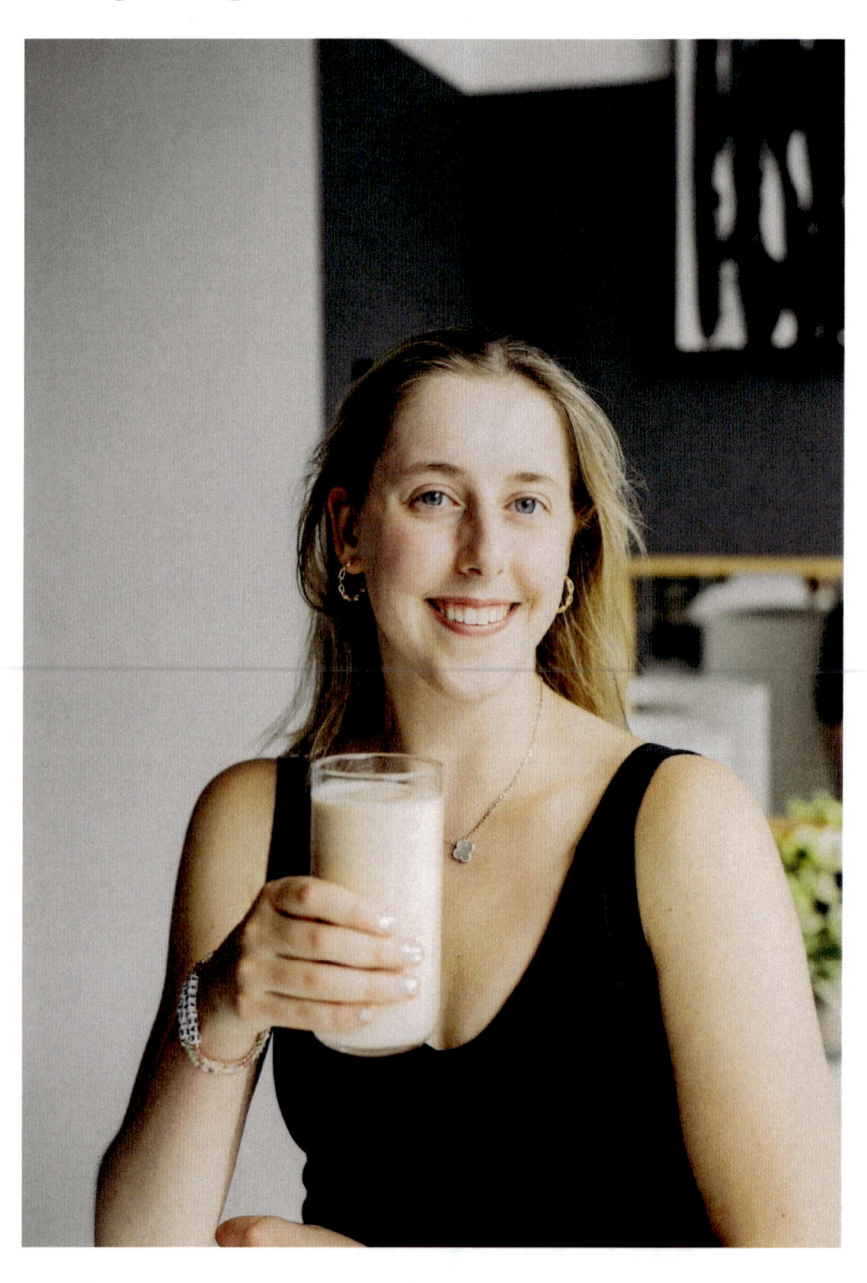

Made in the USA
Columbia, SC
24 June 2024

bafefc13-19db-405a-a826-39776d7a23b3R01